Cor

Ana

Third Editio

Core Topics in Cardiac Anaesthesia

Third Edition

Edited by

Joseph Arrowsmith
Royal Papworth Hospital, Cambridge, UK

Andrew Roscoe
National Heart Centre, Singapore General Hospital

Jonathan Mackay
Royal Papworth Hospital, Cambridge, UK

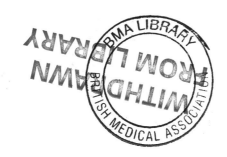

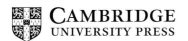

CAMBRIDGE
UNIVERSITY PRESS

CAMBRIDGE
UNIVERSITY PRESS

University Printing House, Cambridge CB2 8BS, United Kingdom

One Liberty Plaza, 20th Floor, New York, NY 10006, USA

477 Williamstown Road, Port Melbourne, VIC 3207, Australia

314–321, 3rd Floor, Plot 3, Splendor Forum, Jasola District Centre,
New Delhi – 110025, India

79 Anson Road, #06–04/06, Singapore 079906

Cambridge University Press is part of the University of Cambridge.

It furthers the University's mission by disseminating knowledge in the pursuit of
education, learning and research at the highest international levels of excellence.

www.cambridge.org
Information on this title: www.cambridge.org/9781108419383
DOI: 10.1017/9781108297783

© Cambridge University Press 2004, 2012, 2020

First published 2004
Second edition 2012
This edition 2020

Printed in Singapore by Markono Print Media Pte Ltd

A catalogue record for this publication is available from the British Library.

Library of Congress Cataloging-in-Publication Data
Names: Arrowsmith, Joseph E., editor. | Roscoe, Andrew,
    editor. | Mackay, Jonathan H., editor.
Title: Core topics in cardiac anaesthesia / edited by Joseph
    Arrowsmith, Andrew Roscoe, Jonathan Mackay.
Other titles: Cardiac anaesthesia
Description: Third edition. | Cambridge, United Kingdom ;
    New York, NY : Cambridge University Press, 2019. | Includes
    bibliographical references and index.
Identifiers: LCCN 2019037040 | ISBN 9781108419383 (hardback) |
    ISBN 9781108297783 (epub)
Subjects: MESH: Anaesthesia, Cardiac Procedures | Cardiac Surgical
    Procedures | Cardiovascular Diseases–surgery | Cardiopulmonary Bypass |
    Heart–drug effects
Classification: LCC RD87.3.C37 | NLM WG 460 | DDC 617.9/6741–dc23
LC record available at https://lccn.loc.gov/2019037040

ISBN 978-1-108-41938-3 Hardback

....

Contents

List of Contributors   ix
Reviews of the First Edition   xiii
Preface to the Third Edition   xv
Preface to the First Edition   xvii
Foreword to the First Edition   xviii
Abbreviations   xix

Section 1   Routine Cardiac Surgery

1   **Basic Principles of Cardiac Surgery**   1
Paolo Bosco and Samer A. M. Nashef

2   **Symptoms and Signs of Cardiac Disease**   6
Joseph E. Arrowsmith

3   **Diagnostic Techniques**   11
Amir Awwad and S. K. Bobby Agarwal

4   **Conduct of Anaesthesia**   24
Andrew I. Gardner and Paul H. M. Sadleir

5   **Principles of Cardiopulmonary Bypass**   30
Timothy Coulson and Florian Falter

6   **Weaning from Cardiopulmonary Bypass**   45
Simon Anderson

7   **Routine Early Postoperative Care**   50
Barbora Parizkova and Aravinda Page

8   **Common Postoperative Complications**   55
Jonathan H. Mackay and Joseph
E. Arrowsmith

Section 2   Anaesthesia for Specific Procedures

9   **Aortic Valve Surgery**   69
Pedro Catarino and Joseph E. Arrowsmith

10   **Mitral Valve Surgery**   75
Jonathan H. Mackay and Francis C. Wells

11   **Tricuspid and Pulmonary Valve Surgery**   82
Joanne Irons and Yasir Abu-Omar

12   **Minimally Invasive and Off-Pump Cardiac Surgery**   91
Ben Gibbison

13   **Thoracic Aortic Surgery**   99
Seema Agarwal and Andrew C. Knowles

14   **Surgery for Cardiomyopathy and Pericardial Disease**   107
Jonathan Brand and Florian Falter

15   **Surgery for Pulmonary Vascular Disease**   113
Choo Y. Ng and Andrew Roscoe

16   **Ventricular Assist Device Implantation**   118
Nicholas J. Lees

17   **Heart Transplantation**   125
Lenore F. van der Merwe and Alan D. Ashworth

Section 3   Cardiac Catheter Laboratory Procedures

18   **Electrophysiological Procedures**   131
Joseph E. Arrowsmith

19   **Procedures for Structural Heart Disease**   137
Cameron G. Densem and Andrew A. Klein

Section 4   Paediatric Cardiac Surgery

20   **General Principles and Conduct of Paediatric Cardiac Anaesthesia**   145
Isabeau A. Walker and Jon H. Smith

21   **Common Congenital Heart Lesions and Procedures**   154
David J. Barron and Kevin P. Morris

vii

22. **Postoperative Paediatric Care**   181
Jane V. Cassidy and Kevin P. Morris

23 **Adult Congenital Heart Disease**   186
Craig R. Bailey and Davina D. L. Wong

Section 5 Cardiopulmonary Bypass

24 **Temperature Management and Deep Hypothermic Arrest**   191
Charles W. Hogue and Joseph E. Arrowsmith

25 **The Effects of Cardiopulmonary Bypass on Drug Pharmacology**   199
Jens Fassl and Berend Mets

26 **Controversies in Cardiopulmonary Bypass**   203
Will Tosh and Christiana Burt

27 **Cardiopulmonary Bypass Emergencies**   210
David J. Daly

28 **Non-Cardiac Applications of Cardiopulmonary Bypass**   215
Joseph E. Arrowsmith and Jonathan H. Mackay

29 **Extracorporeal Membrane Oxygenation**   218
Simon Colah

Section 6 Advanced Monitoring

30 **Cardiovascular Monitoring**   223
Arturo Suarez and Jonathan B. Mark

31 **Neurological Monitoring**   230
Brian D. Gregson and Hilary P. Grocott

Section 7 Transoesophageal Echocardiography

32 **Comprehensive TOE Examination**   239
Justiaan Swanevelder and Andrew Roscoe

33 **Assessment of Ventricular Function**   242
Catherine M. Ashes and Andrew Roscoe

34 **Assessment of Valvular Heart Disease**   248
Massimiliano Meineri and Andrew Roscoe

35 **TOE for Miscellaneous Conditions**   254
Lachlan F. Miles and Andrew Roscoe

Section 8 Miscellaneous Topics

36 **Haematology**   261
Martin W. Besser and Kiran M. P. Salaunkey

37 **Cardiac Surgery during Pregnancy**   269
Savio J. M. Law and Sarah E. Round

38 **Regional Anaesthesia**   274
Trevor W. R. Lee

39 **Pain Management after Cardiac Surgery**   280
Siân I. Jaggar and Helen C. Laycock

40 **Infection**   285
Hannah McCormick and Judith A. Troughton

Index   290

Contributors

Yasir Abu-Omar
Consultant Surgeon
Royal Papworth Hospital
Cambridge, UK

S. K. Bobby Agarwal
Consultant Radiologist
Royal Papworth Hospital
Cambridge, UK

Seema Agarwal
Consultant Anaesthetist
Manchester University NHS
Foundation Trust
Manchester, UK

Simon Anderson
Senior Clinical Perfusion Scientist
Cambridge Perfusion Services
Cambridge, UK

Joseph E. Arrowsmith
Consultant Anaesthetist
Royal Papworth Hospital
Cambridge, UK

Catherine M. Ashes
Consultant Anaesthetist
St Vincent's Hospital
Sydney, NSW, Australia

Alan D. Ashworth
Consultant Anaesthetist
Manchester University NHS Foundation Trust
Manchester, UK

Amir Awwad
Fellow in Radiology
Royal Papworth Hospital
Cambridge, UK

Craig R. Bailey
Consultant Anaesthetist
Guys & St Thomas' Hospitals
London, UK

David J. Barron
Head, Division of Cardiovascular Surgery
The Hospital for Sick Children
Toronto, Canada

Martin W. Besser
Consultant Haematologist
Royal Papworth & Addenbrookes Hospitals
Cambridge, UK

Paolo Bosco
Consultant Surgeon
Guy's and St Thomas' Hospital
London, UK

Jonathan Brand
Consultant Anaesthetist & Intensivist
James Cook University Hospital
Middlesbrough, UK

Christiana Burt
Consultant Anaesthetist
Royal Papworth Hospital
Cambridge, UK

Jane V. Cassidy
Consultant Paediatric Intensivist
Birmingham Children's Hospital
Birmingham, UK

Pedro Catarino
Consultant Surgeon
Royal Papworth Hospital
Cambridge, UK

Simon Colah
Senior Clinical Perfusion Scientist
Cambridge Perfusion Services
Cambridge, UK

Timothy Coulson
Senior Lecturer
The Alfred Hospital
Melbourne, VIC, Australia

David J. Daly
Consultant Anaesthetist
The Alfred Hospital
Melbourne, VIC, Australia

Cameron G. Densem
Consultant Cardiologist
Royal Papworth Hospital
Cambridge, UK

Florian Falter
Consultant Anaesthetist
Royal Papworth Hospital
Cambridge, UK

Jens Fassl
Professor and Chair
Department of Cardiac Anesthesiology
Heart Center Dresden – University Hospital
Technical University of Dresden
Germany

Andrew I. Gardner
Consultant Anaesthetist
Sir Charles Gairdner Hospital
Perth, WA, Australia

Ben Gibbison
Consultant Anaesthetist
University Hospitals Bristol
Senior Lecturer, University of Bristol
Bristol, UK

Brian D. Gregson
Clinical Lecturer in Anaesthesia
University of British Columbia
Vancouver, BC, Canada

Hilary P. Grocott
Professor of Anesthesia & Surgery
Department of Anesthesiology,
Perioperative & Pain Medicine
University of Manitoba
Winnipeg, MB, Canada

Charles W. Hogue
Associate Professor of Anesthesiology
& Critical Care Medicine
The Johns Hopkins Hospital
Baltimore, MD, USA

Joanne Irons
Consultant Anaesthetist
Royal Prince Alfred Hospital
Clinical Senior Lecturer
University of Sydney School of Medicine
Sydney, NSW, Australia

Siân I. Jaggar
Consultant Anaesthetist
Royal Brompton Hospital
London, UK

Andrew A. Klein
Consultant Anaesthetist
Macintosh Professor of Anaesthesia
Royal Papworth Hospital
Cambridge, UK

Andrew C. Knowles
Consultant Anaesthetist
Lancashire Cardiac Centre
Blackpool, UK

Savio J. M. Law
Consultant Anaesthetist & Intensivist
James Cook University Hospital
Middlesbrough, UK

Helen C. Laycock
Clinical Lecturer in Pain Medicine
Imperial College London
London, UK

Trevor W. R. Lee
Associate Professor
Department of Anesthesia & Perioperative Medicine
Max Rady College of Medicine
Rady Faculty of Health Sciences
University of Manitoba
Winnipeg, MB, Canada

Nicholas J. Lees
Consultant Anaesthetist
Harefield Hospital
Middlesex, UK

Jonathan H. Mackay
Consultant Anaesthetist
Royal Papworth Hospital
Cambridge, UK

Jonathan B. Mark
Professor of Anesthesiology
Duke University Medical Center
Veterans Affairs Medical Center
Durham, NC, USA

Hannah McCormick
Specialty Registrar in Microbiology
Royal Victoria Hospital
Belfast, UK

Massimiliano Meineri
Deputy Director
Department of Anaesthesia
Leipzig Heart Center
Leipzig, Germany

Berend Mets
Eric A. Walker Professor and Chair
Department of Anesthesiology
Penn State College of Medicine
Penn State Milton S. Hershey Medical Center
Hershey, PA, USA

Lachlan F. Miles
Consultant Anaesthetist
Austin Hospital
Melboune, VIC, Australia

Kevin P. Morris
Consultant Paediatric Intensivist
Birmingham Children's Hospital
Birmingham, UK

Samer A. M. Nashef
Consultant Surgeon
Royal Papworth Hospital
Cambridge, UK

Choo Y. Ng
Consultant Surgeon
Royal Papworth Hospital
Cambridge, UK

Aravinda Page
Specialty Registrar in Surgery
Royal Papworth Hospital
Cambridge, UK

Barbora Parizkova
Consultant Anaesthetist
Royal Papworth Hospital
Cambridge, UK

Andrew Roscoe
Consultant Anaesthetist
National Heart Centre
Singapore General Hospital

Sarah E. Round
Consultant Anaesthetist
James Cook University Hospital
Middlesbrough, UK

Paul H. M. Sadleir
Consultant Anaesthetist
Sir Charles Gairdner Hospital
Senior Lecturer, University of Western Australia
Perth, WA, Australia

Kiran M. P. Salaunkey
Consultant Anaesthetist
Royal Papworth Hospital
Cambridge, UK

Jon H. Smith
Consultant Anaesthetist
Freeman Hospital
Newcastle upon Tyne, UK

Arturo Suarez
Anesthesiology Fellow
Duke University Medical Center
Durham, NC, USA

Justiaan Swanevelder
Professor and Head
Department of Anaesthesia
and Perioperative Medicine
University of Cape Town
Groote Schuur Hospital
Cape Town, South Africa

Will Tosh
Locum Consultant Anaesthetist
University Hospital Birmingham
Birmingham, UK

Judith A. Troughton
Consultant Microbiologist
Royal Victoria Hospital
Belfast, UK

Lenore F. van der Merwe
Consultant Anaesthetist
Prince Charles Hospital
Brisbane, QLD, Australia

Isabeau A. Walker
Consultant Anaesthetist
Great Ormond Street Hospital
London, UK

Francis C. Wells
Consultant Cardiothoracic Surgeon
Royal Papworth Hospital
Cambridge, UK

Davina D. L. Wong
Consultant Anaesthetist
Guys & St Thomas' Hospitals
London, UK

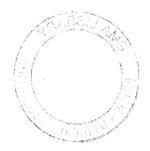

Reviews of the First Edition

"The book has set itself clear objectives and very largely achieves them. Whilst trying not to be all-encompassing nor the only reference book required for this burgeoning field, it covers all the necessary and relevant areas to provide a sound basis and grounding in good clinical practice."

"The extensive list of abbreviations . . . reduces confusion and enhances the flow of the text"

"There is little cross-over between chapters and each chapter covers the topic in sufficient detail to make it useful as a stand-alone reference text."

" . . . a thoughtfully produced and well-written book."

Jonathan J Ross, Sheffield, UK.

British Journal of Anaesthesia *2005; 94(6): 868*

"the book relies heavily on tables and figures, which makes it an effective didactic teaching tool."

"The pharmacology section includes a succinct summary of the drugs used every day in the cardiac operating rooms."

" . . . the chapter on signs and symptoms of cardiac disease is one of the best this reviewer has seen."

" . . . an excellent introductory text book for the trainee in cardiac anesthesia"

" . . . likely to become a classic in the resident or fellow library."

Pablo Motta MD, Cleveland Clinic Foundation, USA.

Anesthesia & Analgesia *2006; 102(2): 657*

" . . . the ubiquitous use of well-labeled diagrams, photographs and clinical tracings adds understanding at every level . . . a delight to use as a teaching device."

" . . . a rare text that is without institutional bias or personal beliefs."

" . . . I would advise curious learners to save their time and money until they have absorbed all that this book has to offer!"

J Cousins, London, UK

Perfusion *2006; 21(3): 193*

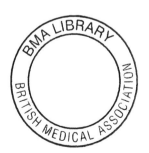

Preface to the Third Edition

In the words of one of our contributors (Sam Nashef*), "There is no such thing as a good cardiac anaesthetist". Recently published** evidence, however, suggests that the variability in cardiac anaesthetists' performance is much lower than that of cardiac surgeons. This may reflect widespread uniformity in training and standardised clinical practice.

As with many textbooks, it was inevitable that the second edition was fatter and heavier than the first as we sought to cover more topics in greater detail. In considering a third edition, the consistent feedback (sometimes blunt) was to delete less frequently read chapters and return to the original remit – a small, concise, portable reference focusing on key points for trainees in the first 6 months of subspecialty training.

We warmly welcome Andy Roscoe, a recognized international authority on transoesophageal echocardiography, as an editor. Under Andy's stewardship, we are confident that future editions of this book will be in safe hands.

In the third edition, we cover many of changes that have occurred since publication of the second edition – a huge expansion in ECMO (a *four-letter word* in many centres), increased numbers of cardiology procedures undertaken in cardiac catheter laboratory and hybrid operating theatre, and the tentative return of aprotinin into clinical practice.

In larger cardiac surgical centres there has been a gradual separation of cardiothoracic anaesthesia from critical care, with the latter becoming a specialty in its own right. Many intensive topics are well covered in a sister publication, *Core Topics in Cardiothoracic Critical Care, Second Edition* and these are referenced in the text.

We are extremely grateful to our contributors for their forbearance and to Cambridge University Press for their seemingly endless patience.

Joe Arrowsmith
Jon Mackay
December 2018

---

* Nashef S. *The Naked Surgeon: The Power and Peril of Transparency in Medicine.* London: Scribe; 2016.
** Papachristofi O, *et al.* The contribution of the anaesthetist to risk-adjusted mortality after cardiac surgery. *Anaesthesia* 2016; 71(2): 138–46.

Preface to the First Edition

This book is primarily aimed at anaesthetic trainees in the first 3–6 months of subspecialty training in cardiac anaesthesia and critical care. It is our response to the many trainees who have regularly asked us to recommend a small textbook on cardiac anaesthesia.

We realize that it is impossible to produce a truly comprehensive review of cardiac anaesthesia in ~120,000 words but hope that this book provides a sound grounding in all of the core topics. The content of this book has been very much guided by The Royal College of Anaesthetists' *CCST in Anaesthesia* manual, The Society of Cardiovascular Anesthesiologists' *Program Requirements for Resident Education*, and recent examination papers from the United Kingdom, North America and Australasia.

Our instructions to contributing authors and editorial aims were simple; produce a concise yet comprehensive overview of the subject emphasizing pathophysiology, basic scientific principles and the key elements of practice. We hope that the use of a presentation format that relies on figures and tables in preference to text will aid comprehension and recall.

We have endeavoured to avoid repetition of information, long lists of references and institutional bias. We trust that the curious trainee will turn to the larger textbooks and the Internet for more detailed discussions and exhaustive literature reviews. Finally, we hope that many sections of this book will also appeal to those preparing trainees for examinations and to clinical nurse specialists working in the field of cardiothoracic intensive care.

We would like to thank all of those who have made the publication of this volume possible; our international panel of contributors for taking the time to share their knowledge and expertise; Gill Clark and Gavin Smith of Greenwich Medical Media for their encouragement, advice and patience; and our Specialist Registrars for their advice and proof reading. Last, we wish to thank our families for their willing, and occasionally unwilling, support during this enterprise.

Jon Mackay
Joe Arrowsmith
January 2004

Foreword to the First Edition

Cardiac anaesthesia brings many divergent disciplines into one unifying practice, making it one of the most complex anaesthetic subspecialties. It requires an understanding of pathology, physiology, pharmacology, internal medicine, cardiology, cardiac surgery and intensive care. The ever-expanding nature of the specialty presents considerable challenges for both the everyday practitioner and the trainee – for whom this text is particularly targeted.

In this day and age, when a vast amount of information is already available both in print and on-line, one may be forgiven for questioning the need for yet another printed textbook. By way of an answer, the Editors (both of whom have worked in the UK and the USA) have produced a textbook (rather than a *cookbook*) that addresses a relatively unfulfilled need—a source that is specifically directed towards those who represent the future of our specialty. By incorporating contributions from authors from many countries, the Editors have largely avoided national and institutional bias.

Today's anaesthetic trainees are confronted with the seemingly impossible task of assimilating, understanding and memorizing an almost infinite body of information. Those who succeed in this task are invariably those who can confidently identify core principles without getting distracted by minute details. The Editors never intended to produce an exhaustive reference and the need to consult other sources of detailed information has, therefore, not been completely eliminated. This book does, however, provide the trainee with a very convenient framework onto which further knowledge can be added as it is acquired. The manner in which the authors have organized and presented information in this book should help the reader to more quickly see the 'bigger picture' and appreciate the subtleties of cardiac anaesthesia.

Hilary P. Grocott, MD, FRCPC
Associate Professor of Anesthesiology
Mark F. Newman, MD
Merel H. Harmel Chair and Professor of Anesthesiology
Duke University, Durham, NC, USA

Abbreviations

A

2D two-dimensional
3D three-dimensional
A_2 aortic valve component of second heart sound
AAA abdominal aortic aneurysm
AAGBI Association of Anaesthetists of Great Britain and Ireland
AATS American Association for Thoracic Surgery
ABG arterial blood gas
ACA anterior cerebral artery
ACC American College of Cardiologists
ACCF American College of Cardiology Foundation
ACE angiotensin converting enzyme
ACHD adult congenital heart disease
ACoA anterior communicating (cerebral) artery
ACP American College of Physicians
ACS acute coronary syndrome(s)
ACT activated clotting time
ADH antidiuretic hormone
ADP adenosine diphosphate
AE air embolism
AECC American–European Consensus Conference
AEP auditory evoked potential
AF atrial fibrillation
AHA American Heart Association
AKI acute kidney injury
ALI acute lung injury
ALS advanced life support
AMVL anterior mitral valve leaflet
AP action potential
APTT activated partial thromboplastin time
AR aortic regurgitation (incompetence)
ARDS acute respiratory distress syndrome
ARF acute renal failure
ARVC arrhythmogenic right ventricular cardiomyopathy
AS aortic stenosis
ASA American Society of Anesthesiologists
ASD atrial septal defect
AT antithrombin
ATP adenosine triphosphate
AV aortic valve
A-V atrioventricular
AVA aortic valve (orifice) area
AVR aortic valve replacement
AVSD atrioventricular septal defect
AXC aortic cross-clamp

B

BA basilar artery
BAER brainstem auditory evoked response
BAS balloon atrial septostomy
BCPS bidirection cavopulmonary shunt
BIS bispectral (index)
BIVAD biventricular assist device
BP blood pressure
BPEG British Pacing and Electrophysiology Group
bpm beats (breaths) per minute
B–T Blalock–Taussig (shunt)
BTT bridge to transplantation

C

CABG coronary artery bypass graft
CAD coronary artery disease
CAJ cavo-atrial junction
CBF cerebral blood flow
CCS Canadian Cardiovascular Society
CFD colour-flow Doppler (sonography)
CHARGE coloboma, heart, atresia, retardation, genital, ear
CHD congenital heart disease
CI cardiac index
CK-MB creatinine kinase MB (isoenzyme)
CMR cardiac magnetic resonance imaging
$CMRO_2$ cerebral metabolic rate (for oxygen)
CNS central nervous system
CO cardiac output
CoA coarctation of the aorta
CP cavopulmonary (shunt)
CPAP continuous positive airway pressure
CPB cardiopulmonary bypass
CPR cardiopulmonary resuscitation
CRA chronic refractory angina
CRT cardiac resynchronization therapy
CSF cerebrospinal fluid
CT computed tomogram/tomography
CTA CT angiography
CTEPH chronic thromboembolic pulmonary hypertension
CVA cerebrovascular accident
CVP central venous pressure
CVVHF continuous veno-venous haemofiltration
CWD continuous-wave Doppler (sonography)
CXR chest X-ray/radiograph

D

DA ductus arteriosus
DASI Duke Activity Status Index
DBD donation after brain death
DC direct current
DCCV direct current cardioversion
DCD donation after circulatory-determined death
DCM dilated cardiomyopathy
DDAVP desmopressin (1-desamino-8-d-arginine vasopressin)
DFT defibrillation (energy) threshold
DHCA deep hypothermic circulatory arrest
DH dorsal horn
DI dimensionless index
DIC disseminated intravascular coagulation
DM diabetes mellitus
DNA deoxyribonucleic acid
DNAR do not attempt resuscitation
DO$_2$ oxygen delivery
DOA depth of anaesthesia
DOAC direct-acting oral anticoagulant
DSCT dual-source computed tomography
DVT deep vein thrombosis

E

EBCT electron-beam CT
ECC extracorporeal circulation
ECG electrocardiograph
ECLS extracorporeal life support
ECMO extracorporeal membrane oxygenation
EDM early diastolic murmur
EDV end-diastolic volume
EECG exercise ECG
EEG electroencephalograph
EMI electromagnetic interference
ESC European Society of Cardiology
ESPVR end-systolic pressure–volume relationship
ET endothelin
EuroSCORE European System for Cardiac Operative Risk Evaluation

F

FAC fractional area change
FBC full blood count
FDA Food and Drug Administration (USA)
FDG fluorodeoxyglucose
FDPs fibrin(ogen) degradation products
FFP fresh-frozen plasma
FFR fractional flow reserve
FiO$_2$ fraction of inspired oxygen
FS fractional shortening

G

Gd-DTPA gadolinium diethylene triamine pentaacetic acid
GFR glomerular filtration rate

GI gastrointestinal
GP glycoprotein
GTN glyceryl trinitrate

H

Hb haemoglobin
Hb-SS haemoglobin-SS (homozygous sickle)
HFSA Heart Failure Society of America
5-HIAA 5-hydroxyindoleacetic acid
HIT heparin-induced thrombocytopenia
HITTS heparin-induced thrombotic thrombocytopenic syndrome
HLHS hypoplastic left heart syndrome
HOCM hypertrophic obstructive cardiomyopathy
HR heart rate

I

IABP intra-aortic balloon pump
ICA internal carotid artery
ICD implantable cardiodefibrillator
ICM implantable cardiac monitoring
ICU intensive care unit
Ig immunoglobulin
IHD ischaemic heart disease
IJV internal jugular vein
IMA internal mammary artery
INR international normalized ratio
INTERMACS Interagency Registry for Mechanically Assisted Circulatory Support
IPC ischaemic preconditioning
IPPV intermittent positive-pressure ventilation
IRI ischaemia reperfusion injury
ITP intrathecal pressure
IV intravenous
IVC inferior vena cava
IVS interventricular septum
IVUS intravascular ultrasound

J

JET junctional ectopic tachycardia

L

LA left atrium/atrial
LAA left atrial appendage
LAD left anterior descending (coronary artery)
LAP left atrial pressure
LAX long axis
LBBB left bundle branch block
LCOS low cardiac output state
LDM late diastolic murmur
LHB left heart bypass
LHC left heart catheterization
LIMA left internal mammary artery
LLSE left lower sternal edge
LMS left main stem (coronary artery)
LMWH low-molecular-weight heparin

LPA left pulmonary artery
LSM late systolic murmur
LSV long saphenous vein
LUSE left upper sternal edge
LV left ventricle/ventricular
LVAD left ventricular assist device
LVEDP left ventricular end-diastolic pressure
LVEDV left ventricular end-diastolic volume
LVEF left ventricular ejection fraction
LVESV left ventricular end-systolic volume
LVID left ventricular internal diameter
LVH left ventricular hypertrophy
LVOT left ventricular outflow tract

M

MAC minimal alveolar concentration
MAO monoamine oxidase
MAP mean arterial pressure
MAPCAs major aorta pulmonary collateral arteries
MCA middle cerebral artery
MCS mechanical circulatory support
MDCT multidetector row CT
MDM mid diastolic murmur
ME mid-oesophageal
MEP motor evoked potential
MI myocardial infarction
MICS minimally invasive cardiac surgery
MIDCAB minimally invasive direct coronary artery bypass
MPA main pulmonary artery
mPAP mean pulmonary artery pressure
MR mitral regurgitation (incompetence)
MRA magnetic resonance angiography
MRI magnetic resonance imaging
MRSA meticillin-resistant *Staphylococcus aureus*
MS mitral stenosis
MSM mid systolic murmur
MV mitral valve
MVR mitral valve replacement
MW molecular weight

N

N_2O nitrous oxide
NASPE North American Society of Pacing and Electrophysiology
NCC non-compaction cardiomyopathy
NEC necrotizing enterocolitis
NG nasogastric
NIBP non-invasive blood pressure
NICE National Institute for Health and Care Excellence
NIRS near-infrared spectroscopy
NMDA N-methyl-D-aspartate
NO nitric oxide
NPV negative predictive value
NSAID non-steroidal anti-inflammatory drug
NSR normal sinus rhythm

NSTEMI non-ST-elevation myocardial infarction
NYHA New York Heart Association

O

OPCAB off-pump coronary artery bypass
OS opening snap

P

P_2 pulmonary valve component of second heart sound
PA pulmonary artery
PaCO$_2$ arterial partial pressure of carbon dioxide
PaO$_2$ arterial partial pressure of oxygen
PAD pulmonary artery diastolic
PAFC pulmonary artery floatation catheter
PAP pulmonary artery pressure
PAWP pulmonary artery wedge pressure
PBF pulmonary blood flow
PBMV percutaneous balloon mitral valvotomy
PCA posterior cerebral artery
PCC prothrombin complex concentrate
PCI percutaneous coronary intervention
PCoA posterior communicating (cerebral) artery
PD peritoneal dialysis
PDA patent ductus arteriosus
PDE phosphodiesterase
PE pulmonary embolus/pulmonary embolism
PEA pulseless electrical activity
PEEP positive end-expiratory pressure
PET positron emission tomography
PF_4 platelet factor 4
PFO patent foramen ovale
PGE_2 prostaglandin E_2
PGI_2 prostaglandin I_2/prostacyclin/epoprostenol
PH-T pressure half-time
PHT pulmonary hypertension
PISA proximal isovelocity surface area
PO *per os* (by mouth)
PPB plasma protein binding
ppm parts per million
PPM permanent pacemaker
PPV positive predictive value
PR pulmonary regurgitation (incompetence)
PS pulmonary stenosis
PSM pan systolic murmur
PSV pressure-support ventilation
PT prothrombin time
PTE pulmonary thromboendarterectomy
PV pulmonary valve
PVC polyvinyl chloride
PVL paravalvular leak
PVR pulmonary vascular resistance
PWD pulsed-wave Doppler (sonography)

Q

Q_P pulmonary flow
Q_S systemic flow

R

RA right atrium/atrial
RBBB right bundle branch block
RBC red blood cell
RCA right coronary artery
RCP retrograde cerebral perfusion
REMATCH Randomized Evaluation of Mechanical Assistance for the Treatment of Congestive Heart Failure
RHC right heart catheterization
RNA ribonucleic acid
RPA right pulmonary artery
rpm revolutions per minute
RR respiratory rate
RRT renal replacement therapy
rSO2 regional cerebral oxygen saturation
RV right ventricle/ventricular
RVAD right ventricular assist device
RVEDA right ventricular end-diastolic area
RVEDP right ventricular end-diastolic pressure
RVEF right ventricular ejection fraction
RVESA right ventricular end-systolic area
RVFAC right ventricular fractional area change
RVH right ventricular hypertrophy
RVOT right ventricular outflow tract
RWMA regional wall motion abnormality

S

S_1 first heart sound
S_2 second heart sound
S_3 third heart sound
S_4 fourth heart sound
SACP selective antegrade cerebral perfusion
SAM systolic anterior motion (of the anterior mitral valve leaflet)
SaO_2 arterial oxygen saturation
SAVR surgical aortic valve replacement
SAX short axis surgical AV replacement (SAVR)
SCA Society of Cardiovascular Anesthesiologists
SIMV synchronized intermittent mandatory ventilation
SIRS systemic inflammatory response syndrome
$SjvO_2$ jugular venous oxygen saturation
SPECT single photon emission computed tomography
SSEP somatosensory evoked potential
SSFP steady-state free-precession
SSI surgical site infection
STEMI ST-elevation myocardial infarction
STS Society of Thoracic Surgeons
SV stroke volume
SVC superior vena cava
SvO_2 mixed venous oxygen saturation
SVR systemic vascular resistance
SVT supraventricular tachycardia

T

T_3 triiodothyronine
T_4 thyroxine
TAPSE tricuspid annular plane systolic excursion
TAPVD total anomalous pulmonary venous drainage
TAVI transcatheter aortic valve implantation
TB tuberculosis
TCD transcranial Doppler (sonography)
TCPC total cavopulmonary connection
TEA thoracic epidural analgesic
TEG thromboelastogram/ thromboelastography
TENS transcutaneous electrical nerve stimulation
TG transgastric
TGA transposition of the great arteries
TOE transoesophageal echocardiography
tPA tissue plasminogen activator
TPG transpulmonary gradient
TR tricuspid regurgitation (incompetence)
TS tricuspid stenosis
TT thrombin time
TTE transthoracic echocardiography
TV tricuspid valve
TXA tranexamic acid

U

UFH unfractionated heparin
uPA urokinase plasminogen activator

V

VA vertebral artery
VACTERL (syndrome) vertebral anomalies, anal atresia, cardiovascular anomalies, tracheoesophageal fistula, esophageal atresia, renal, limb defects
VAD ventricular assist device
VA-ECMO veno-arterial extracorporeal membrane oxygenation
VAP ventilator-associated pneumonia
V_D volume of distribution
VEP visual evoked potential
VF ventricular fibrillation
VO_2 oxygen consumption
VOT ventricular outflow tract
VSD ventricular septal defect
VT ventricular tachycardia
V_T tidal volume
VTI velocity–time integral
VV vitelline vein
VV-ECMO veno-venous extracorporeal membrane oxygenation

W

WHO World Health Organization

Basic Principles of Cardiac Surgery

Paolo Bosco and Samer A. M. Nashef

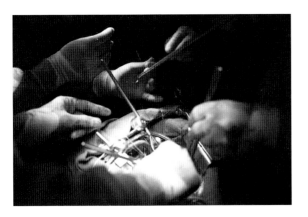

The art of surgery involves doing everything
as gracefully and efficiently as possible
Denton Arthur Cooley (1920–2016)

Cardiac surgery has made extraordinary progress in
the last few decades. This is largely the result of
dedicated effort and almost perfect teamwork among
cardiac surgeons and the allied specialty groups
(anaesthesists are obviously part of it). The creativ-
ity, imagination and skills that have given rise
to numerous technical innovations and surgical
procedures have brought to reality the surgical treatment of the majority of the congenital malformations and the acquired lesions of the heart. The basic
principles of patient selection and surgical technique
in current adult cardiac surgical practice are
outlined below.

Patient Selection

It is debatable whether there is such a thing as 'patient
selection'. Doctors do not have a treatment in their
pocket for which they select patients: they have
patients for whom they should select the best

treatment. Be that as it may, for any medical treatment to be of use, it should provide one of two things:
it should either improve the symptoms or improve
the prognosis. The decision to proceed with a cardiac
operation is therefore based on weighing the advantages (as indicated on symptomatic or prognostic
grounds or both) against the main disadvantage,
which is the risk of the operation.

The symptomatic indication is always the same
whatever the surgery: the failure of medical treatment
adequately to control the symptoms.

Prognostic indications are a little more complicated
and differ between the various cardiac conditions.
Some lesions have such an obvious impact on prognosis that the surgical option is virtually mandatory
unless the risk is truly prohibitive. An example would
be acute aortic dissection involving the ascending
aorta. This carries a cumulative mortality of 1% for
every hour of conservative treatment, so that by two
days nearly half the patients would have expired. Luck-
ily, most cardiac conditions are not like that, and the
risk of conservative management needs to be assessed
carefully and weighed against the risk of surgery. In
some areas that information is still poorly defined, but
in others there are clear guidelines based on quite good
evidence. Some of these are outlined below.

Ischaemic Heart Disease

The evidence for IHD comes from two aging but
still valid studies carried out first in America and
then in Europe, where patients with angina were
randomized to either medical treatment or surgical
treatment. With passing time, those treated surgically
began to show a survival advantage. This was particularly marked in the groups shown in Table 1.1,
listed in descending order of greater prognostic
importance.

1

Table 1.1 Prognostic impact of CABG surgery

Survival benefit	Indication
+++	>50% stenosis of the main stem of the left coronary artery (LMS)
++	Proximal stenosis of the three major coronary arteries: LAD, circumflex and right coronary arteries
+	>50% stenosis of two major coronary arteries including high-grade stenosis of the proximal LAD

It can be seen from the above that coronary angiography is essential to assess the prognostic implications of IHD, and makes decision-making relatively straightforward. On prognostic grounds alone, a young, otherwise fit, patient with a 90% LMS stenosis should be offered surgery, whereas an old, unfit diabetic arteriopath with single vessel disease affecting only a branch of the circumflex coronary artery should not.

Valve Disease

The symptomatic indication is the same as everywhere else: failure of medical treatment adequately to control the symptoms. The prognostic indication in general depends on the valve lesion, the presence of symptoms and changes in the structure and function of the heart (abnormal shape and increased size of the ventricle, ventricular function and AF are markers of an advanced stage of the valve pathology). In other words, regardless of the severity of the stenosis or regurgitation, there is no prognostic indication if the patient is asymptomatic with normal heart function and dimensions.

Risk Assessment

The mortality of cardiac surgery has for over 40 years been measured and incorporated into decisions about clinical care. Crude mortality, however, is not enough, and even journalists understand that the risk profile of the patient has as much to do with outcome as the quality of surgical care that is given.

Many models of risk in adult cardiac surgery have been developed, but the authors of this chapter are particularly (and understandably) biased toward the European System for Cardiac Operative Risk Evaluation (EuroSCORE). This was originally developed in 1999 and rapidly became the most widely used risk model in cardiac surgery. The Euro-SCORE originated from the analysis of data of more than 13,000 consecutive cases performed in more than 100 European centres in 1995. Progress in surgical techniques and postoperative care made the original data set outdated and led to the development of a new model: the EuroSCORE-II. The core of risk factors is almost the same although some definitions are more precise. These variables include patient-related factors (age, gender, lung disease, renal impairment, extracardiac arteriopathy, poor mobility, previous cardiac surgery, active endocarditis, critical preoperative state, DM on insulin), cardiac-related factors (functional class, recent MI, LV function, PHT) and operative-related factors (priority, weight of surgical procedure, surgery on the thoracic aorta). The EuroSCORE calculator is available online.

Operative Principles

Setting Up

Most cardiac operations are carried out with a standard set-up, which follows the patient surgical safety checklists. Once key factors associated with reduction of postoperative morbidity and mortality such as timely antibiotic administration, acknowledgement of allergies, blood availability and sterility have been verified, surgery begins.

Median sternotomy is the preferred access for most cardiac operations. Before dividing the sternum, it is useful to deflate the lungs to mitigate the risk of opening the pleural cavities. This minor event can be easily treated by placing a drain in the opened pleura, but in patients with reduced respiratory reserve it can be beneficial to keep the pleural intact. If the procedure includes the coronary surgery (CABG) the next step will be conduit harvesting (usually the left internal mammary artery (LIMA) and long saphenous vein (LSV). The LIMA is a precious conduit in coronary surgery: it is an ideal graft to the LAD coronary artery, which stays patent virtually forever and seems immune to atherosclerosis. If required, a segment of the LSV is harvested simultaneously. Once this part of the set-up is complete, the patient is fully heparinized and the ACT used to confirm the adequacy of anticoagulation. Cannulation of the ascending aorta and RA will follow. A double purse-string suture is used to secure the aortic cannulation site and further purse-string sutures are placed in the RA to secure the venous cannula or cannulae, which drain blood into the heart–lung machine. Another purse-string suture will be placed lower in the ascending aorta for the cardioplegia line, which will be essential to stop and intermittently perfuse the heart during the 'cross-clamp time'. Additional cannulation sites can be the right superior pulmonary vein for the LV vent insertion, the RA for the retrograde cardioplegia cannula or the PA for further venting. Venting the heart chambers and great vessels provide a relaxing bloodless field, which is an important aspect of a good set-up. Once everybody is happy with the ACT and the conduits are ready, the patient is 'put on bypass': blood is drained from the RA into the oxygenator, by simple gravity or vacuum-assisted. Oxygenated blood is then pumped into the aorta and the ventilator is switched off.

Myocardial Protection

During the central part of the operation, the aorta is clamped between the site of insertion of the aortic cannula and the origin of the coronary arteries. This produces a bloodless field, and makes intricate surgery possible, but during that time the heart will be ischaemic and will need protection.

The strategies used to minimize the ischaemic insult rely on the reduction of the myocardial metabolism and oxygen consumption by cooling the heart and achieving cardiac arrest, and this is achieved by infusing a 'cardioplegic' solution into the coronary arteries. The combination of cooling and cardiac arrest can reduce the myocardial oxygen consumption by more than 95%. There is no fixed time for delivering the cardioplegic solution during the operation but usually this is done every 15–20 minutes. Be aware that long cross-clamp time can be tolerated with an appropriate myocardial protection, which implies meticulous administration of regular doses of cardioplegia. On the other hand, if the surgeon's strategy for saving time is to skip the myocardial protection cardioplegia, the price to pay when the cross-clamp is released could be high, with a globally ischaemic heart and the need of pharmacological or mechanical support.

Coronary Surgery

The standard triple bypass (for triple vessel disease) involves the use of the LIMA and two segments of LSV. The LIMA is routinely anastomosed to the LAD

coronary artery. The LIMA-to-LAD graft is considered a major quality indicator in coronary surgery and is associated with high long-term patency rates. Total arterial revascularization (using also the right mammary or radial arteries) might be beneficial in younger patients since the long-term patency of the vein graft is not ideal. Pooled analysis of observational studies suggests that, at 10 years, there are better outcomes with bilateral internal mammary grafting than with single internal mammary grafting.

Technically, after the cardioplegia, with the heart arrested and vented through the aortic root, the target coronary artery is opened longitudinally, distally to any stenosis. The coronary anastomosis is then constructed with fine continuous sutures. The time required to perform a coronary anastomosis can be variable according to the coronary artery characteristics and the talent and expertise of the surgeon. It should take between 5 and 15 minutes. Precision is essential and should be prioritized over speed. Additional cardioplegia may be given into the aortic root or via the grafts or both as the case proceeds. The LIMA anastomosis, usually to the LAD, is constructed last.

Aortic Valve Surgery

The aorta is opened above the sinuses of Valsalva. If the patient has moderate to severe AR, cardioplegia must be administered directly into the coronary ostia, which are visible through the open aortotomy, or alternatively in a retrograde fashion (being aware that retrograde cardioplegia mainly acts on the LV for anatomical reasons, therefore the RV is poorly protected when only retrograde cardioplegia is used). Direct administration via the aortic root would simply distend the LV and the raised intraventricular pressure would reduce the effectiveness of the cardioplegic solution. AVR is carried out by removing the diseased valve, inserting sutures first into the annulus then into the sewing ring of the prosthesis, sliding the prosthesis on the sutures down into the annulus and tying the sutures. The aorta is then closed with a continuous suture. The intraoperative TOE is accepted as an essential tool to confirm good positioning and function of the prosthetic valve and to exclude any paravalvular leaks.

Mitral Valve Surgery

Mitral repair involves many different manoeuvres, such as leaflet resection, artificial chords, annular plication or annuloplasty. Most units carrying out mitral repair rely heavily on TOE to analyze the nature of the mitral lesion and to confirm the success of the repair. Mitral repair has better short- and long-term outcome if compared to MVR and, in high volume centres, the rate of repair for degenerative MR may be close to 100%. Replacement follows the same pattern as AVR. Bicaval cannulation is required to decompress the RA and permit access to the LA. Once the mitral repair or replacement is completed, the left atriotomy, which represents the standard access, is closed with a continuous suture.

De-airing

If a main heart chamber (atrium, aorta, PA or ventricle) has been opened as part of the procedure, it is important to evacuate air from the heart, especially the left side, before the heart is put back into the circulation and the air escapes to the brain. This may involve a fair amount of vigorous physical activity by the surgeon while the heart, and sometimes the entire patient, is shaken, stirred and repositioned to optimize the process. This, together with a request for restarting ventilation briefly, to expel air from the pulmonary veins, is usually sufficient to rouse the sleepiest anaesthetist from deepest torpor. It is also a reliable signal that the end, though not quite close enough, is now at least in sight. TOE is useful for detecting residual air and determining the adequacy of de-airing.

Clamp-Off

The AXC is then removed, allowing perfusion of the coronary arteries and the heart then begins to come to life. If myocardial protection has been optimal, the heart often reverts to NSR. If not, VF is the commonest dysrhythmia seen and internal cardioversion is carried out. Any proximal anastomoses (so-called 'top ends') of coronary grafts are then carried out using a partially occluding or 'side-biting' aortic clamp; alternatively, top ends can be performed with the AXC on, depending on surgeon preference and on the quality of the aorta (multiple aortic clamping seems to be associated to higher incidence of stroke). The patient is then prepared for 'coming off bypass'. The lungs are ventilated and the perfusionist gradually occludes the RA cannula, thus allowing more blood to return to the heart and be pumped. The arterial pressure line begins to show pulsation as the

heart gradually takes over the circulation. The heart-lung machine is then stopped and the atrial or caval cannulae removed. In this phase of the operation some residual air bubbles can embolize into the right coronary artery, which originates in the anterior part of the aortic root (highest point in a supine patient). The typical sign of this fairly common complication is distension of the RV, global (and usually transient) hypokinesia and obviously, hypotension. The expert anaesthetist will promptly recognize this condition. The first manoeuvres consist in increasing the perfusion pressure in order to get rid of the air through the capillary circulation. Calcium chloride and various vasoconstrictors are usually used. If hypotension and low CO do not resolve promptly the next step is to restart the CPB and assist the heart until the RV recovers.

The End

Heparin is reversed using its antidote, protamine, which often produces hypotension. This can be treated by transfusing blood from the pump into the patient via the aortic cannula. Haemostasis is secured (what a long and tedious process these three simple words describe!) and the chest is closed over the appropriate number of drains and epicardial pacing wires. Achieving perfect haemostasis is both a surgical and a medical task. Checking the ACT and bringing it back to the baseline, administering further doses of protamine to treat heparin rebound and the judicious use of blood products are as important as careful attention to surgical bleeding. A patient who bleeds in the postoperative period is exposed to many risks related to haemodynamic instability, surgical re-exploration and transfusion, and faces an overall higher mortality.

Off-Pump Surgery

In an effort to avoid the potential adverse effects of CPB, some surgeons perform coronary surgery without it, using clever contraptions to steady the bit of heart they are working on. There is no cannulation, extracorporeal circulation or cross-clamping of the aorta. Despite the theoretical advantages of avoiding the use of CPB (aortic cannulation and manipulation, inflammatory response), there is still a controversy in its effectiveness and indication. As a result, off-pump surgery is not the first choice in Europe and the United States for routine surgical revascularization. Furthermore, the outcome seems related to the volume of operations performed, since off-pump surgery is a technically challenging exercise for the surgeon. The absence of CPB means that these operations are more demanding of the anaesthetist as well, who will need to work constantly on optimizing haemodynamics as the heart is mobilized, retracted and stabilized while continuing to support the circulation (see Chapter 12). In general, off-pump CABG has fewer early complications but less complete revascularization and possibly less good long-term graft patency.

Minimally Invasive Cardiac Surgery

Efforts to reduce the invasiveness of cardiac surgery continue apace. What is called 'minimally invasive' does not always truly represent a smaller surgical burden for the patient. In minimal invasive mitral surgery, the surgeon performs the same operation through a small right thoracotomy using long instruments and a camera. Peripheral cannulation sites (jugular and femoral vein for venous drainage and femoral artery for the arterial return may be used and a TOE-guided endo-aortic balloon clamp occludes the ascending aorta and delivers cardioplegia). Often, the cross-clamp and bypass time are prolonged because of the increased difficulty of completing the procedure. The patient avoids a full sternotomy but may have a longer procedure. Minimally invasive mitral surgery requires dedicated training and a regular caseload in order to achieve good and consistent results. Some centres offer AVR through a mini-sternotomy (upper third) or a small right thoracotomy. All the above procedures have outcomes that are strongly volume-related. Valve technology has also evolved and sutureless AV prostheses are now available. Transcatheter AV implantation (TAVI) is also developing, and in the UK it is routinely used for patients requiring AVR who are considered unsuitable for conventional surgery. The reader may wish to speculate on the motivation for all these developments at a time when cardiac surgery is phenomenally successful and has an enviable safety record. Are we motivated by a true desire to help the patients by reducing the invasiveness of our procedure, a desperate attempt to claw back from the cardiologists the large number of patients now treated by percutaneous intervention or do surgeons, like little children, get bored with their predictable old 'toys' and want new ones?

Key Points

- Surgery is indicated on symptomatic grounds when symptoms are not adequately controlled by maximal medical therapy.
- Surgery is indicated on prognostic grounds in situations such as aortic dissection and LMS coronary disease, regardless of the severity of symptoms.
- The use of validated risk models, such as EuroSCORE-II, allows rapid risk assessment at the point of care and helps the surgeon in the decision-making process.
- Most routine cardiac surgical procedures follow a predictable and well-defined path.
- Myocardial protection and surgical accuracy are cornerstones of modern cardiac surgery.
- Haemostasis is the result of medical and surgical efforts.

Further Reading

CASS principal investigators and their associates. Myocardial infarction and mortality in the coronary artery surgery randomized trial. *N Engl J Med* 1984; 310: 750–8.

ESC/EACTS joint task force members. Guidelines on the management of valvular heart disease. *Eur Heart J* 2012; 33: 2451–96.

Lamy A, Deveraux PJ, Prabhakaran D, *et al.* Rationale and design of the coronary artery bypass grafting surgery off or on pump revascularization study: a large international randomized trial in cardiac surgery. *Am Heart J* 2012; 163: 1–6.

Nashef SA, Roques F, Michel P, *et al.* European system for cardiac operative risk evaluation (EuroSCORE). *Eur J Cardiothorac Surg* 1999; 16: 9–13.

Taggart DP, Altman DG, Gray AM, *et al.* Randomized trial of bilateral versus single internal thoracic artery grafts. *N Eng J Med* 2016; 375: 2540–9.

Chapter

2

Symptoms and Signs of Cardiac Disease

Joseph E. Arrowsmith

Despite the widespread availability of investigational tests and imaging techniques for the diagnosis and management of cardiac disease, eliciting a comprehensive history and performing a systematic physical examination remain essential clinical skills.

Symptoms

The presence or absence of specific symptoms should be sought in a systematic fashion. Symptoms should be described in terms of their nature (using the patient's own words), onset, duration and progression, as well as any modifying factors or associations.

Overall functional status: The NYHA functional capacity classification provides an assessment of the impact of symptoms (dyspnoea, angina, fatigue, palpitation) on physical activity. An objective assessment of severity of cardiovascular disease, added in 1994, recognizes the fact that severity of symptoms (i.e. functional capacity) may not reflect the severity of the underlying cardiovascular disease.

Dyspnoea: The sensation of uncomfortable breathing. It is essential to make the distinction between cardiac and respiratory causes. Mechanisms include: hypoxia, hypercarbia, bronchoconstriction, bronchial mucosal oedema, reduced lung compliance (increased work of breathing), reflex hyperventilation and reduced vital capacity (hydrothorax, ascites, pregnancy).

> Cardiac causes include: Elevated pulmonary venous pressure, reduced pulmonary blood flow (right-to-left shunt), and a low CO (RV failure). An acute onset may suggest papillary muscle or MV chordal rupture, whereas a more insidious onset may suggest gradually worsening ventricular function.

Associated symptoms: Especially chest pain, palpitation, diaphoresis and (pre)syncope.

Postural: Supine (orthopnoea, paroxysmal noctural dyspnoea), other (atrial myxoma).

Haemoptysis: Not uncommon in cardiac disease. Frank haemoptysis may occur in MS (bronchial or pulmonary vein rupture) and pulmonary infarction. In pulmonary oedema the sputum is frothy and often streaked with blood. Pulmonary causes include: TB, bronchiectasis and cancer.

Chest pain: Aetiology may be cardiac (ischaemic and non-ischaemic) or non-cardiac. Enquiry should be made about the quality, location, radiation, timing and duration of pain, as well as any provoking, exacerbating or relieving factors and associated symptoms.

> Non-ischaemic cardiac causes include: aortic dissection ('tearing' central pain, radiating to back), MV prolapse (sharp infra-mammary pain), pericarditis (dull central chest pain, worsened on leaning forward) and PE (pleuritic pain worse on inspiration).

> Non-cardiac causes include: oesophagitis and oesophageal spasm (relieved by nitrates), biliary and pancreatic disorders, pleural inflammation and musculoskeletal disorders of the chest wall and spine.

Angina pectoris: Typically described as 'choking', 'tightening' or 'heaviness'. Levine's sign (hand clenched against the chest) may be present. Usually diffuse in nature, located to mid chest or xiphisternum with radiation to the left chest and arm, epigastrium, back or jaw. Typically lasting <10 minutes (duration >20 minutes may indicate ACS – infarction or unstable angina). Provoked by exertion, cold exposure, eating and emotional stress. May be worsened, or paradoxically relieved, by continuing exertion. Relieved by cessation of activity or nitrates. Typically graded using CCS angina scale.

Syncope: Transient loss or near loss (pre-syncope) of consciousness secondary to reduced cerebral blood flow – a low CO or cerebral perfusion pressure. The patient may describe 'drop attacks', a 'funny turn', dizziness or tinnitus. The presence of associated symptoms, such as a premonitory aura, palpitation or chest pain should be actively sought. The differential diagnosis includes: postural hypotension, neurological disorders and cardiac disease.

> Postural hypotension may be drug-induced (e.g. β-blockers, vasodilators), vasovagal (e.g. micturitional), orthostatic (>20 mmHg fall in systolic BP on standing) or secondary to aortocaval compression when supine in pregnancy. DM and Parkinson's disease may cause autonomic dysfunction.

> A witnessed seizure may indicate epilepsy as the cause, whereas pre-syncope associated with transient dysphasia, blindness (amaurosis fugax) or paresis suggests a thromboembolic or vasculopathic cause.

> *Stokes–Adams attacks*: Causes include sinus arrest, heart block and VT.

> *Exertional syncope*: This may suggest AS, coronary artery disease (CAD), PHT or a congenital anomaly of coronary artery anatomy. A family history of syncope may indicate hypertrophic obstructive cardiomyopathy, takotsubo cardiomyopathy or an inherited cardiac conduction defect (long QT syndrome, Wolff–Parkinson–White syndrome).

Oedema: 'Anasarca', the accumulation of interstitial fluid in dependent areas such as the lower limbs and sacral area. Sodium and water retention may occur in cardiac failure, renal failure and malnutrition. Facial oedema may suggest myxoedema or SVC obstruction.

Palpitations: *Awareness of heartbeat*. 'Thumping' sensation in chest, neck or back; 'missed', 'jumping' or 'extra' beats; or 'racing' of the heart. A common symptom in the absence of cardiac disease. It may indicate significant dysrhythmia or abnormal cardiac function. Any relationship to exertion or ingestion of alcohol, caffeine or nicotine should be sought, as should symptoms suggestive of thyrotoxicosis.

Fatigue: A distinction should be made between lethargy or general malaise, and effort tolerance limited by chest pain, dyspnoea, claudication or leg weakness. As static measures of cardiac (ventricular) performance often give no indication of functional reserve, it is essential to obtain a measure of maximal functional capacity and the rapidity of any decline. The Duke Activity Status Index (DASI) is often used to grade functional capacity.

Miscellaneous: These include nausea, anorexia, dry mouth (disopyramide), nocturia and polyuria (diuretics), cough (ACE inhibitors), xanthopsia (digoxin toxicity), tinnitus and vertigo (chinchonism), headache (nitrates), photosensitivity (amiodarone), nightmares (propranolol), abdominal swelling/pain (ascites/hepatomegaly).

Physical Signs

Physical examination is conducted with the patient supine and reclining at 45°. The patient may be required to turn to the left, sit forward, stand or perform isometric exercise.

Observation (Inspection)

General appearance: Conscious level, nutritional status, diaphoresis, xanthelasmata, systolic head nodding (de Musset's sign – AR) and signs of conditions associated with cardiac disease (Marfan, Cushing and Down syndromes, acromegaly, systemic lupus erythematosus, rheumatoid arthritis, ankylosing spondylitis, muscular dystrophy).

Skin: Cyanosis, orange fingers (tobacco use), anaemia, jaundice (hepatic congestion), malar flush, erythema (pressure sores, cardioversion burns), haemorrhagic palmar/plantar lesions (Janeway lesions – endocarditis), bruising and phlebitis (venepuncture, IV therapy and drug abuse).

Surgical scars: These include sternotomy (cardiac surgery), thoracotomy (mitral valvotomy, repair of coarctation or patent ductus arteriosus (PDA)), subclavian (pacemaker or cardiodefibrillator insertion), cervical (carotid endarterectomy), antecubital (coronary angiography), abdominal (aortic aneurysm repair).

Nail beds: Clubbing, cyanosis, splinter haemorrhages, arterial pulsation (Quinke's sign – AR), Osler's nodes (tender finger-tip nodules – endocarditis).

Cyanosis: Cyanosis is blue skin discolouration. May be peripheral (hypovolaemia, low CO) or central (mucous membranes). The latter indicates a deoxygenated Hb concentration >5 g dl^{-1}. May not be manifest in severe anaemia.

Respiratory rate: Tachypnoea may indicate anxiety or underlying dyspnoea. Episodic (Cheyne–Stokes) breathing is suggestive of severe cardiac failure.

Neck: Goitre, carotid abrupt carotid distension and collapse (Corrigan's sign – AR), and jugular veins.

Jugular veins: Pressure level *and* waveform. Level rarely 2 cm above sternal angle when patient reclined at 45° and falls on inspiration. Inspiratory rise suggests pericardial constriction (Kussmaul's sign). Elevated by anxiety, pregnancy, anaemia, exercise, right heart failure and SVC obstruction (non-pulsatile). Giant a-wave (TS, PS, RVH, RA myxoma), cannon a-wave (complete heart block, VT, junctional rhythm, pacing anomaly), systolic cv-wave (TR), slow y-descent (TS), sharp/short y-descent (pericardial constriction), increased x-descent (RV volume overload, tamponade).

Mouth: Foetor oris, mucous membrane dryness, state of dentition, palate, systolic uvular pulsation (Müller's sign – AR).

Fundi: Hypertensive and diabetic changes, Roth spots (endocarditis).

Palpation

Skin: Temperature, capillary refill, pitting oedema.

Pulse: Rate, rhythm, character/volume (bounding, anacrotic, collapsing, thready, irregular), respiratory variation, condition of vessel, radio-femoral delay.

> *Pulsus alternans*: amplitude varies on alternate beats – indicative of severe LV dysfunction.
>
> *Pulsus bisferiens*: combined anacrotic and collapsing pulse.
>
> Irregular pulse may indicate AF, sinus arrhythmia, multiple atrial or ventricular premature beats or SVT with variable atrioventricular block.

'Waterhammer' pulse of AR detected by palpating radial artery as arm is elevated – more easily appreciated in calf muscles when elevating leg.

An arteriovenous fistula (dialysis, severe Paget's bone disease, PDA) may also produce a collapsing pulse.

Delayed/absent femoral pulses (coarctation, dissection, AAA).

Neck: Tracheal deviation, carotid thrill, radiated cardiac thrill. Suprasternal/manubrial pulsation (coarctation).

Praecordium: Apex beat is impulse of ventricular systole normally felt in fifth intercostal space in midclavicular line. S$_4$ may be palpable in LVH. Thrills in MR, VSD, AS, PS, MS and PDA. Left parasternal (RV) heave in PS, PHT and MS.

Lung fields: Vocal fremitus.

Abdomen: Hepatic enlargement/pulsation, splenomegaly (endocarditis), ascites.

Percussion

Praecordium: A crude estimate of cardiac size. Area of dullness increased by pericardial effusion and decreased by emphysema.

Lung fields: Pleural effusion, lobar collapse and pneumothorax.

Abdomen: Hepatomegaly and ascites.

Auscultation

Listen all over. Bell best for low frequencies, rigid diaphragm best for high frequencies. Murmurs exaggerated by inspiration (right heart origin), expiration (left heart origin), posture (left lateral, sitting forward), squatting, standing and isometric exercise (MR in MV prolapse). Classical anatomic areas for auscultation of individual valves unreliable.

Peripheral vessels:

> *Brachial arteries*: BP measurement (by sphygmomanometer), estimation of respiratory paradox.
>
> *Carotid arteries*: Bruit, radiated murmurs.
>
> *Abdominal arteries*: Murmurs normal in 50% young patients and 5% over 50 years old. Renal or coeliac and artery stenosis, splenic artery compression (tumour) or aneurysm.

Femoral arteries: Traube's sign (booming systolic and diastolic 'pistol shot' sounds over the artery in AR), Duroziez's sign (diastolic flow murmur heard in AR when artery partially compressed by stethoscope diaphragm).

Lungs: Vesicular (normal) breath sounds. Bronchial breath sounds, crackles (crepitations) and wheeze (rales, rhonchi). Whispering pectoriloqy, broncophony and egeophony.

Praecordium – heart sounds: Low-pitched sounds of short duration believed to be created by closing valve leaflets, opening valve leaflets and structures 'shuddering' under sudden tension. Amplitude reduced by obesity, emphysema, pericardial effusion, AS, PS, a low CO and dextrocardia; increased by hyperdynamic circulation and in arterial hypertension/PHT; and varies in AF and complete (third-degree) heart block.

First sound (S_1) = closure of TV and MV (loudest). Loudness of M_1 increased with sinus tachycardia, inotropes, thyroxine and delayed MV closure (reduced PR interval and early MS). Splitting not usually audible – may indicate AV opening sound or myocardial injury (e.g. acute MI).

Second sound (S_2) = closure of AV followed by PV. Splitting increased on inspiration as PV closure delayed. Inspiratory splitting increased with PHT, PS and RBBB. Splitting reduced on expiration, and with LBBB, aging, early PHT and AS. Fixed splitting in an ASD, VSD, massive PE. Paradoxical splitting (increases on expiration) by delayed AV closure – AS, LBBB, hypertension.

Third sound (S_3) = rapid early diastolic filling (protodiastolic gallop). May be normal in the young, otherwise pathological. Present in LV/RV failure, MR, TR, pregnancy, left-to-right shunts and anaemia. Shorter and earlier in diastole in constrictive pericarditis.

Fourth sound (S_4) = late diastolic filling (atrial systole). May be present in some tall athletes; otherwise pathological. May indicate reduced LV compliance (LVH, amyloid, ischaemia). Precludes AF and severe MS.

Summation gallop = S_3+S_4 superimposed. May occur in tachycardia.

Ejection click: AS, PS and PHT (reduced on inspiration).

Late systolic click: MV prolapse.

Opening snap (OS): MS. Audible over whole praecordium. Indicates mobile MV leaflets, louder on expiration. Interval between A_2 and OS falls as LA pressure increases and rises with increased aortic pressure. Pneumothorax may produce systolic 'clicking'.

Praecordium – cardiac murmurs: Vibrations caused by turbulent blood flow – more likely with high velocity blood flow, low blood viscosity and an abrupt change in vessel/chamber diameter. Characterized by relationship to cardiac and respiratory cycles, location, radiation, acoustic quality and intensity (Table 2.1).

Mid ('ejection') systolic murmur (MSM): Follows AV/PV opening (crescendo–decrescendo). May be innocent (Grade $\leq$ 3) or due to AV sclerosis, increased pulmonary flow (ASD, total anomalous pulmonary venous drainage (TAPVD)), AS (harsh MSM in aortic area, soft A_2, split S_2) or PS (soft P_2, opening click, louder on inspiration).

Pan (holo) systolic murmur (PSM). High-pitched apical PSM radiating to axilla with soft S_1 and S_3 in MR. Mid or late systolic click suggests MV prolapse. 'Musical' PSM, louder on inspiration, at left lower sternal edge (LLSE) in TR. Harsh PSM at LLSE with thrill (~90%) suggests a VSD.

Early (immediate) diastolic murmur (EDM): AR – 'blowing' decrescendo murmur at LLSE $\pm$ superimposed S_3. Murmur of functional MS (Austin Flint) may be present. PR – decrescendo murmur at left upper sternal edge (LUSE), louder on inspiration. Graham Steell (PR) murmur associated with MS and PHT.

Mid diastolic murmur (MDM) following OS. MS – rumbling apical MDM radiating to axilla,

Table 2.1 Grading of cardiac murmurs

Grade	Characteristics
1/6	Only just audible, even under good auscultatory conditions
2/6	Soft
3/6	Moderately loud
4/6	Loud
5/6	Very loud
6/6	Audible with stethoscope lifted from chest wall

louder on expiration, loud P_2. Duration proportional to severity. In severe MS the OS occurs earlier ($\leq$70 mS after P_2) and is softer/inaudible and duration of MDM increases. TS – louder on inspiration. MDM may be caused by MV/TV thickening in rheumatic endocarditis (Carey Coombs) or by increased flow in the VSD, PDA (MV) or ASD, TAPVD (TV).

Late diastolic murmur (LDM) or presystolic eccentuation: MS – MV flow in late diastole + atrial systole (S_4). OS typically $\geq$100 mS after P_2 in mild MS. S_4 precluded by AF.

Late systolic murmur (LSM): MR/MV prolapse. May only be apparent after exercise.

Continuous murmur: PDA ('machinery' murmur at LUSE with loud P_2), pulmonary arteriovenous fistula or surgical conduit (e.g. Blalock–Taussig, Waterston, Fontan).

Venous hum: Partial obstruction of neck veins (especially in children). Obliterated by digital compression of veins. Important to differentiate from the PDA.

Other sounds: Friction rub and cardiorespiratory.

Further Reading

Campeau L. Grading of angina pectoris. *Circulation* 1976; 54: 522–3.

Constant J. *Essentials of Bedside Cardiology*, 2nd edn. Totowa, NJ: Humana Press; 2002.

The Criteria Committee of the New York Heart Association. *Nomenclature and Criteria for Diagnosis of Diseases of the Heart and Great Vessels*, 9th edn. Boston, MA: Lippincott Williams and Wilkins; 1994.

Hlatky MA, Boineau RE, Higginbotham MB, *et al*. A brief self-administered questionnaire to determine functional capacity (the Duke Activity Status Index). *Am J Cardiol* 1989; 64: 651–4.

Chapter

3

Diagnostic Techniques

Amir Awwad and S. K. Bobby Agarwal

Non-Invasive Diagnostic Tests

Non-invasive diagnostic tests (Table 3.1) are undertaken to support the clinical impression of and to quantify the extent of cardiac disease. Repeating the investigations over time allows for monitoring of management protocols and follow-up on disease progression. Information may be supplemented with advanced and invasive investigations (e.g. angiography in suspected coronary artery disease (CAD)).

Electrocardiography

The ECG represents the sum of myocardial voltage changes throughout the cardiac cycle along the vector of each of the leads recorded. It may be recorded from the skin surface, from the endocardium in the catheter laboratory or from the epicardium during certain open procedures requiring cardiac mapping. The simplicity of acquisition of the surface ECG makes it one of the most frequent tests performed.

The following processes affect the sum of myocardial voltage changes (Table 3.2):

- The frequency of atrial and ventricular systole
- The mass of the chambers undergoing depolarization
- The route by which depolarization occurs
- Myocardial perfusion
- Metabolic influences

The ECG, in conjunction with markers of myocardial necrosis (e.g. troponin I), helps to establish the diagnosis of ST-elevation myocardial infarction (STEMI) or non-ST-elevation myocardial infarction (NSTEMI).

Exercise ECG

Myocardial oxygen extraction is maximal at rest, so an exercise-induced increase in metabolic demand can only be met by increase in coronary blood flow. It follows therefore that coronary flow limitation in the setting of coronary artery stenosis has a far greater

---

Box 3.1 Limitations of the resting surface ECG

- Temporal changes in the ST segment may be missed with a single recording
- Small non-Q-wave infarcts may fail to meet diagnostic criteria
- Large transmural infarcts may obscure additional electrocardiographic events
- The sensitivity to detect ischaemia is limited by the position of the exploring electrode
- Posterior cardiac events are often missed
- Resting ECG may be normal even in the setting of three-vessel CAD
- May fail to reflect the effect of exercise on myocardial perfusion
- ECG changes lag behind changes in diastolic and systolic dysfunction with ischaemia
- Prone to skeletal muscle myopotentials, obscuring changes

Table 3.1 Classification of non-invasive diagnostic techniques

Electrocardiography	Ionizing radiation	Non-ionizing imaging
Resting 12-lead ECG	CXR	Echocardiography
Exercise stress test	CT	MRI
Ambulatory ECG monitoring	Nuclear scintigraphy	
Intraoperative ECG monitoring		
Intraoperative ST-segment analysis		

Table 3.2 Overview of ECG abnormalities

	Abnormality	Description	Comments
Atrioventricular conduction	First-degree block	PR interval >200 ms One P-wave per QRS	Seen in CAD, acute rheumatic fever, digoxin toxicity and electrolyte disturbance
	Second-degree block	Mobitz type I Progressive lengthening of PR interval Mobitz type II PR interval constant, occasional non-conducted beats 2:1 block: two P-waves per QRS complex, normal P-wave rate	Also known as Wenkebach Usually benign May herald complete heart block May herald complete heart block
	Third-degree block	Normal atrial depolarization, no conducted beats, usually wide QRS with ventricular rate <50 per minute	Ventricles excited by slow 'escape' mechanism. MI, chronic fibrosis around bundle of His and in RBBB. Consider pacing
Intraventricular conduction	LBBB	QRS >120 ms, late R-waves in I, aVL and V_{5-6}, no septal Q-waves, deep S in V_1, tall R in V_6, associated with T-wave inversion in lateral leads	Best seen in V_6 Always pathological, prevents further interpretation of ECG
	Left anterior hemiblock	QRS 100 ms, marked left-axis deviation, deep S in II, III, q in I ± aVL	
	Left posterior hemiblock	QRS 100 ms, right-axis deviation	
	RBBB	QRS >120 ms, RSR in V_{1-2}, dominant R and inverted T-wave in V_1, usually normal axis,	Best seen in V_1 May indicate RV problems, may be normal variant Bifasicular block: RBBB with left anterior hemiblock
Ischaemia		ST depression >2 mm	
Infarction		Raised ST segments, ± Q-waves (>3 mm, >30 ms), normalization of ST segments, T-wave inversion	
Hypertrophy	RA	Peaked P-wave	
	LA	Bifid P-wave	
	RV	Right axis deviation, tall R in V_1, T-wave inversion V_{1-2}, deep S in V_6, ± RBBB	
	LV	R in V_{5-6} >25 mm or R in V_{5-6} + S in V_{1-2} >35 mm	

effect during exercise than at rest; thereby increasing the sensitivity of the ECG to detect ischaemia.

Exercise ECG (EECG) testing, using a treadmill or static cycle ergometer, is to investigate 'cardiac-type' chest pain or exertional breathlessness. Both treadmill and cycle-based testing are limited to patients with the ability to exercise. In the Bruce protocol both the speed and gradient of the treadmill are increased at each stage, whereas in the modified Bruce protocol the treadmill speed remains constant during the first three stages. In the Naughton protocol, however, only the treadmill gradient is altered. HR and BP are recorded at each increase in workload and the ECG examined for evidence of ST-segment depression. Myocardial ischaemia is suggested by the development of chest pain, ST-segment changes, failure to increase the BP or arrhythmias. Results are defined as positive, negative, equivocal and uninterpretable.

EECG testing is relatively cheap and can be performed in the outpatient setting. It has low specificity and sensitivity (65–70%) for CAD, although simultaneous TTE detection of regional wall motion abnormalities (RWMAs) improves specificity. Low-grade stenoses (<50%) are difficult to detect as are fixed stenoses with collateral blood flow. Contraindications to EECG included: ACS, severe congestive cardiac failure and severe AS. It may also be unsuitable for patients with physical disability, respiratory disease, peripheral vascular disease, LBBB, or atrioventricular (A-V) conduction abnormalities.

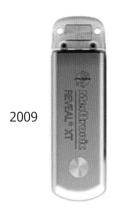

2009   2014

Figure 3.1 The Medtronic Reveal® ICM latest models. Recording electrodes at the top in each model

Ambulatory ECG

Ambulatory ECG monitoring, also known as Holter or continuous 24-hour recording, is a method used to aid the diagnosis of chest pain, palpitations or syncope that occur intermittently during normal daily activities. The ECG electrodes are applied to the chest and attached to a recording device which is carried by the patient for a period of 24–48 hours. Some devices comprise a patient-activated event monitor. Patients are required to complete a log of events to aid analysis and correlate physical activities with contemporaneous ECG changes. The recorder is interrogated to produce a printout or computer analysis of events.

Longer-term implantable ECG recorders are nowadays used to increase event detection rate. They may record data continuously or intermittently. Integral electrodes are placed subcutaneously in the left subclavian position. Over the past decade, a generation of the Reveal® devices has become the most commonly used implantable cardiac monitoring (ICM) systems. Those are capable of up to 3 years of cardiac monitoring, indicated for patients at increased risk of cardiac arrhythmias and/or experiencing transient dysrhythmic symptoms (e.g. dizziness, palpitation, syncope and chest pain). Reveal LINQ® ICM is the latest and smallest (about 1 ml in volume) programmable model that continuously monitors ECG and other physiological parameters (Figure 3.1). It records cardiac information (up to 30 minutes) triggered by either automatic detection of arrhythmias or upon patient activation. The device then communicates wirelessly to a linked secure network that daily transmits data to the clinic (scheduled or by clinician's request). The device is also MRI conditional (1.5 and 3 Tesla) and both insertion and removal procedures are conducted under local anaesthesia.

Transthoracic Echocardiography

TTE is relatively quick and straightforward to perform and provides qualitative and quantitative assessment of cardiac structure and function. Although TTE is an extremely useful tool, it does have several limitations. Certain patient factors reduce echogenicity and therefore make image quality poor or unobtainable. These include obesity, pulmonary emphysema, interference from the ribs, an inability to lie in the lateral position and the presence of surgical drains and anterior chest wall dressings. Findings are relatively operator-dependent and technical difficulties may limit both the quality and completeness of an examination. Spatial resolution is restricted to one wavelength (0.3 mm at 5 MHz) and depth resolution to 200 wavelengths (60 mm at 5 MHz). TTE is poor at imaging posterior structures and Doppler can only be used to estimate flow accurately if the angle of incident ultrasound is <20° (see Chapters 32–35).

Stress Echocardiography

Echocardiography can be combined with exercise testing or dobutamine-induced (40–60 mg kg^{-1} min^{-1}) stress in patients unable to exercise to allow qualitative assessment of ventricular performance with increase in HR. Occasionally, pacing or atropine is required to obtain an adequate HR response. Imaging dynamic changes in LV outflow obstruction in hypertrophic obstructive cardiomyopathy (HOCM) is also possible. Stress echocardiography is more sensitive than stress ECG at detecting ischaemia. The value of the test rests in the visualization of functional changes with increased myocardial demand.

Contrast Echocardiography

Contrast agents can be employed to improve image quality by delineating the border between endocardium and ventricular cavity. Sonographic contrast agents are suspensions of microspheres filled with perfluorocarbon gas, which enhance image resolution by acting as intravascular tracers. The insonated gas bubbles pulsate, with compression occurring at the peak of the ultrasound wave and expansion at the nadir. SonoVue® is a stabilized aqueous suspension of sulphur hexafluoride (2.5 µm microbubbles) within a shell of polyethylene glycol (macrogel 4,000). After peripheral IV injection of 0.2–0.4 ml, the microbubbles traverse the pulmonary vascular bed to opacify the ventricular cavity. Further refinements allow quantification of coronary microcirculation by assessment of subendocardial opacification. This is particularly powerful during stress echocardiography as a reduction in opacification is often easier to appreciate than a new RWMA. Allergic reactions to contrast agents have occurred and therefore contrast is contraindicated in patients with recent unstable cardiac symptoms, a recent (<7 days) coronary intervention, class III and IV heart failure or serious arrhythmias.

Cardiovascular Imaging

Over the years, new cardiovascular radiological imaging modalities have been developed to assess the beating heart. A comprehensive non-invasive cardiac examination is now possible. The anaesthetist must be aware of the indications and limits of each technique.

Chest Radiography

A posteroanterior and lateral CXR provide information about the heart, the lungs, the great vessels and the thoracic skeleton (Box 3.2). A plain preoperative CXR provides a baseline against which to judge postoperative images.

Nuclear Cardiology

Scintigraphy, positron emission tomography (PET) and single photon emission computed tomography (SPECT) detect gamma rays emitted by a radionuclide tracer administered to the patient. In contrast to scintigraphy imaging (planar 2D), PET and SPECT can provide information in three dimensions.

Box 3.2 Assessment of the preoperative chest radiograph before cardiac surgery

Cardiac silhouette
Cardiothoracic ratio ('normal' $\leq$50%)
LA enlargement
Calcification – LV wall, valvular, pericardial
Prostheses/pacing wires

Mediastinal silhouette
Calcification – aortic arch
Mediastinal widening
Tracheal deviation

Hila
Pulmonary arteries and veins
Lymphadenopathy and other masses

Lung fields
Upper lobes blood diversion
Interlobular septal (Kerley B) lines
Perihilar ('Bats Wing') opacities

Diaphragm
Pleural effusion

Skeleton
Sternal wires – previous surgery
Rib notching
Retrosternal space – in redo-surgery

The radionuclide tracers thallium (^{201}TI), technetium-sestamibi (^{99m}Tc-sestamibi) and ^{99m}Tc-tetrofosmin are routinely used for SPECT and scintigraphy. Due to its shorter half-life (^{99m}Tc, 6 hours versus ^{201}TI, 72 hours), a higher dose of ^{99m}Tc can be administered. Superior image quality at a lower radiation dose makes ^{99m}Tc the preferred tracer. The radionuclide tracers rubidium (^{82}Rb) and N-ammonia (^{13}N-ammonia) are used for PET.

In contrast to SPECT, PET is now increasingly penetrating clinical cardiac applications with advanced insights into pathophysiology and biology owing to several recent developments. PET current applications allow assessment of myocardial blood flow, myocardial viability and, when ECG-gated imaging is used, global and regional ventricular function. The main limitations of these techniques are

Table 3.3 Clinical significance of radionuclide tracer uptake during myocardial perfusion

Tracer uptake pattern	Significance
Homogeneous	Normal myocardial perfusion (except when severe three-vessel disease: homogeneous uptake associated with poor LV function) Low risk of cardiac event (0.6% per year)
Reversible defect	Defect on stress study only Indicates reversible ischaemia/viable myocardium High risk of cardiac event (~7–13% per year) Indication of revascularization therapy
Fixed defect	Defect on rest and stress study Indicates MI

Box 3.3 Indications for myocardial perfusion imaging

- Preoperative evaluation
- Myocardial viability assessment
- Risk stratification
- Evaluation after percutaneous coronary intervention (PCI) or coronary artery grafting
- Medical therapy monitoring

relatively poor spatial resolution, soft tissue attenuation artefacts and delivery of a significant dose of ionizing radiation. Recent trends, however, have introduced novel developments into cardiac nuclear imaging, such as dedicated cardiac SPECT cameras (faster, dynamic with lower radiation dose), hybrid nuclear imaging (PET/MRI) and advanced molecular imaging (metabolism and sympathetic innervation).

Stress Imaging

Myocardial imaging at rest and during exercise (stress) permits the assessment of myocardial perfusion (Table 3.3). Pharmacological stress, induced using a vasodilator (adenosine or dipyridamole) or an inotrope (dobutamine), can be used in patients unable to exercise. Multiple or severe inducible ischaemic defects represent significant scintigraphic findings. ECG-gated acquisition gives improved diagnostic accuracy by allowing better distinction between true perfusion abnormalities and artefacts. It also allows evaluation of ventricular function (Figure 3.2).

Furthermore, viable myocardium can be identified either by perfusion (^{201}TI or ^{99m}Tc-sestamibi; assessment of cellular membrane integrity) or metabolic (fluorodeoxyglucose (^{18}FDG)) tracers. Myocardial viability is an important determinant of the likely benefits of revascularization therapy. The indications and effectiveness of myocardial perfusion imaging are summarized in Box 3.3 and Table 3.4.

Computed Tomography

High temporal and spatial resolution is required to visualize small and moving coronary arteries. This has been made possible by the development of multidetector row CT (MDCT) scanners with fast X-ray tube rotation speed and multiple detector rows. The use of first-generation four-slice MDCT was limited by the need for slow heart rates (to reduce motion artefacts) and a long breath-hold time (up to 40 seconds – difficult for breathless patients). The latest generation of 64-slice, ECG-gated MDCT systems can acquire images of the cardiac anatomy, the coronary vessels and any stenoses in <10 seconds. Nowadays, the prospective ECG-triggered flash spiral mode has been introduced to image the heart in a single heart beat (~0.28 seconds). It reduces radiation dose, contrast volume and eliminates stack artefacts that may occur in prospective sequential mode. Additionally, no editing of reconstruction data is required, which will reduce postprocessing time. It is best used to image the coronaries in a very stable HR (± 60 min^{-1}). Due to the high spatial resolution of 64-slice MDCT (~0.4 mm), more than 90% of coronary segments are evaluable with high sensitivity and good specificity. The presence of severe coronary calcification (Agatston Score >400–600 units) reduces the sensitivity of the modality and makes it difficult to assess intraluminal narrowing. The clinical utility of coronary CT angiography (CTA) is summarized in Box 3.4.

The radiation dose of cardiac MDCT is high (~15–21 mSv) with increased associated lifetime risk of cancer. The risk is greater for women (breast cancer), young patients and combined cardiac and aortic scans. In recent years, electron-beam CT (EBCT) and dual-source CT (DSCT) have been

15

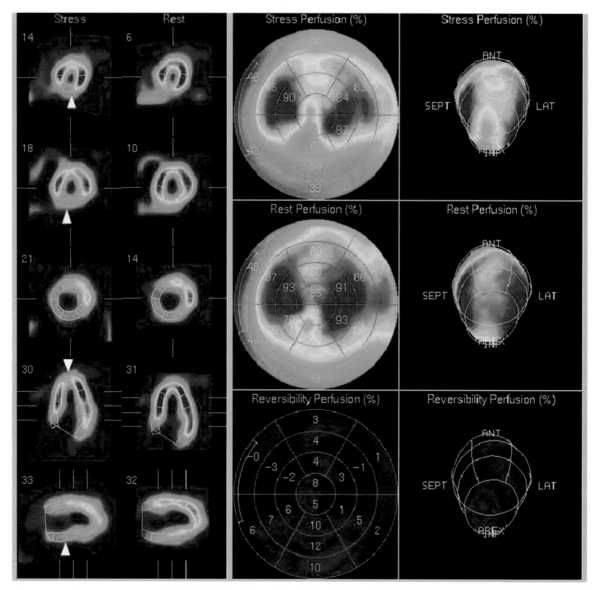

Figure 3.2 99^mTc-sestamibi myocardial perfusion scintigraphy. Example of a patient with reversible apical and inferobasal perfusion defects (white arrows). Analysis of tracer uptake allows quantification and localization (20 myocardial segments) of the lateral (LAT) and septal (SEPT) lesions.

further developed to overcome the temporal limitations and to considerably reduce the radiation dose (~0.7 mSv for DSCT flash).

Coronary Artery Disease

The presence of coronary arterial calcium is a marker of coronary atherosclerosis. Coronary calcium scoring by non-contrast enhanced EBCT and by MDCT is used for risk stratification in patients with CAD. The greater the amount of calcium; the greater

the likelihood of occlusive CAD. The presence or absence of coronary calcification does not, however, allow reliable distinction between stable and unstable plaques. Furthermore, the presence of calcification does not always correlate with coronary stenosis. Thus, calcium scoring has low positive predictive value (PPV).

Since the introduction of 64-slice MDCT in 2004, non-invasive coronary CTA has become an alternative to invasive imaging techniques in many centres.

Table 3.4 Assessment of CAD by non-invasive radiological imaging methods

	CT	MRI	PET/SPECT
Anatomical evaluation			
Non-invasive coronary angiography	Routine application Limited by coronary calcifications (pre-test Ca-scoring), temporal resolution (HR) Sensitivity 98%, specificity 82% High negative predictive value of 99% Limited reliability for treatment decision	Research protocols and specialized centres Sensitivity 93% Specificity 58%	-
Functional evaluation			
Rest and stress perfusion imaging	More experimental Limited by the increasing dose of radiation Underestimate the extent of ischaemia	Routine application Enhancement of perfused tissue during first-pass Gd-ce CMR Detection of CAD with sensitivity 91%, specificity 81%	Gold standard Detection of CAD with sensitivity and specificity >90%
LV function	More experimental	Gold standard Assessment of biventricular ejection fraction, SV, ventricular mass Prognostic value	Gated PET/SPECT Limited by low resolution
Myocardial viability	More experimental	Myocardial scar detection by late gadolinium enhancement in Gd-ce CMR enhancement Prognostic value	Gold standard Prognostic value

Box 3.4   Clinical indications of coronary CT angiography

- Detection of coronary artery stenosis
- Low PPV (60–70%), selected patient (intermediate-risk patient), high NPV
- Coronary artery anomalies
- Origin and course of aberrant coronary arteries, 3D evaluation, high accuracy
- Coronary stent imaging
- Possible to rule out in-stent stenosis, affected by metal artefacts, low PPV
- CABGs
- Visualization of grafts with high accuracy (especially large venous grafts), limited by difficult assessment of native coronary artery, graft occlusion or stenosis diagnosed with high PPV (>92%)

Contrast-enhanced coronary CTA can be performed within 5–10 minutes and fast reconstruction makes the study immediately available for final interpretation (Figure 3.3). With the exception of distal segments and left circumflex coronary artery, evaluation of significant (>50%) coronary stenosis is possible with a high sensitivity and specificity (Table 3.4).

Coronary CTA is particularly useful for ruling out significant CAD. Due to its high negative predictive value (NPV), a normal coronary CTA reliably excludes significant coronary stenosis. The main limitations of MDCT are the inability to assess coronary artery stenoses in the presence of dense calcification and the detection of coronary atherosclerotic lesions that are not flow-limiting. Hybrid systems, linking high-resolution anatomic CT imaging with the functional capability of PET/SPECT, have been developed to overcome the limitations of each technique.

Aortic Disease

MDCT with advanced post-processing techniques or magnetic resonance angiography (MRA) can be used to evaluate the entire spectrum of the aortic disease. These two reference techniques provide crucial information about the aorta and surrounding

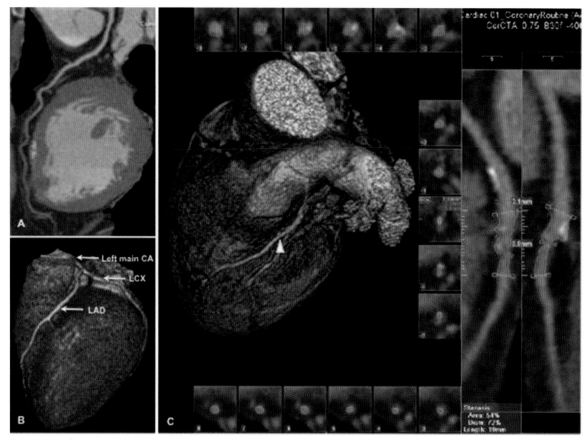

Figure 3.3 Coronary CTA. (A) Curved multiplanar reconstruction image of a normal LAD. Proximal, mid and distal segments are visualized. (B) 3D volume-rendered image of normal coronary artery. LCX = left circumflex artery. (C) Quantitative analysis of RCA stenosis.

structures; helping to display critical anatomical relationships to interventionists and surgeons. CTA remains the preferred technique for evaluation of suspected aortic rupture because of its availability, speed and very high sensitivity and specificity for this complication.

Pericardial Disease

Motion-free MDCT imaging allows better visualization of the pericardium, and thus is regarded a diagnostic tool for pericardial disorders. The main advantage of this CT technique is the high sensitivity for identifying pericardial calcification, making it the best modality for the diagnosis of constrictive pericarditis.

Valvular Disease

Information regarding valvular anatomy and function derived from MDCT is described in Table 3.5.

Cardiac Magnetic Resonance Imaging

Cardiac magnetic resonance imaging (CMR) uses the magnetic properties of atomic nuclei. Hydrogen nuclei (protons) in the body generate local and randomly oriented magnetic fields. The magnet provides a powerful static magnetic field to align the nuclei. Radiofrequency fields are then applied to alter the alignment and then removed. The energy released as the nuclei return to their initial position is detected and used to produce the MRI image. With this technique, both 2D and 3D imaging is possible. A comprehensive CMR examination – static morphological images, ciné CMR sequences, stress and rest perfusion CMR and contrast-enhanced CMR – can be time-consuming (~30 minutes, depending on the sequence and protocol used).

The use of a 1.5- or 3.0-Tesla magnet with a magnetic resonance sequence called steady-state free-precession (SSFP) imaging offers excellent

Table 3.5 Valve assessment with MRI and MDCT

	Ciné MDCT	SSFP ciné MRI
Morphology	Excellent for leaflets, chordae and papillary muscle visualization (high spatial resolution) Accurate quantification of valve calcifications	Moderate Limited for chordae and papillary muscles
Function	Qualitative and quantitative assessment (planimetry) of valve stenosis and regurgitation Good correlation with TTE and TOE Accurate evaluation of valve motion and mechanism of valve disease (cusps prolapse, restrictive cusps motion)	

SSFP: steady-state free-precession.

signal-to-noise and contrast-to-noise ratios, with fast image acquisition and superior image quality.

Injection of the contrast agent gadolinium diethylene triamine pentaacetic acid (Gd-DTPA) improves the sensitivity of CMR. Gadolinium is less nephrotoxic than conventional radiocontrast agents, making Gd-enhanced CMR an option for patients with renal impairment. Perfused tissue appears brighter during the first pass of Gd-DTPA (enhanced signal in spin-lattice relaxation time/T1-weighted images).

CMR is now established as the non-invasive imaging modality of choice for the evaluation of the structure and function of the heart and blood vessels (Table 3.6).

Coronary Artery Disease

CMR can be used to detect CAD by both direct (i.e. angiographic) and indirect (i.e. perfusion) methods (Table 3.4). Low spatial resolution, poor reproducibility and a large percentage of non-assessable segments limit the use of coronary MRA.

The most important use of perfusion CMR is the assessment of myocardial viability (late Gd-ceCMR). The high PPV of perfusion CMR has been validated in several clinical studies. The presence of normal perfusion is predictive of a 99% chance of 3-year event-free survival.

CMR also provides accurate quantification of the cardiac chamber volume and function as well as the myocardial mass and is considered the 'gold standard' for these measurements.

Aortic Disease

MRA is particularly useful in patients with thoracoabdominal aortic aneurysm (oblique sagittal MRA images) and has the advantage of not exposing patients who require regular follow-up to repeated doses of ionizing radiation (Table 3.6).

Table 3.6 Characteristics and common functional and morphological CMR indications

Indications	Myocardial ischaemia and viability Congenital heart disease (morphology, shunt evaluation) Cardiomyopathies (primary and secondary) Cardiac mass and inflammatory disease Heart valve disease Pericardial disease Aortic disease
Advantages	No ionizing radiation No iodinated contrast material Excellent soft-tissue contrast
Contraindications (~20% of patients)	Ferromagnetic foreign body Aneurysm clip Intra-orbital metal Non-MRI compatible implant Claustrophobia

Valvular Disease

Both MDCT and CMR allow accurate evaluation of heart valve function (Table 3.5). CMR planimetric (ciné CMR) or continuity equation-based phase-contrast (PC-CMR) allows measurements of the AV orifice area, directional flow and velocity profiles, regurgitation fraction and pressure gradients. This correlates strongly with TOE and TTE findings, and thus can be an alternative tool for the diagnosis of AS and AR.

Pericardial Disease and Cardiac Masses

High soft-tissue contrast and the ability to acquire multiplanar and SSFP ciné images make CMR the reference method for the evaluation of pericardial diseases and cardiac masses. The pericardium is seen on both T1- and T2-weighted (spin–spin relaxation time) CMR images as a thin band of low signal intensity. CMR can detect small or loculated effusions, acute pericarditis and is useful for treatment follow-up and the differentiation of constrictive pericarditis from restrictive cardiomyopathy.

Invasive Diagnostic Techniques

Cardiac Catheterization

Cardiac catheterization was originally developed as a means to measure pressures within the heart chambers and great vessels (Table 3.7). The introduction of radiopaque contrast media led to the development of ventriculography and coronary angiography. These invasive procedures involve exposure to contrast media and ionizing radiation and may be accompanied by both minor and life-threatening complications. Despite the development of new, non-invasive techniques (e.g. radionucleotide perfusion imaging and MRI), cardiac catherization remains the most widely used method for assessing the severity and distribution of CAD. In addition to diagnostic information, cardiac catheterization permits therapeutic intervention (e.g. angioplasty, valvuloplasty) as well as assessing prognosis and aiding surgical planning.

Right Heart Catheterization

Right heart catherization (RHC) is mainly indicated for patients with a history of unexplained dyspnoea, valvular (particularly mitral) disease or an intracardiac shunt. It is used in combination with left heart catherization in only 10% of patients – arguably too

infrequently given the relatively high incidence of PHT in cardiac disease.

A radio-opaque catheter is inserted under local anaesthesia via a large vein (e.g. femoral, internal jugular) and advanced through the RA and RV to the PA. Plain catheters may be deployed via the femoral vein, while insertion via the jugular or subclavian approach may be aided by the use of a balloon-tipped catheter. Each cavity has a characteristic pressure waveform profile – diastolic pressure rises in the RV whereas it falls in the PA. The PAWP, which can be obtained by wedging a plain catheter in a distal PA or by inflating the balloon, reflects LA and LV filling pressures.

The CO can be measured using either thermodilution or the Fick method (requiring Hb concentration and oximetric measurements in both systemic and pulmonary arterial blood; see Chapter 30)

The anatomic location and haemodynamic significance of left-to-right shunts (i.e. ASD, VSD) can be assessed using oximetry at different vascular and cardiac levels (e.g. SVC, IVC, RA, RV and PA). Abnormally high SO_2 or a step increase in SO_2 will be found where a left-to-right shunt exists. The ratio of pulmonary to systemic blood flow (the shunt fraction; Q_P/Q_S) can be calculated using the shunt equation.

In patients with PHT, the wedge pressure and TPG (i.e. mean PAP – mean wedge) help to determine the origin of PA elevation (pre- versus post-capillary). The rate of distal run-off following balloon occlusion, a technique known as PVR partitioning, may be particularly useful in the management of chronic thromboembolic PHT. In pre-capillary PHT,

Table 3.7 Measurements obtained during left and right heart catheterization, and normal values

	Parameter	Measurement	Normal values	Units
Left	Arterial/aortic pressure	S/D (M)	<140/90 (105)	mmHg
	LV pressure	S/D_E	<140/12	mmHg
Right	RA pressure	(M)	(<6)	mmHg
	RV pressure	S/D_E	<25/5	mmHg
	PAP	S/D (M)	25/12 (22)	mmHg
	PAWP	(M)	(12)	mmHg
	CI		2.5–4.2	l min^{-1} m^{-2}
	D_E volume index		<100	ml m^{-2}
	A-V O_2 content difference		<5.0	ml dl^{-1}
	PVR		~100	dyne s cm^{-5}
	SVR		800–1,200	dyne s cm^{-5}

S/D (M); systolic/diastolic (mean), D_E; end-diastolic.

Table 3.8 Left heart catheterization procedures

Technique	Procedure	Information obtained
Manometry	Pressure measurements are made with the catheter in aortic root and LV cavity	AV gradient LVEDP
Angiography	The ostia or the coronary arteries, vein grafts or internal mammary artery are selectively cannulated and contrast injected	Coronary anatomy, left or right dominance, location and severity of stenotic lesions, presence of collateral circulation, patency of bypass grafts
Ventriculogram	A pigtail catheter is advanced across AV into LV. 40–60 ml contrast is rapidly injected	Ventricular size and function LV ejection fraction LV aneurysm Severity of MR
Aortogram	A catheter is placed in the aortic root, contrast is injected manually	Severity of AR

vasoreactivity testing using NO can be performed to identify patients who may benefit from long-term therapy with calcium channel blockers. PVR and PHT reversibility are routinely assessed in prospective heart transplant recipients as these parameters affect post-transplant outcome. RHC is undertaken after cardiac transplantation to assess graft function and to obtain endomyocardial biopsies.

The LA and LV can be instrumented via transeptal puncture, typically at the site of the fossa ovalis. This permits the acquisition of both diagnostic information (e.g. MS) and therapeutic intervention (e.g. ASD/PFO closure, mitral valvuloplasty).

The major complications of RHC include: dysrhythmias, thrombosis, haemorrhage and cardiac or PA perforation.

Left Heart Catheterization

A comprehensive left heart catherization (LHC) complete examination includes: manometry, coronary angiography, left ventriculography and aortography (Table 3.8).

Coronary Angiography

Almost 60 years after the procedure was first serendipitously performed by F. Mason Sones, selective coronary angiography remains the method most widely used to define coronary arterial anatomy (Figure 3.4). In addition, it provides important information regarding coronary dominance (determined by the origin of the posterior descending artery), congenital anomalies, collateral blood supply and the presence of calcification.

Table 3.9 Complications of LHC

Site	Examples
Access site	Bleeding, haematoma, pseudoaneurysm Vascular injury – distal limb ischaemia Infection
Vascular	Aortic dissection Renal, mesenteric, cerebral embolization
Cardiac	Coronary dissection/occlusion MI Dysrhythmia – including VF
General	Vasovagal syncope Contrast-induced nephrotoxicity Allergic reactions to contrast Radiodermatitis

In adults a 4-6 Fr (1.3-2 mm diameter) sheath is placed in a peripheral (femoral, brachial or radial) artery under local anaesthesia. A series of long catheters are then advanced through the sheath into the proximal aorta and LV cavity. Selective cannulation of the coronary ostia and subsequent injection of radiopaque contrast allows demonstration of the coronary arterial anatomy. A reduction in luminal diameter of >75% (>50% in left main stem) is considered significant.

The technique exposes patients to iodinated contrast media and ionizing radiation, both of which may be associated with complications (Table 3.9). Although PCI during LHC carries greater risk, major complications (e.g. death, stroke, MI and dysrhythmia) occur in less than 0.1% of diagnostic

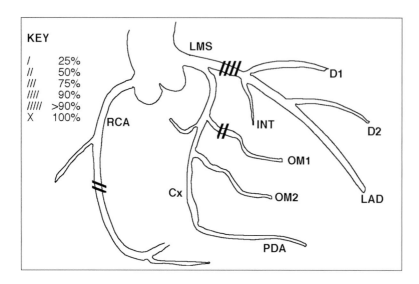

KEY

/	25%
//	50%
///	75%
////	90%
/////	>90%
X	100%

Figure 3.4 An example of a coronary angiogram report showing; left dominance, severe proximal LAD disease and mild disease in the mid right coronary artery (RCA) and the first obtuse marginal branch (OM1) of the circumflex artery (Cx). Other abbreviation: INT, intermediate branch; D1, first diagonal branch; D2, second diagonal branch; LMS, left main stem; PDA, posterior descending artery; OM2, second obtuse marginal branch; Cx, circumflex artery.

procedures. Local vascular and haemorrhagic complications (e.g. haematoma, false aneurysm, distal ischaemia) are the most common adverse events (2–8%), particularly when the femoral approach is used. Because of reduced haemorrhagic complications, use of the radial arterial approach is increasing. Rarer complications include allergic reactions to contrast media, contrast-induced nephropathy and late radiodermatitis.

Conventional coronary angiography has several limitations:

- As coronary angiography produces 2D images, stenoses may be incorrectly evaluated in tortuous and angulated vessels. Moreover, stenoses are often evaluated in comparison with a seemingly normal reference segment that may actually be diseased
- Misinterpretations may be made due to suboptimal contrast media injection, an inadequate number of orthogonal projections or catheter-induced coronary spasm
- There may be some variability in inter- and intra-observer diagnosis and reporting

Some of these limitations can be overcome by assessing the fractional flow reserve (FFR), which provides an index of the physiological significance of a coronary stenosis. A pressure-sensitive guidewire is advanced past the stenosis of interest and the FFR calculated by dividing the mean distal coronary pressure by the mean aortic pressure (measured simultaneously) at maximal hyperaemia - typically induced by IV or intra-coronary adenosine. FFR measurement is useful for the assessment of the haemodynamic impact of intermediate coronary artery lesions. Recent evidence suggests that FFR-guided PCI reduces the rate of stent implantation and decreases the incidence of MI and death at 1 year.

Ventriculography and Aortography

A high-volume contrast injection (35–45 ml) via a 6 Fr pigtail catheter positioned in the LV cavity provides information on LV ejection fraction, regional LV wall function and MR (semi-quantitative). When the pigtail catheter is positioned in the aortic root, the aortic diameter and the presence of AR can be assessed with 45–55 ml contrast injection.

Intravascular Ultrasound

Intravascular ultrasound (IVUS) is an intra-coronary imaging technique that uses miniaturized ultrasound transducers to provide high-resolution (100-150 μm), cross-sectional real-time images, not only of the coronary artery lumen, but also of the vessel wall with differentiation of its layers. In clinical practice, IVUS is used during interventional procedures, to assess angiographically ambiguous lesions and to provide additional information on left main stem (LMS) disease.

In contrast to IVUS, coronary angiography provides a silhouette image of the vessel lumen – a luminogram – which may be confounded by the phenomenon of coronary remodelling. In stenosis of <40%, plaque accumulation is accompanied by an increase in arterial size, resulting in a stable lumen area. IVUS allows assessment of the extent of atherosclerosis through the visualization of plaque disease in the vessel wall, which may not be detected by angiography. IVUS has demonstrated a greater prevalence of atherosclerosis than there was initially thought to be with angiography. Furthermore, the development of the optical analogue of IVUS (optical coherence tomography; OCT) enabled in vivo and in situ cross-sectional imaging, with a resolution 10-fold that of IVUS (15 μm), providing near-histological real-time analysis of plaque disease.

Key Points

- Myocardial perfusion imaging may identify ischaemic myocardium that would benefit from revascularization.

- Contrast-enhanced CMR allows assessment of myocardial viability with a greater accuracy than [18]FDG-PET/SPECT.
- Negative 64-slice MDCT/DSCT coronary angiography reliably excludes significant CAD.
- The development of hybrid PET-SPECT/CT/MRI imaging enables the simultaneous assessment of the anatomic extent and functional consequences of CAD.
- MDCT and MRI are alternative modalities for valvular imaging with good correlation with echocardiography.
- Cardiac catheterization remains the 'gold standard' for imaging the coronary arteries.
- Serious complications are rare but may be life-threatening.
- FFR is useful for the haemodynamic assessment of intermediate coronary artery lesions.
- RHC is an underused investigation.

Further Reading

Dangas GD, Di Mario C, Kipshidze NN, Barlis P, Addo T (eds.). *Interventional Cardiology Principles and Practice*, 2nd edn. Oxford: Wiley Blackwell; 2017.

Garcia MJ. *Non-Invasive Cardiovascular Imaging: A Multimodality Approach*. London: Lippincott Williams & Wilkins; 2012.

Grech ED. *ABC of Interventional Cardiology*, 2nd edn. Oxford: Wiley Blackwell; 2011.

Kern MJ, Sorajja P, Lim MJ (eds.). *The Cardiac Catheterization Handbook*, 6th edn. Philadelphia: Elsevier; 2016.

Kowey P, Piccini JP, Naccarelli G, Reiffel JA (eds.). *Cardiac Arrhythmias, Pacing and Sudden Death*. Cham: Springer; 2017.

Lanccelloti P, Zamorano JL, Habib G, Badano L (eds.). *The EACVI Textbook of Echocardiography*, 2nd edn. Oxford: Oxford University Press; 2017.

Medtronic Inc. *Reveal LINQ insertable cardiac monitoring system*. www.medtronic.com/us-en/healthcare-professionals/products/cardiac-rhythm/cardiac-monitors/reveal-linq-icm.html (accessed December 2018).

Mortensen KH, Barry PA, Gopalan D. Radiology for cardiothoracic intensivists. In Valchanov K, Jones N, Hogue CW (eds.), *Core Topics in Cardiothoracic Critical Care*, 2nd edn. Cambridge: Cambridge University Press; 2018, pp. 44–57.

Moscucci M (Ed.). *Baim & Grossman's Cardiac Catheterization, Angiography and Intervention*, 8th edn. Philadelphia: Lippincott Williams & Wilkins; 2013.

Thelen M, Erbel R, Kreitner K-F, Barkhausen J. *Cardiac Imaging: A Multimodality Approach*. Stuttgart: Georg Thieme Verlag; 2009.

Topol EJ, Teirstein PS. *Textbook of Interventional Radiology*, 7th edn. Philadelphia: Elsevier; 2016.

Chapter

4

Conduct of Anaesthesia

Andrew I. Gardner and Paul H. M. Sadleir

The aims of anaesthesia for cardiac surgery are: prevention of perioperative cardiac ischaemia and arrhythmias, tight haemodynamic control, avoidance of non-cardiac complications and early tracheal extubation. This chapter deals with the management of low-risk patients undergoing elective CABG surgery.

Preoperative Assessment

For the majority of elective patients, preoperative assessment should take place several days before surgery in a pre-admission clinic. This allows an assessment of the patient's ability to withstand the intended surgical procedure and provides an opportunity to explain anaesthetic procedures, obtain consent for specific interventions and discuss appropriate cessation of medication prior to surgery. Having an interval between assessment and surgery permits the early identification of potential problems, allows additional investigations to be undertaken, and alerts support services, such as transfusion, pacing and critical care, of likely demand. This approach significantly reduces the likelihood of delays or cancellation on the day of surgery. This is particularly important for patients considered suitable for admission to hospital on the day of surgery.

The presence of previously documented symptoms and signs (see Chapter 2) should be verified, the results of preoperative investigations (in particular coronary angiography and echocardiography) reviewed and any new or undiagnosed problems excluded.

In addition to a routine systematic preoperative history and examination, specific areas of interest include:

- Intended conduit harvest sites: may restrict placement of monitors and cannulae
- Recent history of anticoagulant therapy (see below)
- Permanent pacemaker/implantable defibrillator: may need reprogramming before induction of anaesthesia
- Oesophageal pathology: may be a relative or absolute contraindication for TOE
- Religious or cultural beliefs: (e.g. Jehovah's Witness and blood product transfusion)

All regular anti-anginal, antihypertensive and anti-cardiac failure medications should be continued in the preoperative period (Table 4.1).

Oral hypoglycaemic agents should be managed according to institutional protocols to maintain normoglycaemia during the fasting periods. It is recommended that sodium-glucose co-transporter-2 inhibitors be stopped two days before surgery to reduce the risk of perioperative euglycaemic diabetic ketoacidosis. This may require the introduction of

Table 4.1 A guide to which regular medications should be continued until the day of surgery

Continue	Controversial	Discontinue
Statins (decreases in-hospital mortality and need for RRT)	Aspirin	Thienopyridines (e.g. clopidogrel, prasugrel)
β-blockers (reduced risk of post-CABG AF)	ACE inhibitors	GP IIb/IIIa inhibitors (e.g. tirofiban)
Nitrates	Angiotensin receptor blockers	DOACs (e.g. rivaroxaban)
Calcium antagonists		Diuretics
Potassium channel openers		NSAIDs
Corticosteroids		MAO inhibitors
Antidysrhythmics		Biguanides (metformin)
Bronchodilators		

RRT, renal replacement therapy; GP, glycoprotein; DOAC, direct-acting oral anticoagulant; MAO, monoamine oxidase.

other diabetic therapies to ensure normoglycaemia between preoperative assessment and surgery.

The optimal timing of cessation of antiplatelet and anticoagulant therapy is determined by balancing the risk of perioperative bleeding against the risk of thrombotic complications.

Thienopyridines should be discontinued at least 5 days before surgery.

Aspirin withdrawal remains controversial: continuation of therapy during the 5 days before surgery may reduce early (in-hospital) mortality and improve graft patency without increasing the risks of reoperation for bleeding or transfusion. However, published evidence is inconclusive; in many centres concern about the risk of haemorrhagic complications still prompts aspirin cessation 7-10 days before surgery, while in other centres aspirin therapy is continued up until the day of surgery, particularly in patients with critical coronary artery stenoses.

Direct-acting oral anticoagulants (e.g. dabigatran, rivaroxaban, apixaban) should be discontinued 72 hours before surgery.

Other antithrombotic agents used in secondary prevention, such as tirofiban or unfractionated heparin by infusion, are typically withdrawn 2-4 hours before surgery.

Premedication

Despite trends in other anaesthetic subspecialties, sedative premedication remains common in cardiac anaesthetic practice. The stated goals are: minimization of the

---

Box 4.1 Examples of premedicant drugs in cardiac anaesthesia

Oral (90–120 minutes prior to induction of anaesthesia):
Lorazepam 2–4 mg
Temazepam 10–20 mg
Clonidine 100–150 µg
Pregabalin 75–150 mg
Methadone 0.1–0.2 mg kg^{-1}

Intramuscular (45–60 minutes prior to induction of anaesthesia):
Morphine sulphate 0.2–0.3 mg kg^{-1} + hyoscine hydrobromide 200–400 µg
Patients are often given supplemental oxygen after the administration of sedative premedicants

---

risk of cardiac ischaemia secondary to anxiety, hypertension and tachycardia while at the same time avoiding respiratory depression. Although opioids, benzodiazepines and antihistamines are commonly prescribed, the final choice of drugs is subject to institutional variability (Box 4.1). The use of gabapentanoids as premedication is increasing, for both attenuation of sympathetic response during general anaesthesia and reduction of acute and chronic pain after cardiac surgery. Longer acting amnestic drugs have the advantage of covering the early ICU period. As respiratory depression is a known sequel of sedative premedication, supplemental oxygen should be prescribed and administered until induction of anaesthesia.

Preparation

As for all anaesthetic procedures, the availability of drugs, equipment and staff (surgeon, nursing staff, perfusionist) should be checked prior to the patient's arrival in the operating suite. Drugs that should be immediately available include: inotropes, antidysrhythmics, calcium, magnesium, heparin and protamine (Box 4.2).

Anaesthetic/Operating Room

On arrival, the identity of the patient should be verified and consent for surgery confirmed in accordance with the WHO 'Safe Surgery' checklist. The availability of cross-matched blood should also be checked. The operative site should be clearly marked if appropriate (e.g. thoracotomy, radial artery harvest site). Non-invasive monitoring (ECG, NIBP and pulse oximetry) is then instituted prior to any anaesthetic procedures.

Vascular Access and Invasive Monitoring

Cannulae are sited under local anaesthesia in a forearm vein (14 G) and the non-dominant radial artery (20 G). In the case of non-dominant radial artery harvest, either the dominant radial artery or femoral artery may be cannulated. An IV infusion is then commenced, and arterial pressure transduced and monitored. Femoral arterial pressure monitoring is used when both radial arteries are required for conduits.

Insertion of central (i.e. internal jugular or subclavian) venous cannulae may then be undertaken; however, in many centres this is deferred until after induction of anaesthesia. With appropriate training, the use of ultrasound to guide internal jugular vein

25

cannulation has been shown to reduce complications and the number of attempts required.

Inserting a PAFC in low-risk CABG surgery patients has little impact on clinical management or outcome, and routine use of the device is declining. A PAFC sheath may, however, be inserted for central vascular access, and has the advantage of facilitating subsequent PAFC insertion if indicated after separation from CPB. Many cardiac anaesthetists use a PAFC sheath in combined or complex procedures, and in patients with poor LV function.

Depth-of-anaesthesia monitoring by processed EEG devices may reduce the incidence of awareness in this group of elective CABG patients long considered to be at high risk. An additional advantage of using these devices is that it is possible to reduce the dose of anaesthetic agents and consequently reduce drug-induced cardiovascular depression and cost.

Box 4.2 Preparation for cardiac anaesthesia

Equipment

Anaesthetic machine, laryngoscopes and intubation aids, suction apparatus

Monitoring (standard anaesthetic monitoring plus pressure transducers, depth-of-anaesthesia monitoring, TOE, ABG, ACT)

Infusion pumps and transfusion apparatus

Arterial and venous cannulae

Defibrillator and external pacemaker box

Ultrasound for venous access

Drugs to be drawn up

Anaesthetic

Local anaesthetic (lidocaine)

Analgesic (e.g. fentanyl, sufentanil, remifentanil, alfentanil)

Muscle relaxant (e.g. pancuronium, rocuronium)

Induction agent (e.g. etomidate, propofol, midazolam)

Cardiovascular

Vagolytic (atropine, glycopyrrolate)

Vasopressor (metaraminol, phenylephrine)

β-blockers

Other

IV fluids

Prophylactic antibiotics

Anticoagulant (heparin)

Antifibrinolytic agents (tranexamic acid, ε-aminocaproic acid)

Epidural

Thoracic and cervical epidural analgesia have been used for postoperative analgesia in cardiac surgery. This controversial aspect of cardiac anaesthesia is discussed in Chapter 38.

Induction

In some centres, induction of anaesthesia takes place in a separate anaesthetic room. The benefits of a quiet environment, patient privacy and reduced 'turnover' time have to be balanced against the risk of cardiovascular collapse requiring urgent CPB.

Many techniques have been described for the induction and maintenance of anaesthesia for cardiac surgery. There is no ideal single agent and there is no place for a 'mono-agent' technique. The characteristics of an ideal cardiac anaesthetic agent include:

- Unaltered haemodynamics
- Lack of myocardial depression
- Lack of coronary vasoconstriction or steal
- Non-anaesthetic cardioprotective effects
- Residual analgesia
- Rapid onset, offset and titration

Following a period of preoxygenation, balanced anaesthesia is induced with a combination of induction hypnotic, opioid and neuromuscular blocking drugs (Box 4.3). Moderate doses of opioid attenuate

---

Box 4.3 Drugs for the induction of anaesthesia

Induction agents

Etomidate 0.15–0.30 mg kg^{-1}

Propofol 1.0–1.5 mg kg^{-1}

Midazolam 0.05–0.10 mg kg^{-1}

Thiopental 3–4 mg kg^{-1}

Opioids

Fentanyl 5–10 μg kg^{-1}

Sufentanil 0.5–1.0 μg kg^{-1}

Remifentanil 0.5–2.5 μg kg^{-1} → 0.05–0.50 μg kg^{-1} min^{-1}

Alfentanil 50 μg kg^{-1} → 1 μg kg^{-1} min^{-1}

Neuromuscular blockers

Pancuronium 0.10–0.15 mg kg^{-1}

Rocuronium 0.5–0.9 mg kg^{-1}

Vecuronium 0.1 mg kg^{-1}

Atracurium 0.6 mg kg^{-1}

Box 4.4 Procedures following induction of anaesthesia

Tracheal intubation	Secure tube to side of mouth and exclude tongue compression
Mechanical ventilation	Tidal volume 6–8 ml kg^{-1} to maintain normocapnea FiO$_2$ of 0.6 in air Although theoretically possible to use N$_2$O in early pre-CPB period, failure to switch to air could increase risk of air embolus. Most anaesthetists now avoid N$_2$O
Maintain anaesthesia	Volatile or IV agents
Secure additional vascular access	Central venous – if not undertaken prior to induction. Use short internal jugular lines (10–12 cm) or do not insert >12 cm from skin puncture
Urinary catheterization	A suprapubic catheter may be inserted at end of case and before transfer to ICU if transurethral catheterization is not possible
Antibiotic prophylaxis	Covering skin organisms to prevent surgical site infection (sternal wound infection and mediastinitis) and dictated by local protocols (usually ß-lactam or glycopeptide antibiotics)
Temperature monitor	Nasopharyngeal/bladder
Patient protection	Eyes closed and taped, heels padded, knees slightly flexed Protect ulna and radial nerve pressure points
TOE probe	If indicated, it is easier to insert before the patient is prepared and draped for surgery
Gastric tube	NG/orogastric tube is used in some centres to reduce postoperative nausea and vomiting. May be used to vent stomach prior to insertion of TOE if it is suspected that the stomach has been insufflated during induction
Confirm patency of peripheral lines	Peripheral and central venous lines should run freely. Arterial line should aspirate easily
Depth of anaesthesia monitoring	If not applied prior to induction

the response to direct laryngoscopy and tracheal intubation while causing minimal myocardial depression and allowing a reduction in the dose of hypnotic anaesthetic agent required. Muscle relaxants provide ideal intubating conditions, prevent patient movement or shivering, and reduce oxygen consumption. Contrary to traditional teaching, many anaesthetists administer the muscle relaxant early to patients without obvious airway problems to prevent opioid-induced coughing or chest-wall rigidity. Pancuronium is commonly used because of its long duration of action and sympathomimetic action, which attenuates the bradycardia associated with high-dose opioid anaesthesia and β-blockade. Rocuronium has the advantage of rapid onset (decreasing the risk of stomach insufflation, which may result in degradation of TOE images), and the useful property that it can be reversed with a selective relaxant binding agent (sugammadex) if residual blockade is present at the time of emergence. Procedures undertaken after induction of anaesthesia are summarized in Box 4.4.

Transfer to Operating Room

When an anaesthetic room has been used for induction it is necessary to transfer the patient to the operating room. Although this procedure has the potential for complications (e.g. accidental avulsion of lines and tubes), observing simple precautions can minimize them (Box 4.5).

On arrival in the operating room, the patient should first be reconnected to the ventilator, the

Box 4.5 Anaesthetic checklist prior to start of surgery

- Ventilation
- Zero monitoring lines
- The five 'A's

   Access

   Anaesthesia

   Arterial gas

   ACT (baseline)

   Antibiotics

- Check cross-matched blood

Table 4.2 Degrees of anaesthetic and surgical stimulation

High	Low
Direct laryngoscopy	Post tracheal intubation
Tracheal intubation	Preparing and draping
TOE probe insertion	Surgical 'delays'
Skin incision	Mammary artery harvesting
Sternotomy	
Sternal retraction	
Sternal elevation	

capnograph, pulse oximeter and ECG. Pressure areas are checked and padded. A temperature probe should be inserted, and TOE probe if indicated. Pressure transducers are then reconnected and re-zeroed. Venous lines are checked for patency, and access to three-way taps are confirmed before the patient is prepared and draped for surgery. To avoid inadvertent intra-arterial drug administration, it is essential that arterial and venous injection ports are physically separated and clearly labelled.

Drug infusion lines should be checked, and correct functioning of infusion pumps should be confirmed.

Maintenance

Both volatile agents (0.5–1 MAC) and propofol (3-4 mg kg^{-1} h^{-1} or target-controlled infusion 1.5–3 µg ml^{-1}) are commonly used for the maintenance of anaesthesia prior to the onset of CPB.

Volatile agents are known to confer a degree of cardioprotection by virtue of ischaemic pre- and post-conditioning, however this has not been demonstrated an improved clinical outcome (see Chapter 5). There appears to be no difference in outcome between commonly used inhalational agents in low-risk cases.

The use of dexmedetomidine in cardiac surgery patients is becoming more common, as it may reduce the incidence of postoperative delirium, haemodynamic instability and length of intensive care stay.

A supplemental dose of opioid is frequently administered a few minutes before sternotomy, and anaesthetic requirements may vary according to surgical stimulation (Table 4.2). When assessing volume status, the anaesthetist should be aware that the harvest of bypass graft conduits may result in a significant concealed haemorrhage.

The ECG, and TOE if present, should be monitored for evidence of myocardial ischaemia. The use of surgical retractors and retrocardiac swabs may make ECG interpretation difficult. The surgeon should be alerted if there is doubt about the presence of ischaemia. Attempts may be made to treat these changes pharmacologically with systemic administration of GTN or a β-blocker (e.g. esmolol). CPB should be instituted if ischaemic changes persist or circulatory collapse ensues. Completion of conduit harvesting can then continue during 'non-ischaemic' CPB – i.e. prior to application of the AXC.

Following pericardiotomy, the anaesthetist should observe the heart to gain an appreciation of its size, filling and contractility. Fluid administration is guided by MAP, CVP and TOE findings. There appears to be little to choose between crystalloid and colloid solutions, although glucose-containing solutions are best avoided.

Key Points

- Although patients are extensively investigated from a surgical point of view, preoperative anaesthetic assessment will often identify issues that require further attention.
- The goals of cardiac anaesthesia are tight haemodynamic control and avoidance of perioperative cardiac ischaemia.
- Supplemental oxygen should be administered to the patient when sedative premedication is given.
- Good communication between the anaesthetist, surgeon and perfusionist is vital for safe transition to CPB.

Further Reading

Aboul-Hassan SS, Stankowski T, Marczak J, *et al*. The use of preoperative aspirin in cardiac surgery: a systematic review and meta-analysis. *J Card Surg* 2017; 32: 758–74.

Kappeler R, Gillham M, Brown NM. Antibiotic prophylaxis for cardiac surgery. *J Antimicrob Chemother* 2012; 67: 521–2.

Peacock SC, Lovshin JA. Sodium-glucose cotransporter-2 inhibitors (SGLT-2i) in the perioperative setting. *Can J Anaesth* 2018; 65: 143–7.

Reich DL, Fischer GW. Perioperative interventions to modify risk of morbidity and mortality. *Semin Cardiothorac Vasc Anesth* 2007; 11: 224–30.

Saugel B, Scheeren TWL, Teboul J-L. Ultrasound-guided central venous catheter placement: a structured review and recommendations for clinical practice. *Crit Care* 2017; 21: 225.

Shaw JR, Woodfine JD, Douketis J, Schulman S, Carrier M. Perioperative interruption of direct oral anticoagulants in patients with atrial fibrillation: a systematic review and meta-analysis. *Res Pract Thromb Haemost* 2018; 2: 282–90.

Wang G, Niu J, Li Z, Lv H, Cai H. The efficacy and safety of dexmedetomidine in cardiac surgery patients: A systematic review and meta-analysis. *PLoS One* 2018; 13: e0202620.

World Health Organization. WHO guidelines for safe surgery 2009. who.int/patientsafety/safesurgery/en/ (accessed December 2018).

Xia Z, Li H, Irwin MG. Myocardial ischaemia reperfusion injury: the challenge of translating ischaemic and anaesthetic protection from animal models to humans. *Br J Anaesth* 2016; 117: ii44–ii62.

Principles of Cardiopulmonary Bypass

Timothy Coulson and Florian Falter

Introduction

The ideal operating conditions to enable cardiac surgery are a bloodless and motionless field. This requires both cardiac arrest and the drainage of blood from the heart. In order to provide these conditions a separate means of maintaining nutrient supply to the rest of the body is needed. In addition, the heart must be prevented from becoming sufficiently ischaemic as to infarct previously viable muscle. The two core tenets, therefore, of CPB are:

1. Protect the heart (myocardial protection).
2. Protect the patient (preservation of the patient brain, kidneys and other vital organs while the heart is stopped).

Myocardial Protection

Determinants of Myocardial Supply and Demand

Under normal circumstances myocardial oxygen supply is determined by blood flow and blood oxygen content. Blood flow is determined by Ohm's law, such that flow is directly proportional to the driving pressure gradient and inversely proportional to the resistance to flow.

Blood flow = Driving pressure/Resistance

In the LV, intramyocardial pressure during systole limits coronary blood flow, such that the majority of flow occurs during diastole. The effect is that the oxygen delivery is significantly reduced during periods of tachycardia as a result of a reduced diastolic time. Increased resistance may also be encountered as a result of ventricular hypertrophy, reduced coronary artery calibre (which may be affected by extrinsic and intrinsic regulation) and increased blood viscosity (Poiseuille's law). Blood oxygen content is determined by Hb concentration, oxygen saturation and (to a very small extent) dissolved oxygen.

Myocardial oxygen demand is determined by the HR, contractility and wall tension – a 'stretched' heart will consume more oxygen. In addition to these factors there is a basal metabolic demand, even when the heart is arrested.

Optimizing Supply and Demand

In the initial phase of CPB, blood is still supplied by the coronary arteries and the mechanical pump replacing the heart reduces myocardial work. However, in order to provide a bloodless and motionless field, the blood supply must be interrupted, and the heart stopped. Minimal energy consumption occurs in diastolic arrest. The heart subsequently only requires basal metabolic demands to be met. The prevention of ventricular dilation using a LV vent may also reduce oxygen demand. Basal cellular metabolic demand may be further reduced using hypothermia. Both cardiac arrest and the supply of metabolic substrate are facilitated using a 'cardioplegia' solution. Cold cardioplegia can be used with external cardiac cooling to further reduce myocardial oxygen demand (Figure 5.1).

While it is also possible to achieve a relatively motionless field by inducing VF, in combination with intermittent cross-clamping and moderate hypothermia, the electrical activity results in a higher oxygen requirement and may result in significant myocardial ischaemia. Cross-clamp/fibrillation is uncommon in contemporary practice.

Myocardial Ischaemia and Injury

Myocardial Hibernation and Stunning

Interruption of myocardial blood supply will eventually cause cardiomyocyte death and MI. However, when the interruption is shorter, periods of ischaemia

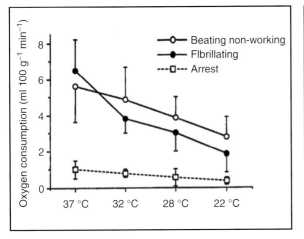
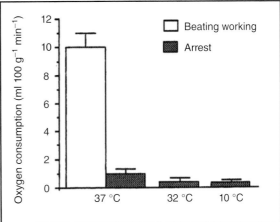

Figure 5.1 Temperature versus oxygen consumption with varying myocardial activity

may result in reduced mechanical function that recovers over minutes to hours. This depression in myocardial function has been termed 'stunning'. In general, the period of stunning lasts significantly longer than the original ischaemic insult. When the limitation of coronary blood flow is chronic, but insufficient to cause infarction, myocardial hibernation may occur. Function may be restored by inotropic support or restoration of blood flow. The former helps distinction between non-viable and viable tissue that may recover after revascularization.

Ischaemia Reperfusion Injury

Perfusion of a previously ischaemic region of myocardium can lead to significant injury over and above the injury caused by the original insult. This occurs after surgery as well as percutaneous intervention. Clinical presentations include arrhythmias, myocardial stunning, microvascular obstruction and lethal myocardial reperfusion. Myocardial injury after cardiac surgery is likely to be multifactorial, relating to myocardial handling, perioperative inflammation and arterial manipulation, as well as classical ischaemia reperfusion injury (IRI) itself. Mechanisms of IRI relate to cellular calcium overload, oxidative stress, rapid pH change and opening of a transmembrane pore with irreversible cardiomyocyte hypercontracture and cell death.

Ischaemic Conditioning

Ischaemic conditioning refers to the process of rendering myocardium less vulnerable to ischaemic

injury – essentially another form of cardioprotection. It was first observed more than 30 years ago when it was noted that intermittent occlusion of the LAD artery for four 5-minute periods before a prolonged period of occlusion was associated with reduced infarct size in dogs. This phenomenon became known as 'ischaemic preconditioning' (IPC) and appeared to be an endogenous method of preserving myocardium in response to ischaemia. Since then, it has been shown there are two 'windows' of myocardial protection after IPC. The first occurs 2–3 hours after IPC and is known as 'classical IPC', the second occurs after 48–72 hours and is known as 'delayed IPC' (Figure 5.2). The cellular mechanisms underlying IPC have not been fully elucidated.

One of the challenges in IPC is that myocardial events occur without prior warning, such that by the time they have occurred it is too late to institute IPC. In addition, in the case of cardiac surgery, clamping and unclamping of the aorta in order to provide IPC may have significant adverse thromboembolic effects. The process of intermittent reperfusion of an ischaemic territory before complete reperfusion has been termed ischaemic postconditioning and is most feasible in the cardiac catheter laboratory. However, despite promising early trials, later trials showed mixed effects and the results of the largest randomized trials have failed to demonstrate benefit. Given these findings and the increased risk of thromboembolism with external arterial occlusion it seems unlikely that postconditioning will be useful in adult cardiac surgery.

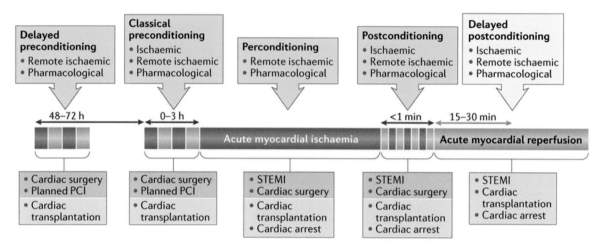

Figure 5.2 Types and timing of ischaemic conditioning in relation to the original ischaemic and reperfusion episode. Dark shading represents clinical situations in which conditioning has been tested, while light shading represents potential conditioning applications. Reprinted from Hausenloy DJ, Yellon DM. Ischaemic conditioning and reperfusion injury. *Nat Rev Cardiol* 2016; 13: 193–209 with permission from Macmillan Publishers Ltd.

The application of ischaemic conditioning stimulus to the heart itself limits the application and feasibility of IPC. However, there is evidence that application of an ischaemic stimulus remote to the heart can induce cardioprotection. This so-called remote ischaemic preconditioning (RIPC) is most commonly induced by using an inflatable tourniquet to produce 5–20 minutes of limb ischaemia. Like IPC, the mechanisms underlying RIPC are only partially understood, although it appears that both neural and humoral components are required. The relative simplicity of the technique has led to a number of large trials in cardiac surgery; however, to date no large trial has demonstrated efficacy.

Pharmacological Preconditioning

Arguably, the most attractive form of preconditioning would use a pharmacological agent to activate myocardial protection. Volatile agents were found to reduce IRI in animal models in the 1970s and 1980s. The proposed mechanisms of cardioprotection share IPC pathways. Multiple proof-of-concept clinical studies have shown reductions in surrogate markers of myocardial ischaemia (e.g. troponin) using volatile anaesthesia versus propofol and/or midazolam. Retrospective studies have suggested a reduction in mortality with volatile anaesthesia and in a recent meta-analysis mortality was halved. However, all the studies were small, and, given the low conversion rate for positive meta-analyses when repeated in large

randomized trials, this result should be taken with a degree of scepticism.

Cardioplegia

Cardioplegia refers to a range of solutions designed to induce temporary diastolic cardiac arrest. In addition to the chemical induction of cardiac arrest, cardioplegia may also be used to induce myocardial hypothermia and provide additional protection using buffers, metabolic substrates and other pharmacological agents. Most cardioplegia solutions use a concentrated K^+ solution (15–20 mmol l^{-1}) with approximately physiological concentrations of other electrolytes to maintain isotonicity. The hyperkalaemia results in a less negative membrane potential, maintaining cell depolarization. This is known as extracellular cardioplegia. Alternatively, a solution with very low Na^+ content (~15 mmol l^{-1}) may be used to hyperpolarize the membrane and prevent depolarization. This is known as intracellular cardioplegia. There is little evidence to support one cardioplegia type over the other.

Additives may be used to provide cellular nutrition or reduced energy consumption and cellular damage. The most common additive used is blood. There is reasonable evidence that the addition of blood to cardioplegia provides superior myocardial protection versus crystalloid solution alone. Blood is usually added to crystalloid in a 4:1 ratio (4 parts blood: 1 part crystalloid) with final electrolyte concentrations similar to those described above. Other additives used include antiarrhythmic agents, calcium channel blockers, β-blockers, amino acids and bicarbonate. There is little high-quality evidence to support or refute their use. Cardioplegia may be delivered cold (<20 °C) or warm (21–37 °C). Of studies that have examined the question of warm versus cold cardioplegia many are small and of poor quality. Meta-analysis of these studies found no difference in major adverse cardiac events, although some indices of myocardial function and injury were improved in the warm cardioplegia group. Where cold cardioplegia is used, a 'hot-shot' of warm cardioplegia is sometimes given before removal of the AXC and myocardial reperfusion. Small studies have suggested that this may reduce myocardial injury on reperfusion.

Cardioplegia may be delivered via the coronary arteries (antegrade) or via the venous system using the coronary sinus (retrograde). Most commonly, the antegrade cardioplegia is delivered using a cannula placed between the AXC and the heart (Figure 5.3A). A pressure of 80–100 mmHg is used, and providing the AV is competent, all flow will be delivered into the coronary arteries. In the case of an incompetent or open aorta, cardioplegia can be delivered by direct coronary ostial cannulation. Alternatively, a balloon-tipped cannula can be placed in the coronary sinus to deliver blood via the venous system. This may be done 'blind' or guided using TOE. Delivery pressures are lower to avoid damage to the sinus. The theoretical advantage of retrograde cardioplegia is protection of myocardium rendered more vulnerable by coronary artery disease and ventricular hypertrophy. However, a significant proportion of the retrograde blood is lost to the Thebesian system (requiring larger cardioplegia volumes to be given), and RV protection may be inferior. In practice, a combined retrograde and antegrade approach may provide the best protection (Figure 5.3B).

The Cardiopulmonary Bypass Circuit

The CPB circuit provides protection for the patient by maintaining blood flow to the rest of the body while the heart is stopped. The key components of CPB are: a venous drainage line, a reservoir for drained blood, a pump, a heat exchanger and oxygenator and an arterial line to return blood to the patient. However, modern CPB machines include many more components. A schematic diagram is shown in Figure 5.4.

Components

Tubing

Tubing is required to connect the components of the system to one another. Flow characteristics are determined by the length and width of the tubing (Poiseille's law). Larger-diameter pipes allow higher flow rates but carry the disadvantage of a higher prime volume and greater haemodilution. A variety of materials are available, including polyvinyl chloride (PVC), silicone and rubber. PVC has the advantages of relative strength and flexibility (although flexibility is reduced with lower temperatures), and is used in the majority of the circuit. PVC can be bonded with heparin to reduce the occurrence of clot formation in the circuit. Silicone may be used in the roller pumps due to a reduced tendency to cause haemolysis; however, prolonged use may cause spallation (release of silicone into the lumen).

Arterial Cannula

Blood is returned to the patient via an arterial cannula, usually placed in the ascending aorta (an easily accessible location at sternotomy with a low incidence of cannulation-related injury). Other common sites of return include the femoral, subclavian and innominate arteries. The arterial cannula should be designed to provide optimal blood flow, minimize arterial wall trauma and be easily secured. The flow properties of the numerous different types of cannulae available can be compared using their performance index, which is defined as the pressure gradient versus the outer diameter at any given flow. A variety of cannula designs are available (Figure 5.5).

Venous Cannula

The venous cannulae drain blood from the heart into the venous reservoir. While they can be placed peripherally they are most commonly placed centrally. A two-stage cannula may be inserted via the RA into the IVC. The tip drains blood from the IVC while proximal holes drain blood from the SVC (Figure 5.6). Alternatively, single-stage cannulae can be inserted into each of the IVC and SVC, allowing complete drainage of venous return and better access for open-heart valvular procedures. Flow of blood into the CPB circuit is achieved by gravity-driven (siphon) drainage or by using vacuum-assisted drainage. Siphoning venous blood relies on air-free tubing to avoid accumulated air stopping drainage ("air lock")

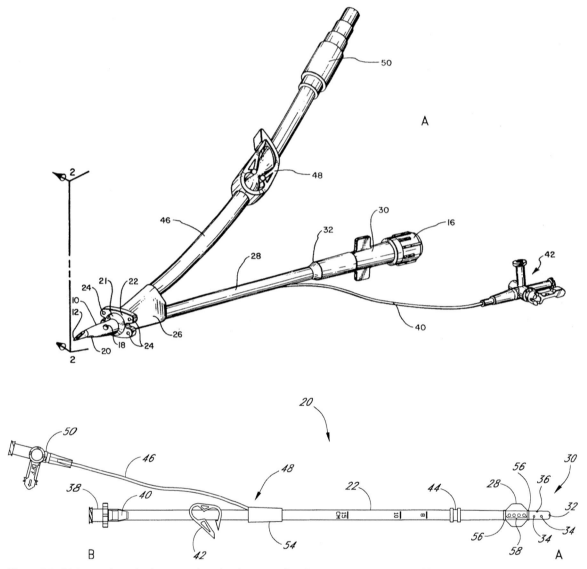

Figure 5.3 (A) Antegrade cardioplegia cannula with side-port to allow function as a vent. From Buckberg GD, Todd RJ. Patent US 5013296 A. May 1991. (B) Retrograde cardioplegia cannula with rigid, curved introducer to allow placement in coronary sinus, balloon-tip for secure placement and side-port for continuous pressure monitoring. From Bicakci M, Higgins SW. Patent US 6500145 B1. December 2002.

and on the bypass reservoir being placed below the level of the patient's thorax. Venous drainage is largely determined by the patient's CVP, the height difference between the thorax and the reservoir and the diameter of the venous cannula.

Venous Reservoir

The venous reservoir receives blood from the venous lines. It allows a margin of safety by maintaining a level of fluid in the reservoir when venous drainage is temporarily impeded. Drainage from the lowermost part prevents any air in the venous line from entering the arterial side of the circuit. The majority of venous reservoirs are rigid and 'open'. This allows easier filtering and addition of cardiotomy sucker blood (Figure 5.7). 'Closed' reservoirs are collapsible and tend to require more attentive management. They are commonly used in 'mini-bypass'. A vacuum assist may be added to the drainage line to improve drainage, although this may increase the likelihood of air entrainment.

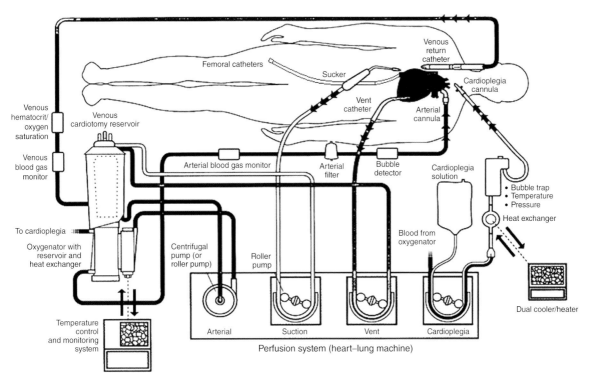

Figure 5.4 Schematic diagram of CPB machine components and connections

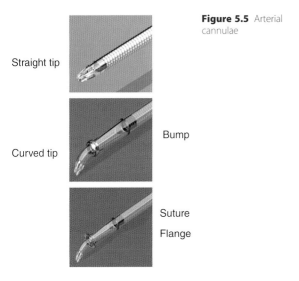

Figure 5.5 Arterial cannulae

Straight tip

Curved tip

Bump

Suture

Flange

Pumps

Two types are in widespread use: roller pumps and centrifugal pumps. Roller pumps have been used since the early days of CPB and remain the most commonly used device. They typically consist of a rotating head with two rollers that compress the tubing mounted in a circular track ('raceway'). Rotation generates a positive pressure after the roller and a negative pressure behind, resulting in forward flow of blood (Figure 5.8). Rapidly altering the rate of pump head rotation can produce pulsatile blood flow. While this is more 'physiological' than constant (non-pulsatile) flow, evidence of improved outcome is sparse. Roller pumps are robust, relatively cheap and largely insensitive to preload and afterload. Disadvantages include more haemolysis than centrifugal pumps, and the potential for pumping large volumes of air if entrained into the circuit. Sudden venous occlusion may result in 'cavitation' within the circuit (the formation of gas bubbles due to a reduction in pressure).

Centrifugal pumps consist of an impeller suspended within a plastic shell through which blood can flow (Figure 5.9). The impeller spins in response to the rotation of an external magnet, resulting in the generation of a pressure differential and forward movement of blood. Because of their cost, centrifugal pumps are typically reserved for longer and more complex cases and ECMO. Unlike roller pumps, they are preload and afterload dependent and do not

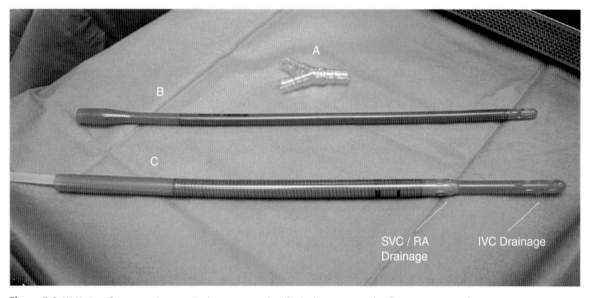

SVC / RA
Drainage

IVC Drainage

Figure 5.6 (A) Y-piece for connecting two single-stage cannulae; (B) single-stage cannula; (C) two-stage cannula

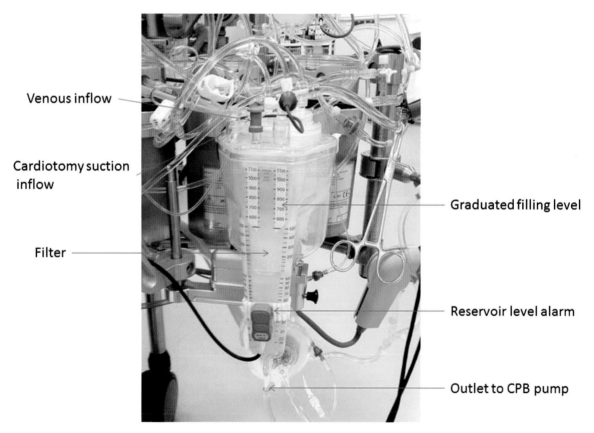

Venous inflow

Cardiotomy suction
inflow

Filter

Graduated filling level

Reservoir level alarm

Outlet to CPB pump

Figure 5.7 Rigid, 'open' venous reservoir

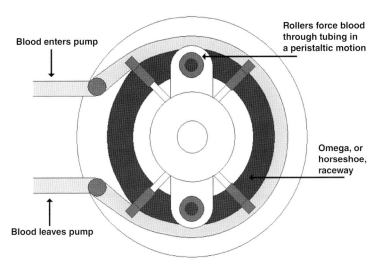

Figure 5.8 Schematic diagram of a CPB roller pump

Blood enters pump

Rollers force blood through tubing in a peristaltic motion

Omega, or horseshoe, raceway

Blood leaves pump

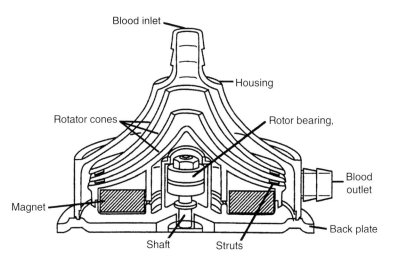

Figure 5.9 Schematic diagram of a centrifugal pump

Blood inlet

Housing

Rotator cones

Rotor bearing,

Blood outlet

Magnet

Back plate

Shaft   Struts

prevent retrograde blood flow when switched off. As a result, air entrainment into the arterial cannula is possible on cessation of flow and arterial air on recommencement of flow. Centrifugal pumps cannot generate excessive pressure and tend to cause less haemolysis than roller pumps.

Oxygenator

Oxygenators are a key component of the CPB circuit and act as the patient's 'lungs'. Notably, carbon dioxide, other gases and anaesthetic agents are exchanged with the blood at this point, in addition to oxygen. Early 'bubble' oxygenators, in which gas was passed through the blood phase before draining into a reservoir, have been superseded by membrane oxygenators which incorporate a gas-permeable material to separate the gas and blood phases. Modern membrane oxygenators use multiple microporous hollow polypropylene fibres to maximize the surface area available for gas exchange. Typically, blood travels outside the fibres, with gas inside (although the opposite configuration is also possible). Although blood comes into contact with the gas phase at the onset of CPB, protein deposits on the fibres quickly separate the two phases. Surface tension of the blood prevents a significant volume of water leaking into the fibre, or gas leaking out. After a number of hours (usually 6–8) evaporation and condensation of serum leaking through the fibres results in reduced efficiency and the oxygenator must be changed. In a situation analogous to native lungs, oxygenation of blood is regulated by the partial pressure of oxygen delivered

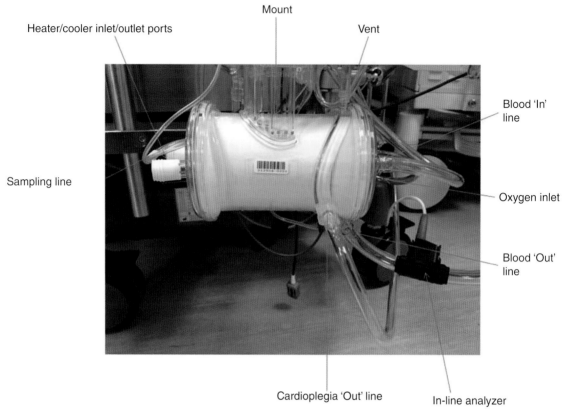

Heater/cooler inlet/outlet ports

Mount

Vent

Blood 'In' line

Sampling line

Oxygen inlet

Blood 'Out' line

Cardioplegia 'Out' line

In-line analyzer

Figure 5.10 Combined oxygenator and heat exchanger

to the gas phase, while carbon dioxide removal is regulated by the rate of gas flow (sometimes called 'sweep' gas). Although the surface area for gas transfer is significantly less than the lungs, efficiency is improved by increased blood transit time to allow longer for diffusion and multiple passes through the membrane.

Most oxygenators also have an integrated heat exchanger, comprising a highly thermally conductive material in contact with the blood (Figure 5.10). This is cooled or heated by an external heater/cooler that pumps water through the heat exchanger. Recently, heater–cooler units have been implicated in the airborne transmission of *Mycobacterium chimaera* in patients, with a latency period of up to 3.6 years after cardiac surgery. At the time of writing most centres have established an elaborate cleaning routine.

Filters and Bubble Traps

The return of arterial blood distal to the heart and lungs exposes the patient to the risk of the delivery of

gaseous and particulate emboli to the systemic circulation. Screen filters may be added to the circuit (most commonly in the arterial line position) to reduce this risk. Screen filters consist of a microporous (20–40 μm) material that allows the passage of blood but traps particles and gas. They can be combined with a bubble trap to allow venting of collected gas. Here, blood enters the side of the cylindrical trap. The blood moves in a circular fashion, such that the less-dense gas bubbles become trapped in the centre, rising to the top while the blood exits from the lowermost part. Gas can then be vented through the top of the device. Although it is clear that these devices reduce microemboli, evidence of organ protection is lacking.

Leucocyte depleting filters may also be used in the circuit. The theoretical benefit is a reduced systemic inflammatory response syndrome (SIRS) and, hopefully, improved outcomes postoperatively. However, results of trials have been mixed and the translation of theory to evidence of improved important outcomes has not been consistently demonstrated.

Cardiotomy Suction

Cardiotomy suction returns anticoagulated blood from the surgical field to the circuit, maintaining an adequate reservoir volume and haematocrit. While this is clearly a necessary component, the act of suctioning causes blood trauma and risks the introduction of emboli to the circuit. Haemolysis, platelet damage and activation of the coagulation and complement systems may occur, contributing to post-bypass coagulopathy and systemic inflammation. While some degree of blood trauma is inevitable, minimizing this may ameliorate adverse effects. This may be carried out by reducing the volume of air co-aspirated with blood, lowering suction volumes and time and keeping negative pressures low (low flow rate suction, large sucker tips and avoidance of sucker occlusion). Cell salvage may be used to 'wash' the blood and remove microaggregates, cytokines and other unwanted proteins, but it will result in depletion of plasma coagulation factors and platelets.

Vents

Vents may be used to suction blood and air from cardiac cavities, preventing ventricular distension and reducing gross air emboli. LV distension may result in a decreased DO_2 and ensuing ischaemia. It may occur as a result of AR (which may occur after aortic cannulation and cardiac distortion even in previously competent valves), Thebesian vein drainage, shunt flow, bronchial blood supply and blood not drained by the CPB venous cannulae. Vents may be inserted via the right superior pulmonary vein, aortic root (which may double up as a cardioplegia delivery cannula), PA or ventricular apex. The latter is less commonly used in contemporary practice. Air may be entrained any time the heart or great vessels are opened and may be removed by de-airing procedures, chamber and aortic root vents.

Minimally Invasive Extracorporeal Circulation (MiECC) Techniques

MiECC (sometimes referred to as 'mini-bypass') refers to a range of surgical, perfusion and anaesthesia techniques aimed at minimizing the deleterious effects of CPB. These include haemodilution, coagulopathy, inflammation and microembolism. Circuit components required for classification as MiECC include a closed circuit without a reservoir, biologically inert surfaces, lower prime volume, centrifugal pump, venous

bubble trap and a cell-saver system. The addition of a soft-shell reservoir to capture blood displaced by the prime allows a small degree of blood-volume management, while a modular hard-shell reservoir can be made available for emergency adverse event management.

There is evidence to suggest MiECC results in reduced haemodilution, improved coagulation, reduced postoperative bleeding, improved renal function and superior myocardial protection. Evidence for other improved outcomes, such as mortality and neurological outcome, is available but weaker. Despite these positive outcomes, uptake of MiECC has been low, with concerns relating to the possible adverse event of massive air entrainment and embolism, as well as technical difficulties in blood-volume management. Advocates for MiECC have asserted that these concerns are not backed up by the favourable safety profile described in available literature.

Safety Standards

A number of safeguards within the circuit aim to eliminate error as much as possible. Specialist societies of clinical perfusion scientists, cardiac anaesthetists and surgeons in the UK have designed a set of minimum safety standards for the CPB circuit:

- Power failure alarm, backup power and hand cranks
- Torch next to bypass machine
- Bubble detector in arterial and cardioplegia lines; pump cut-off if bubbles are detected
- Level alarm with cut-off attached to venous reservoir
- Overpressure alarms in arterial and cardioplegia lines with cut-off/flow reduction
- Retrograde flow alarm and occlusion device if using centrifugal pump
- Gas scavenging for anaesthetic agents
- Arterial limb temperature alarm
- Additional perfusion staff member available
- Sucker and vent check by perfusionist plus additional staff member

Conduct of Cardiopulmonary Bypass

Communication

The temporary replacement of a patient's heart and lungs with an external machine requires the interaction of multiple teams and is arguably one of the most team-orientated tasks faced in anaesthesia. Communication is paramount to patient safety. A good understanding of the mechanics and physiology of CPB helps to decrease risk. The use of closed-loop communication or call-outs and check-backs are commonly used at key stages and may prevent mis-communication. They also allow all team members to be aware of the procedural stage. A number of key events must be acted on and recognized by all team members:

- Heparin administration
- Institution of CPB and announcement of 'full flow' (when the target flow is achieved)
- 'Lungs off', or 'lungs on', at the beginning and end of CPB, and when requested to facilitate surgical access
- CPB termination
- Administration of protamine and cardiotomy suction/vents off ('suckers off')

Preparation for CPB

Prior to starting the procedure, a team briefing allows dissemination of information, including cannulation sites, myocardial protection strategies, equipment and any patient-specific risks. The perfusion team assembles and checks the CPB machine. The venous and arterial lines are typically supplied in continuity, to prevent contamination and to facilitate fluid priming. Institutional preference generally dictates which fluid(s) are used to prime the circuit. Primes include crystalloid (saline, lactate-containing solutions and balanced crystalloids) and colloid (gelatin, albumin or blood) solutions. Prime additives may also be used, and include heparin, mannitol, steroid, calcium, magnesium, antifibrinolytics, corticosteroids and antibiotics. There is insufficient evidence to recommend any type of pump prime or additive. Unfractionated heparin is probably the most widely used additive and is used to reduce the effect of dilution when the prime volume is added to the circulating volume. The volume of pump prime also affects haemodilution. With low body mass or low starting Hb concentration blood may need to be added to the prime. Key patient demographics are collected to enable the calculation of required pump flows and other variables. An additional perfusionist, using a standardized checklist, then checks the machine. Of particular importance is the configuration of the cardiotomy suction and

vents, which if set up to pump rather than suck could result in fatal gas embolus.

Anticoagulation

Systemic anticoagulation of the patient is required to prevent activation of the clotting system within the circuit or within the surgical field. Heparin (300–400 IU kg^{-1}) is by far the most commonly used anticoagulant for CPB. Point-of-care coagulation testing is almost universal and is usually achieved using the ACT test. Whole blood is added to an activator such as kaolin and the time taken for a clot to form measured. The target ACT for CPB varies by institution but is usually between 350 and 550 seconds. There is some evidence that a higher ACT results in reduced coagulopathy due to reduced activation of coagulation during CPB. Heparin resistance may occur, requiring higher doses of heparin to achieve the desired ACT. This is more common in patients with recent heparin use where antithrombin (AT) may become depleted or inactive. If the target ACT can't be achieved despite high doses of heparin (e.g. >500 IU kg^{-1}), exogenous AT in the form of FFP or AT concentrate should be considered. Some evidence exists (from small, retrospective studies) that failure to correct AT deficiency may result in worse outcomes.

Another potential consequence of previous heparin use is the heparin-induced thrombotic thrombocytopenic syndrome (HITTS). In this case an alternative to heparin may be required. Possible alternatives include bivalirudin, lepirudin and danaparoid but limited experience in their use and perioperative clotting disorders mean that they should be avoided if possible, usually by delaying surgery.

Cannulation

Arterial cannulation typically occurs first to allow direct administration of CPB prime in the case of hypotension. For a catastrophic incident, such as major haemorrhage or circulatory collapse, or in the event of difficulty in placing the venous line, shed anticoagulated blood can be recovered using cardiotomy suction and returned to the patient until venous cannulation is achieved (so-called 'sucker bypass'). Prior to cannulation, arterial pressure should be reduced to a systolic pressure of 90–100 mmHg (MAP 60–70 mmHg) to reduce the chances of iatrogenic arterial dissection. In some centres epiaortic ultrasound is used to identify an appropriate site for cannulation, avoiding atherosclerotic plaques. The tip of the arterial cannula is placed 1–2 cm into the lumen of the aorta, and is clamped and secured with purse-string sutures. Once tied in safely, the cannula is connected to the arterial limb of the CPB circuit, taking care not to introduce any air. The intraluminal position is confirmed by releasing the clamp and finding a pulsatile pressure waveform in the arterial line. This is usually called out by the perfusionist ('good swing' or similar).

The aortic cannula is usually the narrowest part of the CPB circuit. This results in high pressure, high resistance and turbulence if not placed with great care. A pressure gradient in excess of 100 mmHg between the arterial limb of the CPB circuit and the MAP should be avoided as this may cause haemolysis or aortic wall injury. High arterial line pressure may indicate line misplacement (e.g. aortic branch), equipment error or an elevated SVR.

Two single-stage cannulae or one two-stage venous cannula are placed in the vena cavae or RA, respectively. These are connected to the venous limb of the circuit. A retrograde cardioplegia cannula may also be placed at this time (and guided using TOE), or subsequently after institution of bypass.

Initiation of CPB

The pump is started and release of the arterial clamp allows flow to begin. The venous clamp is then released allowing drainage from the right side of the heart. This order of events prevents exsanguination of the patient if there is a problem with CPB and full flow cannot be established. Once full flow has been established the perfusionist usually calls this out. Subsequently, ventilation of the lungs can be halted, anaesthetic cardiorespiratory alarms switched off and cardiorespiratory management handed over to the perfusion team. Prior to the placement of an AXC, the surgeon checks that the perfusion team are satisfied with the CPB function. Cardioplegia is given immediately after cross-clamping of the aorta, often resulting in transient hypotension and requiring a vasopressor such as metaraminol or phenylephrine to be given.

Physiological Management during CPB

Haemodynamic Management

Ideal physiological conditions for CPB are controversial. Where the heart is not ejecting, standard physiological principles apply, whereby the MAP is directly proportional to the SVR and the blood flow or CO. Given that preload, afterload, contractility and HR are taken out of the equation for CO, only the pump flow and SVR remain as variables. Both the MAP and the CO are important determinants of global and regional blood supply, but the optimal balance between the two is not known.

A MAP target of 50–70 mmHg is commonly used; with a higher end of the range often targeted where there are concerns about effective cerebral perfusion (such as in carotid stenosis or a reduction in cerebral oximetry value). The flow rate is indexed to body surface area and is analogous to the CI. Flows of 2.2–2.5 l min^{-1} m^{-2} are typically used. Brief periods of low flow are usually well tolerated, particularly during hypothermia. Adequacy of flow may be assessed using evidence of target organ perfusion (urine output, cerebral oximetry or lactate production) and oxygen extraction (SvO$_2$). A low SvO$_2$ during CPB indicates an imbalance between DO$_2$ and VO$_2$ and should trigger a change in the perfusion strategy by addressing one or several of:

- Pump flow
- Haematocrit
- SaO$_2$
- Depth of anaesthesia
- Temperature

Urine production can be used as a measure of renal perfusion, which in turn can serve as a surrogate for systemic perfusion. When using urine output as a monitor, the patient's preoperative renal function needs to be taken into account. Visual inspection of urine can be important when considering the use of mannitol in the presence of significant haemoglobinuria.

The haematocrit is reduced on institution of CPB due to haemodilution. The putative benefits of reduced blood viscosity and improved microvascular flow are offset by reduced oxygen carrying capacity and reduced oncotic pressure, possibly resulting in worse tissue oedema. The haematocrit and other haemodynamic targets are shown in Table 5.1.

During bypass, the CVP should be close to zero or no more than low single figures. Overly liberal drainage with an excessively negative CVP can lead to collapse of the structures around the venous cannula with impaired drainage and the formation of gaseous emboli, a phenomenon known as cavitation.

Table 5.1 Target parameters during CPB

Parameter	Target range
Indexed pump flow rate	2.2–2.5 l min^{-1} m^{-2}
MAP	50–70 mmHg
CVP	0–5 mmHg
SvO_2	>65%
Haematocrit	0.2–0.25
Glucose	5–10 mmol l^{-1}
Base excess	−5 to 5 mmol l^{-1}

An increase in the CVP during bypass is often caused by obstruction of the cannula or tubing or by an insufficient gradient between the table and the pump. If not corrected elevated venous pressure can lead to impaired perfusion of vital organs. If not immediately correctable, the patient's head and eyes should be monitored for sign of engorgement during periods of high CVP. The venous reservoir is equipped with a 'level alarm'. The level sensor is generally placed at the 400 ml mark to avoid air being pumped into the arterial system of the pump.

Metabolic Management

Mild hypothermia (32–34 °C) during CPB is routinely used in many centres. The rationale for this is a small margin of safety associated with reduced metabolic rate and oxygen consumption. In addition to this, a reduction in the production of hypoxia-induced mediators is thought to contribute to the protective effect of hypothermia. Proponents advocate hypothermia on the grounds that it offers some protection to susceptible organs – the brain, the heart and the kidneys. While the evidence for hypothermia is in equipoise, it is widely accepted that hyperthermia is injurious; particularly to the brain. For this reason, rapid and excessive ('overshoot') rewarming should be avoided. The optimal rewarming rate has not been established, but a rise of less than 0.5 °C min^{-1} and a difference of <4 °C between arterial inflow and venous outflow have been recommended (for rewarming from >30 °C). Similarly, care should be taken with temperature monitoring. As a minimum, temperature-monitoring sites should include the CPB arterial line and a patient site close to the brain (e.g. nasopharyngeal). An additional 'lower perfusion' site such as the bladder may be used

to reflect slower equilibrating sites when more profound hypothermia is used.

The acid–base status should be regularly monitored using ABG analysis. Both pH-stat and α-stat strategies may be successfully used to manage patients. When a patient is managed using a pH-stat strategy, blood pH is maintained at a constant level (blood-gas measurements are corrected to body temperature). During α-stat management, the pH is measured at a standardized temperature of 37 °C. Some centres prefer the use of pH-stat for cases where deep hypothermia is used because the greater cerebral blood flow induced by hypercapnia is thought to improve brain cooling. Others argue that this luxuriant flow may be detrimental, resulting in increased microemboli and raised intracranial pressure. Plasma concentrations of potassium, bicarbonate, calcium and magnesium may all vary widely during CPB and should be kept within a reasonable physiological range.

Anaesthesia

Both volatile and IV anaesthesia can be delivered during CPB. A vaporizer may be used in conjunction with the fresh gas supply, with volatile-agent exchange occurring within the oxygenator. The absence of an 'end-tidal' agent equivalent in the CPB circuit makes accurate estimation of the agent delivery difficult during CPB. For this reason, IV anaesthesia is the most commonly used delivery method, often in combination with a volatile agent (in an effort to activate pharmacological preconditioning). Given the number of available ports for drug delivery during cardiac surgery and the multiple opportunities for distraction, considerable care should be taken to ensure that the anaesthesia delivery line is visible and patent. The anaesthetist should also be aware of the effects of drug interactions, haemodilution, extracorporeal sequestration and hypothermia on plasma drug levels. Processed EEG monitoring may be a useful aid for awareness monitoring but should be taken in the context of its known pitfalls.

Cardiac Rhythm

Removal of the AXC results in reperfusion of the heart. Electrical activity recommences as potassium and metabolites are washed out. It is not uncommon for ventricular dysrhythmia to occur, in which case internal cardioversion is appropriate (10–20 J). In the event of persistent VF/VT, electrolytes and bypass graft patency should be checked and antidysrhythmics considered.

Even in the case of normal pre-CPB ventricular function, there is often impaired relaxation post CPB, rendering the CO relatively rate dependent. Epicardial pacing wires are commonly used to ensure a reliable HR and atrioventricular synchrony, and as a fail-safe against conducting system disturbance and subsequent delayed malignant bradycardias. These risks must be balanced against the small risk of myocardial damage or bleeding associated with their placement. Where the risk of pharmacologically unresponsive bradycardia is small, they may be omitted entirely. During surgery, when diathermy is still in use, a fixed-rate pacing mode may be used. This should be switched to a sensing-mode as soon as electromagnetic interference is ceased, to reduce the chances of inadvertently triggering VF.

Weaning from CPB

Prior to weaning from CPB a list of key parameters should be checked (Box 5.1). When all of the team is

---

Box 5.1   Checklist before coming off CPB

Airway
Endotracheal tube connected
Capnography connected

Breathing
'Lungs on'
Consider 100% oxygen where air entrainment
  a risk

Circulation
Adequate rhythm/reliable pacing
Appropriate inotropes and vasopressors available or
  running
Sufficient Hb concentration
De-airing adequate

Drugs
Anaesthesia running
Emergency drugs available

Electrolytes and metabolism
Potassium concentration 4–4.5 mmol l^{-1}
Temperature 36–37 °C
Acid–base status balanced

---

ready, the perfusionist slowly clamps the venous line, allowing blood to return to the heart. There is a gradual reduction in pump flow until complete cessation, and the heart resumes normal function. The arterial line remains in the aorta and is used for transfusion of blood from the CPB venous reservoir.

Decannulation

Venous cannulae and vents are typically removed first. Remaining blood in the field is returned to the venous reservoir. Before protamine is given, all suction from the field is halted. A small test dose of protamine is usually given (10–30 mg). Assuming no major adverse reaction occurs, the remaining protamine is given slowly. Protamine dosing remains controversial. Traditionally, a dose ratio of 1 mg protamine to 100 units of heparin is used; however, this doesn't take into account the elimination of heparin during the case, and a reduced dose may therefore be appropriate. Transient hypotension is a common occurrence and may be countered using fluid transfusion or judicious doses of vasopressor. After removal of the aortic pipe, blood remaining in the CPB circuit can be transferred to an administration bag and returned to the patient.

Haemostasis and Closure

After administration of protamine, a repeat ACT and ABG are taken. In most cases a return of the ACT to baseline is sufficient to suggest normal coagulation. In more complex cases, with longer CPB times or deep hypothermia, patient co-morbidity or preoperative anticoagulant use, more extensive coagulation tests are warranted. These may include point-of-care tests (such as thromboelastography) and laboratory tests.

After haemostasis has been achieved, the chest is closed using sternal wires. Mild reduction in the CO may occur due to reduced RV filling. Rarely, graft kinking may cause significant instability at this point. Skin closure and transfer of the patient to the ICU follows. The patient should be meticulously monitored throughout this period.

Key Points

- Providing a bloodless and motionless surgical field necessitates protection of the heart from ischaemic injury.

- Cardioplegia is the most commonly used strategy to prevent myocardial injury and is in general highly effective.

- The management of CPB lends itself to standard protocols.

- Communication between all care providers is paramount during CPB.

Further Reading

Anastasiadis K, Murkin J, Antonitsis P, *et al.* Use of minimal invasive extracorporeal circulation in cardiac surgery: principles, definitions and potential benefits. A position paper from the Minimal invasive Extra-Corporeal Technologies international Society (MiECTiS). *Interact Cardiovasc Thorac Surg* 2016; 22: 647–62.

Edelman JJB, Seco M, Dunne B, *et al.* Custodiol for myocardial protection and preservation: a systematic review. *Ann Cardiothorac Surg* 2013; 2: 717–28.

Engelman R, Baker RA, Likosky DS, *et al.* The Society of Thoracic Surgeons, The Society of Cardiovascular Anesthesiologists, and The American Society of ExtraCorporeal Technology: clinical practice guidelines for cardiopulmonary bypass – temperature management during cardiopulmonary bypass. *J Cardiothorac Vasc Anesth* 2015; 29: 1104–13.

Ghosh S, Falter F, Perrino AC Jr (eds.). *Cardiopulmonary Bypass*, 2nd edn. Cambridge: Cambridge University Press; 2015.

Habertheuer A, Kocher A, Laufer G, *et al.* Cardioprotection: a review of current practice in global ischemia and future translational perspective. *BioMed Res Int* 2014; 2014: 1–11.

Hausenloy DJ, Yellon DM. Ischaemic conditioning and reperfusion injury. *Nature* 2016; 13: 193–209.

Kunst G, Klein AA. Peri-operative anaesthetic myocardial preconditioning and protection: cellular mechanisms and clinical relevance in cardiac anaesthesia. *Anaesthesia* 2015; 70: 467–82.

Recommendations for Standards of Monitoring and Safety during Cardiopulmonary Bypass Society of Clinical Perfusion Scientists of Great Britain & Ireland Association for Cardiothoracic Anaesthesia and Critical Care Society for Cardiothoracic Surgery in Great Britain & Ireland; 2016. www.scps.org.uk/pdfs/RSM%20and %20Safety%20during%20CPB% 20Aug%202016%20booklet.pdf (accessed June 2019).

Chapter

6

Weaning from Cardiopulmonary Bypass

Simon Anderson

Failure to wean a patient from CPB at the first attempt after routine cardiac surgery is a relatively uncommon occurrence. Following prolonged, complex or emergency surgery, however, failure to wean is relatively common. In the majority of cases, weaning difficulty can be attributed to myocardial ischaemia secondary to a prolonged AXC time, inadequate myocardial protection, frank MI or coronary embolism. Less common causes include extremes of prosthetic valve malfunction, anastomotic strictures, extremes of vascular resistance and cardiac compression from retained surgical swabs.

The key to successful termination of CPB in this situation is the recognition that there is a problem, the identification of the cause or causes and the timely institution of remedial therapy accompanied by effective communication (Box 6.1). In order to prevent ventricular distension and inadequate coronary perfusion, the surgical team must act before the situation escalates. In certain scenarios the reinstitution of CPB, insertion of an IABP or institution of ECMO should be considered. Generally speaking, conditions impeding successful weaning can be considered as either correctable or non-correctable by the anaesthetist (Box 6.2).

Correctable Causes

Impaired Ventricular Function

Dysfunction may be systolic or diastolic, can affect the LV or RV and may be regional or global. TOE is invaluable in assessing the extent and severity of ventricular dysfunction and the response to intervention. Myocardial stunning secondary to prolonged myocardial ischaemia, or inadequate myocardial protection or revascularization, usually responds to a further period of CPB and inotropes; however, more frequently, ECMO can be used over a 24–48-hour period to allow cardiac function to recover. Preceding any attempt to wean from CPB, a minimum period of 10–15 minutes of coronary reperfusion following removal of the AXC should be observed. A spasm of native coronary arteries or arterial bypass conduits, which may cause significant ventricular dysfunction, usually responds to nitrates.

Box 6.1	Diagnosing a post-CPB low CO state
CI	<2.0 l min^{-1} m^{-2}
SVR	<5 Wood units (<400 dyne s cm^{-5}) >20 Wood units ($>1,600$ dyne s cm^{-5})
LA pressure/ LVEDP	>20 mmHg
Urine output	<0.3 ml kg^{-1} h^{-1}

Box 6.2	Causes of failure to wean from CPB
Correctable by the anaesthetist or perfusionist	
Impaired myocardial function	
Air embolism	
Dysrhythmia	
Hypothermia	
Metabolic/acid–base	
Preload	
Respiratory/airway	
Extremes of SVR and PVR	
Profound haemorrhage	
Gross anaemia	
Monitoring artefact	
Not correctable by the anaesthetist or perfusionist	
Acute MI	
Inadequate surgical correction	
New anatomical defect	
Prosthetic valve malfunction	

Air Embolism

The incidence of air embolism is increased following procedures in which the left heart is opened (e.g. aortic, MV, AV and LV aneurysm surgery). The right coronary artery (RCA) is more commonly affected as its ostium lies superiorly in the supine patient. RV distension and conduction abnormalities may be the first clinical indications of air embolism. TOE may reveal a regional wall motion abnormality (RWMA) and myocardial 'air contrast' (increased echo reflectivity) in the RCA territory. In practice, vasopressors are used to treat mild myocardial dysfunction, whereas allowing the heart to eject while on partial CPB may be necessary if myocardial dysfunction is severe. Ventilation of the lungs with an FiO_2 of 1.0 should, at least in theory, accelerate the absorption of nitrogen from intravascular air.

Dysrhythmia

It is futile to attempt to terminate CPB in the presence of untreated asystole, bradycardia, VT or VF. Atropine and epicardial pacing are the first-line treatments for bradydysrhythmias. Persistent ventricular dysrhythmias require electrical cardioversion in the first instance. An underlying physical or metabolic cause should be actively sought before resorting to antidysrhythmics (e.g. lidocaine, amiodarone). New-onset AF or other SVT may respond to synchronized transatrial cardioversion, whereas unstable nodal rhythms may be converted to sinus rhythm by isoproterenol.

Hypothermia

Ventricular irritability, dysrhythmias and contractile dysfunction are more common at temperatures <34 °C. Deep hypothermic circulatory arrest (DHCA) is necessary for some complex procedures, affecting the patient blood flow requirements and subsequent complete rewarming both bladder and nasopharyngeal temperatures are necessary if DHCA is utilized. See Table 6.1 for details.

Metabolic/Acid–Base

Increased or decreased $[K^+]$, decreased $[Mg^{2+}]$ and increased $[H^+]$ may induce dysrhythmia, impair myocardial contractility and increase PVR.

Table 6.1 Effect of hypothermia on patient flow index requirements

Hypothermia	Temperature (°C)	Flow Index (l min^{-1} m^{-2})
Normothermia	34–37	2.4
Moderate hypothermia	32–34	2.2
Hypothermia	28–32	1.8–2.0
Profound hypothermia	<28	1.6

Preload

An inadequate ventricular preload leads to a reduced CO. Overenthusiastic elevation of atrial pressures risks ventricular distension, MR, TR and cardiac failure. TOE assessment of the LV end-diastolic area is often a better guide to preload optimization than CVP monitoring.

Respiratory/Airway

Inadvertent failure to restart mechanical ventilation may occur, particular when the surgeon has requested repeated periods of apnoea to facilitate surgical access at the end of a procedure. Severe bronchospasm apparent at the termination of CPB is a rare but potentially lethal complication. The management of this complication requires continuation of CPB, consideration of ECMO, avoidance of lung distension (which may damage an internal mammary artery graft), bronchoscopy (to exclude airway obstruction) and aggressive treatment with several bronchodilators (e.g. isoflurane, epinephrine, β_2-agonists, aminophylline, ketamine, $MgSO_4$) and corticosteroids.

Extremes of SVR or PVR

CPB provides a ready opportunity to accurately calculate the SVR.

SVR = (MAP − CVP)/Pump flow

The resulting figure, in Wood units, can be converted to dyne s cm^{-5} by multiplying by 80. For example: when MAP = 65 mmHg, CVP = 5 mmHg and pump flow = 5 l min^{-1}, the SVR = 12 Wood units or 960 dyne s cm^{-5}. Assuming that the SVR does not markedly change during weaning from CPB, an estimate of CO can be made using the MAP, CVP and calculated SVR. A target SVR of 10–14 Wood units (800–1,120 dyne s cm^{-5}) with a CVP of 5 mmHg will generate a MAP in the range 55–75 mmHg with a CO of 5 l min^{-1}. Reduced tissue perfusion and increased myocardial work secondary to excessive afterload (i.e. SVR >20 Wood units) may lead to acidosis and myocardial ischaemia. In addition, increased vascular sheer stress may cause aortic dissection during decannulation and worsen bleeding from suture lines. An excessively low afterload (i.e. SVR <6 Wood units) may result in inadequate coronary perfusion and a low CO.

PHT secondary to pre-existing disease or new-onset pulmonary vasoconstriction may impede successful weaning, particular in the presence of RV dysfunction. Potentially reversible causes (e.g. incomplete lung inflation, protamine-induced pulmonary vasoconstriction, CPB-induced acute lung injury) should be sought and treated. Therapy should be targeted at both the RV and the pulmonary circulation. The use of inotropes, vasoconstrictors, head-up posture and an IABP may reduce RV end-diastolic pressure and improve RV perfusion and contractility. Haemofiltration and inhaled NO, iloprost or phosphodiesterase inhibitors may reduce PVR.

Profound Haemorrhage

Bleeding from posterior structures or suture lines can be difficult to deal with. Elevating or rotating the heart around its base may impede venous return and dramatically reduce the CO. Assessment and surgical repair may be more safely carried out on CPB.

Gross Anaemia

A haematocrit of <20% is undesirable as low oxygen-carrying capacity coupled with a low CO may lead to tissue hypoxia and acidosis. The haematocrit may be elevated by diuretic administration, red-cell transfusion, reducing crystalloid administration or haemofiltration.

Monitoring Artefact

Unexplained hypotension may be due to problems with invasive monitoring. Zero-drift, damping, line occlusion, transducer misplacement and other causes of inaccuracy must be excluded before the administration of vasoactive drugs. A large discrepancy between peripheral arterial pressure and CPB arterial line pressure (monitored by the perfusionist) should prompt the use of direct aortic pressure monitoring using a 21 G needle and a separate manometer line and transducer.

Non-Correctable Causes
Acute MI

This is a difficult diagnosis to make intraoperatively. The diagnosis is suggested by persistent ECG changes in the presence of a new, irreversible, severe RWMA (i.e. akinesia or dyskinesia) in a coronary artery territory. Causes include distal coronary embolization, graft occlusion and incomplete revascularization. The surgeon may consider further revascularization on CPB; however, re-heparinzation and application of an AXC lead to further cardiac ischaemia.

Inadequate Surgical Correction

This is more common in surgery for congenital heart disease. Incomplete myocardial revascularization may cause problems, particularly in redo surgery.

New Anatomical Defect

Iatrogenic MS, a new ASD or an LVOT obstruction may arise following MV surgery. Similarly, a basal VSD is a recognized complication of surgery for hypertrophic obstructive cardiomyopathy.

Prosthetic Valve Malfunction

Large paravalvular leaks, an impeded leaflet opening due to prolapse of subvalvular tissue, the inadvertent use of a mitral prosthesis in the aortic position (and vice versa) and an incorrect twisted insertion of dacron graft are rare causes of failure to wean from CPB.

Pharmacological Support

Having excluded and treated reversible causes of failed weaning from CPB, administration of inotropic agents should be considered. Both the SVR and PVR, as well as institutional preference, largely dictate drug selection.

Mechanical Support

Intra-aortic balloon counter-pulsation is a common intervention undertaken in all cardiac surgical centres.

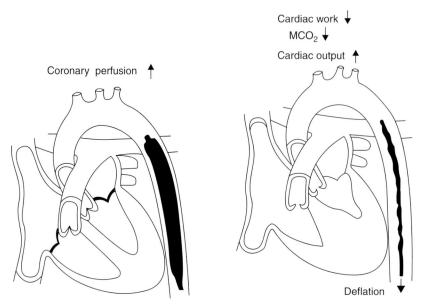

Figure 6.1 The IABP. The balloon is positioned in the descending thoracic aorta just distal to the origin of the left subclavian artery. During diastole, the balloon is rapidly filled with helium and impedes blood flow to the distal aorta. The rise in proximal aortic pressure augments coronary perfusion pressure. The balloon is deflated at the end of diastole (*before* the onset of isovolumic LV contraction) resulting in a reduced LVEDP. (Courtesy of Datascope Corp, NJ, USA.)

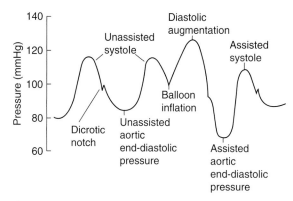

Figure 6.2 Proximal aortic pressure waveforms without and with IABP augmentation. Balloon inflation takes place at the dicrotic notch (AV closure). Balloon deflation takes place before AV opening so as not to impede LV ejection. (Courtesy of Datascope Corp, NJ, USA.)

In contrast, the use of univentricular or biventricular mechanical assist devices and ECMO (Chapters 16 and 29) is usually restricted to designated specialist centres with their use increasing annually.

Intra-Aortic Balloon Pump

The IABP may be used to augment pharmacological therapy or when drugs alone have resulted in failure to wean from CPB. The device consists of an inflatable, sausage-shaped balloon (30–40 ml), which is normally inserted into the descending thoracic aorta via the femoral artery such that the tip lies just distal to the origin of the left subclavian artery (Figure 6.1). Correct positioning may be confirmed by TOE or CXR. The device improves LV performance by augmenting coronary perfusion and reducing the LVEDP (Figure 6.2).

Indications and Contraindications

As the IABP does not interfere with cardiac surgery, insertion may be undertaken before induction of anaesthesia in high-risk patients and in patients with angina despite maximal medical therapy. Other indications are summarized in Box 6.3.

The use of the IABP is contraindicated in the presence of moderate or severe AR, severe peripheral vascular disease and aortic dissection.

Management

Use of an IABP requires systemic anticoagulation with unfractionated heparin to achieve an activated partial thromboplastin ratio of 1.5–2.0. The correct timing of balloon inflation and deflation is critical to optimal operation. On most IABP devices, timings

> **Box 6.3** Indications for IABP insertion
> - Ischaemic myocardium
> - Structural complications of acute MI
> - Cardiogenic shock

can be derived from the ECG (R-wave), pacemaker potentials or the arterial waveform, and adjusted manually. In addition, the extent of balloon inflation ('augmentation') and the ratio of inflations to HR (i.e. 1:1, 1:2 or 1:3) can be altered, aiding the perfusionist with IABP timing. Excessive tachycardia and irregular cardiac rhythms (particularly AF) reduce the effectiveness of the IABP.

Complications

Incorrect IABP positioning may result in left-arm ischaemia (balloon too high/proximal) or renal/GI ischaemia (balloon too low/distal). The most common complications are vascular injury (including dissection and pseudoaneurysm), lower-limb ischaemia and infection at the insertion site.

Balloon rupture is not uncommon, usually in patients with a calcified aorta. The use of helium, which has high blood solubility, reduces the risks associated with gas embolism.

Thrombocytopenia is not uncommon and may be the result of mechanical platelet damage, inadequate anticoagulation or heparin itself.

Key Points

- Myocardial stunning and inadequate myocardial protection or revascularization are common causes of failure to wean from CPB.
- Many of the causes of failure to wean from CPB are amenable to intervention by the anaesthetist and perfusionist.
- Intraoperative MI is difficult to diagnose with confidence.
- The IABP is contraindicated in the presence of significant AR.

Further Reading

Arrowsmith JE. Severe bronchospasm following cardiopulmonary bypass. In: Arrowsmith JE, Simpson J (eds). *Problems in Anesthesia: Cardiothoracic Surgery*. London: Martin Dunitz; 2002, pp. 133–8.

Intra-aortic Balloon Counterpulsation Therapy: Theory Program. Getinge Education Academy. https://getinge.training/d/course/101000 1718/ (accessed December 2018).

Toshner M, Pepke-Zaba J. Pulmonary hypertension in the cardiothoracic intensive care unit. In Valchanov K, Jones N, Hogue CW (eds.). *Core Topics in Cardiothoracic Critical Care*, 2nd edn. Cambridge: Cambridge University Press; 2018, pp. 272–77.

Routine Early Postoperative Care

Barbora Parizkova and Aravinda Page

Early postoperative care is a critical factor in determining successful outcomes following cardiac surgery. With increasing pressure for efficiency while ensuring patient safety is maintained, it is vital that healthcare professionals are familiar with the pathways and protocols designed to allow for rapid recovery of patients. At the same time it is important that complications are detected early, escalated appropriately and intervened upon in a timely fashion.

Fast-Tracking

Determining if a patient is suitable to be fast-tracked or for enhanced recovery versus the need for more advanced care begins early in the patient pathway, during the preoperative assessment by the surgeon and anaesthetist. 'Routine' cardiac cases are 'fast-tracked' in a cardiac recovery unit, which is a part of the ICU. Such clinical areas are often managed by experienced nursing staff who follow institution-specific protocols while being overseen by a responsible physician. These protocols address issues such as the weaning from mechanical ventilation and the management of expected postoperative issues. These strategies have been safely implemented to facilitate early ICU and hospital discharge. It is important to emphasize the need for early involvement of specialized medical staff when there is deviation of a patient's progress from a clearly defined pathway or anticipation of such an incident.

Transfer, ICU Admission and Handover

During the transfer from the operating room, uninterrupted invasive monitoring is essential for the early recognition of haemodynamic instability secondary to fluid shifts during movement and dysrhythmias. On arrival in the ICU it is important that there is a prompt handover to the nurse responsible for ongoing care. This should include anaesthetic and intraoperative details as shown in Box 7.1. This is

---

Box 7.1 Handover checklist

The patient

Demographics: name, age, height, weight

Pre-existing medical conditions

List of preoperative medications

Allergies/drug sensitivities

Cardiac status (ventricular dysfunction, valvular disease)

The procedure

Planned/actual surgical procedure performed

Complications and other significant events

Details regarding weaning from CPB, vasoactive drugs, pacing, IABP

Optimal cardiac filling pressures in theatre

Anaesthesia

Vascular line types and insertion sites (along with any complications that occurred during their placement)

Laryngoscopy grade, difficulties during intubation

Continuous infusions and current rates

Recent ABG (especially potassium and Hb levels)

Blood products administered and ordered for later administration

Fluids administered, urine output and use of haemofiltration during CPB

Recent laboratory investigations (TEG, full blood count, coagulation)

The postoperative plan

Optimal acceptable ranges of MAP, CVP, PAWP as ICU targets

Expected duration of sedation and mechanical ventilation

Need for CXR as indicated

usually performed while the ICU ventilator is being connected and monitoring (usually including capnography, invasive monitoring, oximetry and ECG) is switched from the portable monitor to the fixed ICU monitor. In patients who require epicardial pacing, it is important that the pacing is checked and changed from a fixed rate to demand mode as appropriate. Once the handover has been completed, an initial ABG should be drawn to ensure appropriate oxygenation and ventilation is being achieved. Baseline potassium, Hb and metabolic state should be reviewed and corrected as appropriate. If the patient is bleeding excessively, a baseline full blood count and coagulation screen and/or a thromboelastogram (TEG) should be acquired.

Mechanical Ventilation, Sedation and Analgesia

In the UK, it is widely considered that the risk of bleeding, haemodynamic instability and hypothermia following cardiac surgery outweighs any potential benefits of tracheal extubation in the operating theatre prior to transfer to ICU. Initially, a 'full' mechanical ventilation mode is selected, for example synchronized intermittent mandatory ventilation (SIMV) with an adequate rate (10–12 breaths per minute), tidal volume (6–8 ml kg^{-1}) and a modest PEEP (5 cmH$_2$O) to reduce postoperative atelectasis. As spontaneous respiratory effort returns, lower-rate SIMV with pressure-support ventilation (PSV) can be used. Eventually, ventilation using only PSV (to overcome the resistance of the ventilatory system) with a modest PEEP can be used prior to tracheal extubation.

In the setting of mediastinal bleeding, a higher PEEP (5–10 cmH$_2$O) may be used; however, this may have deleterious haemodynamic effects. Sedation and mechanical ventilation are usually continued for 30–240 minutes post transfer to the ICU to allow for rewarming and to exclude significant bleeding. Use of

forced-air warming blankets can minimize the duration of postoperative hypothermia (<36 °C), which is not uncommon and can have adverse effects (Box 7.2). Many centres routinely use propofol for sedation due to its short and predictable duration of action. The criteria that should be considered prior to switching of sedation with a view to weaning ventilation and extubation are listed in Box 7.3.

Effective postoperative analgesia reduces pain on movement and deep inspiration, facilitating early weaning from ventilation. Commonly used systemic opioids include fentanyl, morphine and, in some centres, alfentanil. Paracetamol 1g IV is administered shortly after arrival, and at 6-hourly intervals thereafter. Once oral intake has been established, commonly used oral analgesics (e.g. oxycodone, codeine, dihydrocodeine and paracetamol) should be introduced and IV opioids ceased.

NSAIDs can be helpful in managing postoperative pain following cardiac surgery, albeit at the risk of increased bleeding (inhibition of the platelet function), upper GI ulceration and renal impairment. The use of the epidural analgesia is discussed in Chapter 38.

Haemodynamics

Hypotension

The most frequently encountered problem after cardiac surgery is hypotension. This is usually caused by hypovolaemia secondary to fluid shifts during transfer, excessive diuresis, bleeding or peripheral vasodilatation. Hypotension not responding to an IV fluid challenge (250–500 ml) or requiring multiple fluid challenges is an indication for escalation and further assessment.

Myocardial Ischaemia

Haemodynamic instability that is thought to be due to myocardial ischaemia should be verified with a 12-lead ECG for ST-segment analysis. Echocardiographic (TOE)

Box 7.2   Adverse effects of hypothermia

- Increased SVR and hypertension
- Predispose to atrial and ventricular arrhythmias
- Precipitate shivering, which increases peripheral O$_2$ consumption and CO$_2$ production
- Produce platelet dysfunction and generalized impairment of the coagulation cascade
- Prolongs the time to tracheal extubation

Box 7.3   Criteria for withdrawing sedation and weaning from mechanical ventilation

- Haemodynamically stable
- Able to make a valid respiratory effort
- Able to protect their airway
- Fully rewarmed
- Normalization of ABG
- Acid–base balance within specified range

detection of a segmental wall motion abnormality represents the most sensitive early detector of myocardial ischaemia and can initiate further investigation (e.g. angiography to confirm graft patency) or surgical re-exploration and revascularization.

Ventricular Dysfunction

Inadequate myocardial protection, myocardial hyperthermia, impaired coronary graft flow, incomplete revascularization and reperfusion injury can all contribute to postoperative ventricular dysfunction. The CO may be optimized by increasing the HR to 80–90 bpm in the early postoperative period. Atrial demand pacing (AAI mode) is preferable to ventricular demand (i.e. VVI) because of the contribution of the 'atrial kick', which amounts to 15–30% of the SV. β_1-agonists, such as dopamine, dobutamine and adrenaline, are the most frequently used inotropes. Phosphodiesterase inhibitors such as enoximone or milrinone may also be considered, although secondary vasodilatation often requires the addition of a vasoconstrictor such as noradrenaline. In the case of hypotension refractory to inotropic support, IABP placement should be considered as it reduces myocardial oxygen demand and improves coronary perfusion.

Tachycardia

Haemodynamically unstable tachyarrhythmia should be cardioverted without delay by pharmacological or electrical means according to Cardiac Advanced Life Support (CALS) guidelines. Postoperative AF occurs in up to 30% of patients following CABG. The prompt correction of electrolyte disturbances (e.g. hypokalaemia and hypomagnesaemia) and the early reintroduction of β-blockers can reduce the incidence of postoperative AF. The administration of antidysrhythmics such as digoxin or amiodarone should be considered.

Arterial Hypertension

Perioperative hypertension (MAP >90 mmHg) can be caused by:

- Weaning from anaesthesia
- Intolerance of the endotracheal tube
- Pain – inadequate analgesia
- Hypercarbia and hypoxaemia

- Hypothermia
- Inappropriate use of vasoconstrictors
- Withdrawal from preoperative antihypertensive medication (β-blockers, central α_2-agonists)

If hypertension persists, commencing an infusion of GTN to control BP (MAP 60–80 mmHg) may be considered. Where appropriate, the reintroduction of regular antihypertensive medication (e.g. calcium channel blockers, β-blockers) may be indicated.

Fluid and Electrolyte Management

Cardiac procedures involving CPB usually result in a positive fluid balance with excessive fluid intake and fluid sequestration into third spaces. Patients with good cardiac and renal function typically correct these imbalances through diuresis over the first two postoperative days. Elderly patients with cardiac and renal dysfunction may require diuretics to promote excretion of this excess fluid. Fluid intake (crystalloid and colloid), urine output and chest tube drainage should be recorded hourly. In adults, total crystalloid intake (oral and IV) is typically restricted to 750 ml m^{-2} in the first 24 hours, and 1,000 ml m^{-2} in the following 24-hour period. Colloids or blood products in the case of bleeding may be administered in response to hypotension, low CVP or oliguria.

Hypokalaemia is more common than hyperkalaemia, and it is commonly associated with preoperative diuretic therapy, dilution or ion shifts, associated with hyperventilation (iatrogenic) and high urinary output. The serum potassium concentration should be maintained at 4.5–5.5 mmol l^{-1}. IV potassium supplementation via a central venous catheter should not exceed 20 mmol over 30–60 minutes. Rapid potassium infusion can induce lethal arrhythmias mandating continuous ECG monitoring. Hyperkalaemia ([K$^+$] >6.5 mmol l^{-1}) in the absence of cardiac dysfunction may be treated with furosemide (20–40 mg) or 50% dextrose (50 ml) mixed with soluble insulin (15 IU) infused over 30 minutes. A bolus of calcium chloride (10 mmol) or calcium gluconate may be used in the presence of cardiac dysfunction. Hypomagnesaemia should be corrected with magnesium sulphate (2–4 g), administered intravenously over 30–45 minutes. Hyperglycaemia (glucose concentration >10 mmol l^{-1}) will require an insulin infusion to be commenced as per local protocols.

Common Postoperative Complications

Further discussion of postoperative complications can be found Chapter 8.

Respiratory Failure

Frequent pulmonary toilet and incentive spirometry should be used to prevent atelectasis. If hypoxaemia develops, facemask CPAP can be used to improve the atelectasis-related shunt. If ventilation also becomes impaired with rising $PaCO_2$, non-invasive ventilation via a facemask can be employed in an attempt to avoid the need for tracheal intubation.

Bleeding

Many patients with 'non-surgical bleeding' will drain 50–100 ml h^{-1} for the first few hours after surgery. Drain output must be measured accurately to guide management and determine the need for re-exploration. Bleeding may be considered to be excessive if it is:

- >3 ml kg^{-1} h^{-1} in the 1st postoperative hour
- >2 ml kg^{-1} h^{-1} in the 2nd to 4th postoperative hours
- >1 ml kg^{-1} h^{-1} in the 5th to 12th postoperative hours

Broadly speaking, chest tube drainage of 500 ml h^{-1} or sustained drainage >200 ml h^{-1} justifies consideration of surgical re-exploration.

There are many reasons for bleeding: residual heparin effect, platelet dysfunction, thrombocytopenia, surgical issues, hypothermia, hypertension and fibrinolysis. Most cardiac centres routinely use antifibrinolytics (tranexamic acid or ε-aminocaproic acid). A suggested protocol for the management of bleeding in the setting of coagulopathy is shown in Figure 7.1.

Transfusion of platelet concentrates may be considered when there is the suspicion that bleeding may be a result of platelet dysfunction secondary to either preoperative platelet inhibitors or prolonged CPB.

Early re-exploration of a bleeding patient has been shown to be associated with improved outcome. Excessive mediastinal bleeding with inadequate drainage or sudden massive bleeding may cause cardiac tamponade.

Oliguria

Urine output <0.5 ml kg^{-1} h^{-1} for two consecutive hours should prompt immediate investigation and treatment. An adequate CO and MAP with appropriate filling pressures has to be achieved. A fluid challenge with 250–500 ml of colloid may be administered; if there is no response and the patient is well filled with adequate BP, a bolus of furosemide should be considered.

First Postoperative Day

The timing of chest drain removal is a surgical decision, and typically occurs when there is no air leak and drainage is <25 ml h^{-1} for at least two consecutive hours. The peripheral arterial cannula is removed prior to transfer to the ward but may be retained if the patient is transferred to a step-down unit with

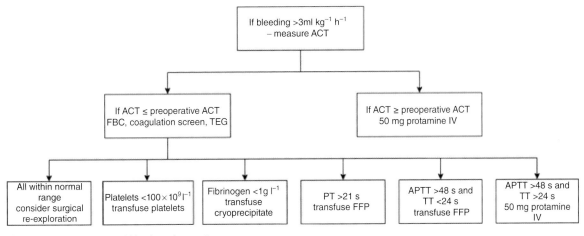

Figure 7.1 Management of bleeding after cardiac surgery

invasive monitoring facilities. Pacing wires are usually removed on the fourth postoperative day on the ward. The central venous catheter is removed not earlier than the second postoperative day. The urinary catheter is retained for at least two days.

Family Involvement in the Postoperative Period

It is a good practice for either the medical or nursing staff to contact relatives within the first hour of ICU admission to update them with a brief report. Family members should be encouraged to assist with adequate pulmonary toilet, coughing, deep breathing and mobility of their relatives.

Key Points

- Problems in the early postoperative period are common. Most can be successfully managed by applying locally developed protocols.
- Demand pacing should be used in preference to fixed-rate pacing to reduce the risk of VF.
- A high level of vigilance is required to detect occult bleeding and cardiac tamponade.
- Good communication between anaesthetists, intensivists, surgeons and nursing staff is essential.

Further Reading

Abu-Omar Y, Farid S. Intensive care unit management following valve surgery. In Valchanov K, Jones N, Hogue CW (eds.), *Core Topics in Cardiothoracic Critical Care*, 2nd edn. Cambridge: Cambridge University Press; 2018, pp. 317–23.

Bojar RM. *Manual of Perioperative Care in Adult Cardiac Surgery*, 5th edn. Hoboken, NJ: Wiley-Blackwell; 2010.

Hensley FA, Gravlee GP, Martin DE. *A Practical Approach to Cardiac Anesthesia*, 5th edn. Philadelphia, PA: Lippincott Williams & Wilkins; 2012.

Lighthall GK, Olejniczak M. Routine postoperative care of patients undergoing coronary artery bypass grafting on cardiopulmonary bypass. *Semin Cardiothorac Vasc Anesth* 2015; 19: 78–86.

Nashef S, Bosco P. Management after coronary artery bypass grafting surgery. In Valchanov K, Jones N, Hogue CW (eds.), *Core Topics in Cardiothoracic Critical Care*, 2nd edn. Cambridge: Cambridge University Press; 2018, pp. 313–16.

Common Postoperative Complications

Jonathan H. Mackay and Joseph E. Arrowsmith

A comprehensive review of the complications of cardiac surgery would fill an entire volume. This chapter covers the more common and life-threatening complications. The reader is directed to the publications list under further reading.

Cardiovascular Complications

Haemodynamic instability following CPB is common. The goal of cardiovascular management in the ICU is to maintain adequate oxygen transport to end organs until complete recovery of cardiac function.

Cardiac Arrest

Resuscitation of cardiac arrest after cardiac surgery differs from conventional advanced life support (see Figure 8.1):

- In shockable rhythms, up to three shocks should be administered in rapid succession *before* chest compressions
- In asystole, epicardial pacing should be attempted *before* chest compressions
- In pulseless electrical activity (PEA), pacing-induced VF should be excluded
- Epinephrine administration may be deferred and doses reduced to reduce the risk of hypertension after return of spontaneous circulation
- Chest reopening should be undertaken after two cycles

Initial Optimization

The response to increasing preload can be thought of in three distinct phases (Box 8.1).

In health, preload optimization typically occurs with a PAWP of 10–15 mmHg. Many cardiac surgical patients have reduced LV compliance, which becomes further reduced by the effects of CPB and catecholamines. In these patients, a higher PAWP (i.e. >15 mmHg) is often required to maintain adequate SV.

Heart rate, rhythm and myocardial contractility are the major determinants of myocardial VO_2. Because of its 30% augmentation of end-diastolic volume (EDV), NSR is desirable whenever possible. Atrial or atrioventricular (A-V) pacing at 80–100 bpm can improve endocardial perfusion by shortening the diastolic filling time and reducing the EDV.

VF, and unstable ventricular and supraventricular tachydysrhythmias should be immediately converted by either electrical or chemical cardioversion. Maintenance of normal or supranormal $[K^+]$ (i.e. 4.5–5.5 mmol l^{-1}) and $[Mg^{2+}]$ reduces ventricular irritability.

Cardiodepressant antidysrhythmics should be used with caution in patients with impaired myocardial function.

Afterload can be viewed as the sum of external forces opposing ventricular ejection, of which the SVR is one component (Box 8.2). Laplace's law states that the LV wall tension or stress is directly proportional to the intracavity pressure and cavity radius, and is inversely proportional to the LV wall thickness.

Considering the CO, MAP and PAWP in the patient with optimal preload simplifies haemodynamic management (Box 8.3).

LV Dysfunction

Ventricular function is commonly depressed for 8–24 hours following CPB. The ideal measure of LV performance, the slope of the end-systolic pressure–volume relationship (ESPVR), cannot easily be derived at the bedside. For this reason, surrogate measures of contractility (i.e. RA pressure, PAWP, MAP, PAP and CO) are used. Although echocardiography can be used to assess ventricular function, the findings are generally load-dependent (Figure 8.2).

Decreased contractility can be secondary to metabolic abnormalities, cardiodepressant agents, reperfusion injury and myocardial ischaemia (coronary vasospasm, thrombosis or occlusion). The incidence

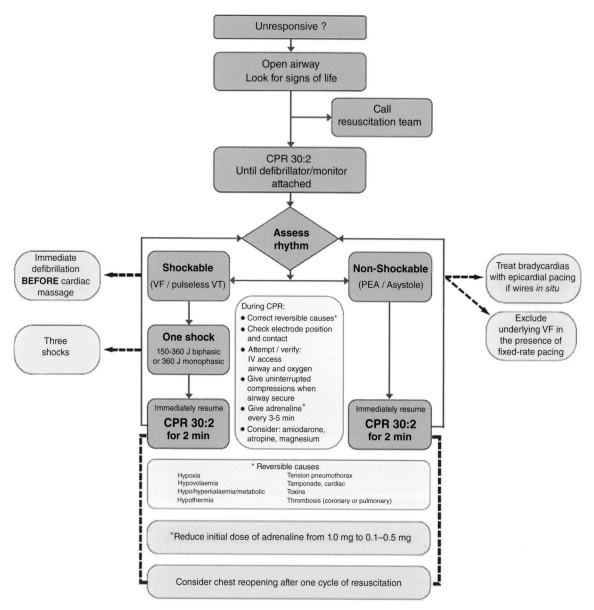

Figure 8.1 Algorithm for resuscitation after adult cardiac surgery. Six suggested modifications to the standard ALS algorithm are highlighted in the bright yellow boxes to the sides and below. Therapeutic hypothermia may be considered after successful resuscitation. (Adapted from the Resuscitation Council (UK) 2010 ALS algorithm)

of perioperative MI (often clinically silent) is thought to be ~5%. The diagnosis of MI in the post-CABG patient may be challenging (Box 8.4).

Before initiating inotropic therapy, all remediable factors (i.e. rate, rhythm, preload and afterload) should be addressed. Indications for use of the IABP and mechanical cardiac support are discussed in Chapters 6 and 16).

RV Dysfunction

RV failure can be difficult to manage because of the dependence of the LV filling on right-sided function. If the RV output falls, the LV filling and therefore the LV output are reduced. The RV is extremely sensitive to increases in afterload (i.e. PVR). Although more effective in LV failure, the IABP may reduce the RV afterload

Box 8.1 The three phases of the response to increasing preload

1	**Intact preload reserve**	↑ EDV → ↑ SV and ↑ CO
2	**Preload optimization**	↑ EDV → CO unchanged
3	**Exhausted preload reserve**	↑ EDV → ↓ CO & ↓ MAP

Box 8.2 Causes of increased afterload in the cardiac surgical patient

- History of preoperative essential or secondary hypertension
- Increased endogenous catecholamines released during CPB
- Hypothermia
- Emergence from anaesthesia
- Response to pain can lead to arteriolar vasoconstriction
- Administration of exogenous vasoconstrictors

Box 8.3 Simplified approach to haemodynamic management in the patient with optimal preload

↑ **MAP and** ↓ **CO**	Afterload is likely to be normal or high, and therapy with an inotrope plus a vasodilator, or with a phosphodiesterase inhibitor might be considered
↓ **MAP and** ↑ **CO**	Afterload is probably low and a vasopressor should be considered
↓ **MAP and** ↓ **CO**	Contractility and afterload are reduced and therapy with both inotropes and vasopressors should be considered

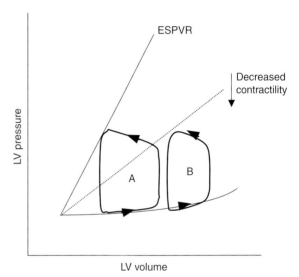

Figure 8.2 LV pressure–volume loops illustrating (A) the normal ventricle, and (B) the decrease in slope of the ESPVR line with decreased contractility. This decrease in contractility can also be accompanied by a decrease in the SV, and an increase in the LVEDP.

Box 8.4 Diagnosis of perioperative MI

ECG	Difficult to interpret in perioperative period -particularly ST and T-wave alterations Reliance on Q-wave formation has a low sensitivity in this setting
Creatinine kinase MB (CK-MB)	Traditional enzyme marker used to confirm MI Found in skeletal muscle and atria Low specificity following cardiac surgery
Troponin I	Adenosine triphosphatase inhibitor of actin-myosin complex Higher sensitivity and specificity than CK-MB Levels >60 µmol l^{-1} correlate with both Q-wave MI and new regional wall motion abnormality

and improve coronary perfusion. Short-term use of an RV assist device may allow time for RV recovery.

Reducing the RV afterload can improve the RV systolic performance and the right heart CO. Drug therapy includes inhaled milrinone, NO (5–10 ppm) and epoprostenol (PGI$_2$); IV PGI$_2$ (2–5 ng kg^{-1} min^{-1}); and oral agents, such as sildenafil and bosentan.

Pericardial Tamponade

Pericardial tamponade is characterized by hypotension, tachycardia and an elevated CVP. Although it typically occurs acutely within 24 hours of cardiac surgery, it can develop chronically over several days. In tamponade, the decrease in the LV filling during inspiration is accentuated. The fall in the SV produces

---

Box 8.5   Clinical signs suggestive of cardiac tamponade

- Oliguria
- Reduced or absent chest tube drainage
- Pulsus paradoxus
- Equalization of the RA pressure, PA diastolic pressure and PAWP
- Loss of the *y*-descent in RA pressure and PAWP
- Low voltage ECG/electrical alternans pattern

Box 8.6   Resuscitation goals in cardiac tamponade

Preload	Elevated – avoid high PEEP
HR	High – because of reduced SV
Rhythm	Sinus preferable but limited atrial kick
SVR	High
Contractility	Normal or elevated

Box 8.7   Causes of respiratory failure after cardiac surgery

Central neurological	CNS depressant drugs, CVA, pain
Spinal cord	Neuraxial anaesthesia, trauma, ischaemia
Peripheral neurological	Trauma
Neuromuscular	Neuromuscular blockers, severe $\downarrow\downarrow$ [K$^+$], [Mg^{2+}], [PO$_4{}^{3-}$], myasthenia gravis, starvation
Airway	Retained secretions, asthma
Chest wall	Flail chest, kyphoscoliosis, ankylosis
Pleural	Pneumothorax, pleural effusion
Lung	Smoking-related disease, atelectasis, pneumonia, aspiration, ARDS, PE
Cardiac	LV failure, low CO state, valve disease, tamponade, right-to-left shunt

---

a reflex increase in HR and myocardial contractility. Diagnostic clues include those described in Box 8.5.

In addition to detecting an obvious extracardiac collection, the most common TOE manifestation is the collapse of the right-sided chambers when their intracavity pressures are at their lowest – i.e. the RV in early diastole and the RA in early systole. Management consists of resuscitation (Box 8.6) and prompt surgical drainage.

Postoperative AF

AF and atrial flutter are the most common postoperative supraventricular tachydysrhythmias following cardiac surgery. New-onset AF occurs within 24–72 hours of surgery in up to 30% patients. Independent predictors of AF include age >65 years, hypertension, male sex, a previous history of AF and valve surgery.

In the absence of contraindications, all patients who develop AF should be anticoagulated within 24–48 hours. If AF has persisted for >48 hours and therapeutic anticoagulation has not been maintained, TOE should be performed to exclude the presence of LA thrombus.

Electrical or chemical cardioversion to NSR is preferred, especially when patients are haemodynamically unstable, symptomatic or unable to receive anticoagulation. Pharmacological ventricular rate control may be acceptable in some cases.

Respiratory Complications

Some degree of impairment of respiratory function occurs in all patients undergoing cardiac surgery. As many as 10% of cardiac surgical patients will have postoperative impairment of gas exchange that is sufficient to cause concern, prolong mechanical ventilation and delay discharge from the ICU. This ranges from transient atelectasis and retained secretions, to overwhelming acute lung injury (ALI) and ARDS. The causes of respiratory complications following cardiac surgery are summarized in Box 8.7. It should be borne in mind that the major determinant of pulmonary outcome following cardiac surgery is cardiac function.

Respiratory Failure

Acute respiratory failure is the inability to perform adequate intrapulmonary gas exchange causing hypoxia *with or without* hypercarbia. The accepted quantitative criteria for the diagnosis are PaO$_2$ <8.0 kPa (60 mmHg) on air and PaCO$_2$ >6.5 kPa (49 mmHg) in the absence of primary metabolic alkalosis.

Atelectasis affects dependent areas of lung – particularly the left lower lobe following internal mammary artery harvest. The combined effects of anaesthesia, mechanical ventilation and sternotomy reduce functional residual capacity, vital capacity and tidal volume (V_T). These effects may be compounded by diaphragmatic dysfunction caused by direct or thermal (cold) injury to the phrenic nerve. Recruitment manoeuvres, such as PEEP and full lung expansion prior to chest closure, may reverse some of the atelectasis that inevitably occurs during surgery. Postoperative atelectasis is best managed by adequate analgesia, physiotherapy, recruitment manoeuvres, incentive spirometry and forced coughing.

Table 8.1 American–European consensus conference (AECC) definitions of ALI and Berlin definitions of ARDS

ALI	PaO_2/FiO_2 <40 kPa (300 mmHg)
ARDS	Bilateral pulmonary infiltrates on CXR
	PAWP <18 mmHg
	Mild
	PaO_2/FiO_2 26–40 kPa (201–300 mmHg)
	PEEP/CPAP ≥ 5
	Moderate
	PaO_2/FiO_2 <26 kPa ($\leq$200 mmHg)
	PEEP/CPAP ≥ 5
	Severe
	PaO_2/FiO_2 13 kPa (<100 mmHg)
	PEEP/CPAP ≥ 5

J Crit Care 1994 Mar; 9: 72–81. *JAMA* 2012; 307: 2526–33.

ALI and ARDS

Hypoxia with bilateral pulmonary infiltrates and low LA pressure following cardiac surgery used to be known as 'pump lung'. The clinical features, which resemble those of sepsis with severe hypoxaemia, include increased PVR, increased vascular permeability and an elevated alveolar–arterial O_2 gradient. This ALI usually resolves within 48 hours or progresses to ARDS (Table 8.1).

The incidence of ARDS following CPB is reported to be as high as 2.5% in some series. Predisposing factors include redo cardiac surgery, hypotension, sepsis and massive transfusion. The aetiology and subsequent complications, rather than respiratory failure itself, dictate mortality from ARDS. Death is usually due to *multiple* organ dysfunction. The avoidance of CPB does not eliminate the risk of ALI or ARDS. The management of ARDS following cardiac surgery is summarized in Box 8.8.

Gastrointestinal Complications

The reported incidence of GI complications after cardiac surgery is low (<3%). The morbidity and mortality associated with GI complications, however, are disproportionately high. The pathogenesis of GI complications after cardiac surgery is multifactorial. Apart from the stress of major surgery, anaesthesia, anticoagulation and hypothermia, cardiac surgery is associated with a reduction and redistribution in systemic blood flow. GI complications are summarized in Box 8.9.

Box 8.8 General principles of the early management of ARDS following cardiac surgery

General	Predominantly supportive
	Resuscitation, identification and treatment of cause, prevention of further organ dysfunction
	Fluid restriction and forced diuresis
	Early institution of RRT should be considered
Ventilation	Most patients require mechanical ventilatory support
	No single ventilation strategy suits all lung regions
	Ventilation with large V_T (10–15 ml kg^{-1}) associated with ventilator-associated lung injury
	Modern lung management strategies based on pressure-controlled, small V_T (5–6 ml kg^{-1}) ventilation, optimal (best) PEEP, manipulation of the inspiratory:expiratory time ratio, permissive hypercarbia, patient posture and proning
Adjuvant therapy	Inhaled NO improves oxygenation by >20% in two-thirds of patients, but appears not to improve survival in ARDS
	Peripheral, veno-venous ECMO
	Extracorporeal technology CO_2 removal

Box 8.9 Common GI complications after cardiac surgery

Ileus	Common and frequently benign and self-limiting
	Presents with large NG aspirates, failure to absorb enteral feed and vomiting
	An NG tube will prevent gastric distension
	Therapy directed at identifiable cause and preventing secondary complications
	Prokinetics may be of use
	Incarcerated hernia, volvulus or obstruction should be considered in persistent cases
	Exploratory or diagnostic laparoscopy or laparotomy may be required
Haemorrhage	Accounts for 30-40% of all GI complications (upper $\gg$ lower)
	Upper: oesophagitis, variceal bleeding, gastritis, gastric ulceration, *Helicobacter pylori*, duodenitis, duodenal ulceration
	Lower: mesenteric ischaemia, antibiotic-associated colitis, haemorrhoids, tumours, diverticulosis, inflammatory bowel disease, angiodysplasia
	Incidence reduced by widespread use of histamine (H_2) receptor antagonists
	In the presence of critical splanchnic ischaemia, enteral feeding may worsen the situation
	Early diagnostic or therapeutic endoscopy is indicated in those patients least able to tolerate the haemodynamic instability
	Proctoscopy, sigmoidoscopy or colonoscopy should be performed if upper GI endoscopy is negative or lower GI haemorrhage is suspected
	Mesenteric angiography or radionuclide scan – performed while the patient is bleeding – allows identification of the bleeding vessel and permits embolization
	Surgical intervention is reserved for patients who fail to respond to medical management and is associated with significant mortality
Mesenteric ischaemia	Accounts for a quarter of GI complications after cardiac surgery
	Usually non-occlusive; due to a low CO or prolonged CPB
	Atherosclerotic embolism and arterial or venous thrombosis is less common
	Persistent metabolic acidosis and worsening lactatemia may be the only suggestive signs
	Abdominal pain is an inconsistent and often late symptom
	Abdominal CT may reveal gut dilatation, gut wall thickening or gas in the intestinal wall
	Mesenteric angiography is of limited use
	A high index of suspicion and a low threshold for an early laparotomy are the most important factors in reducing mortality
	Delays in diagnosis and intervention are inevitably fatal
Perforation	May occur at any point in the GI tract
	May be pathological (e.g. duodenal ulcer, diverticular disease) or iatrogenic (e.g. TOE, chest drain insertion, and sigmoidoscopy)
	Pneumoperitoneum is an unreliable sign in the setting of cardiac surgery
	Perforation secondary to TOE is believed to have an incidence as high as 0.1%
Hepatic dysfunction	Common after cardiac surgery
	Normal preoperative liver function tests do not preclude the development of significant postoperative hepatic dysfunction
	Clinically obvious jaundice is rare
	Progression to hepatitis and hepatic failure is extremely rare
	Hepatic dysfunction usually indicates multiple organ system failure
	Worsening coagulopathy (rising PT) with persistent hypoglycaemia is an ominous sign
Cholecystitis	Accounts for 10–15% of GI complications
	Usually occurs in the absence of gallstones
	Symptoms and signs often vague and non-specific
	A high index of suspicion is required to make an early diagnosis
	Delays in diagnosis and treatment undoubtedly contribute to high mortality (~75%)

Box 8.9 *(cont.)*

Acute pancreatitis	Transient pancreatic hyperamylasaemia is common after cardiac surgery
	The pancreas is highly susceptible to hypoperfusion and inflammation
	Symptoms of subclinical pancreatitis (e.g. anorexia, nausea and ileus) are usually mild and resolve within a few days
	Management is largely supportive
	Broad-spectrum antibiotics reduce the risk of infective complications
	Uncomplicated acute pancreatitis is associated with 5–10% mortality, whereas the mortality from acute necrotizing pancreatitis is up to 50%
	An untreated pancreatic abscess or infected pseudocyst is invariably fatal

Box 8.10 Risk factors for GI complications after cardiac surgery

Demographic

Age >65 years

Poor nutritional status

History of peptic ulcer disease

Preoperative drugs

NSAIDs

Aspirin/clopidogrel/prasugrel

Corticosteroids

Warfarin

Type of surgery

Emergency operations (e.g. aortic dissection)

Redo operations

Valve operations

Combined procedures (e.g. valve and CABG)

Preoperative factors

Peripheral vascular disease

Renal insufficiency

Hepatic impairment

Preoperative LV ejection fraction < 40%

Significant arrhythmia (e.g. AF)

Cardiogenic shock

Intraoperative and postoperative

Profound hypotension/hypoperfusion

Prolonged duration of CPB (>120 minutes)

Significant arrhythmia (e.g. AF)

Inotrope and vasoconstrictor therapy

IABP or TOE use

Haemorrhage and transfusion

Surgical re-exploration within 24 hours

Respiratory failure – requiring prolonged ventilatory support

Renal failure

Sternal/mediastinal infection

Bleeding and mesenteric ischaemia are the most common GI complications. A number of risk factors have been identified (Box 8.10). Despite improvements in perioperative care, anaesthesia and operating techniques, the incidence of GI complications has not changed in recent years due to the older surgical population with more numerous co-morbidities.

The symptoms and signs of GI complications may be subtle; their onset insidious and masked by sedatives and analgesics. Transient, mild GI dysfunction after cardiac surgery needs to be distinguished from more serious conditions requiring medical or surgical intervention. The lack of early signs and delayed diagnosis contributes to the high morbidity and mortality.

Renal Failure

The overall incidence of postoperative ARF requiring renal replacement therapy (RRT) in the adult cardiac surgical population is around 5%. This ranges from <1%, in patients with normal preoperative creatinine concentration, to >40% in patients with preoperative creatinine concentration >200 μmol l^{-1} (2.3 mg dl^{-1}). ARF after cardiac surgery increases the length of ICU and hospital stay. The additional costs associated with ARF are considerable, particularly as a small proportion of patients remain dependent on RRT after hospital discharge. Although rarely a primary cause of death, ARF is an independent risk factor of mortality after cardiac surgery and is associated with 50% mortality.

Definitions

Nowadays, the term ARF has been replaced by the term acute kidney injury (AKI). The RIFLE classification (**R**isk of renal dysfunction, **I**njury to the kidney, **F**ailure of kidney function, **L**oss of kidney function and **E**nd-stage kidney disease) defines AKI according

61

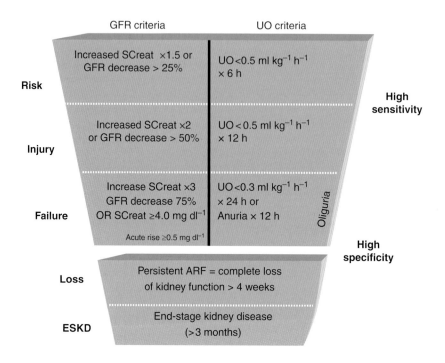

Figure 8.3 The RIFLE classification of ARF includes separate criteria for creatinine and urine output (UO). A patient can fulfil the criteria through changes in serum creatinine concentration (SCreat) or changes in UO, or both. The criteria that lead to the worst possible classification should be used. Note that the F component of RIFLE is present even if the increase in SCreat is under three-fold provided that the new SCreat is greater than 4.0 mg dl^{-1} (350 µmol l^{-1}) in the setting of an acute increase of at least 0.5 mg dl^{-1} (44 µmol l^{-1}). The designation RIFLE-FC should be used in this case to denote 'acute-on-chronic' disease. Similarly, when the RIFLE-F classification is achieved by UO criteria, a designation of RIFLE-FO should be used to denote oliguria. The shape of the figure denotes the fact that more patients (high sensitivity) will be included in the mild category, including some without actually having renal failure (less specificity). In contrast, at the bottom of the figure the criteria are strict and therefore specific, but some patients will be missed. Reproduced from Bellomo *et al.*, *Crit Care* 2004; 8: R204.

to changes in serum creatinine concentration and urine output (Figure 8.3).

Predictors of Acute Perioperative AKI

A variety of perioperative factors have been shown to be associated with renal dysfunction after cardiac surgery (Box 8.11). Post-renal causes of renal dysfunction should be excluded before attempting to differentiate between pre-renal and renal aetiologies.

Mechanisms

The final common pathway of all renal insults is renal tubular cell death, by either apoptosis or necrosis. CPB may cause kidney injury as a result of non-pulsatile blood flow; catecholamines and inflammatory mediators; arterial emboli; free Hb, reduced renal blood flow and reduced DO$_2$ secondary to haemodilution and hypotension.

Cellular inflammation plays an important role in the pathophysiology of postoperative renal

dysfunction. The systemic inflammatory response syndrome (SIRS) is induced by contact of cellular and humoral blood components with the CPB circuit, and is characterized by the activation of the clotting, kallikrein and complement systems.

Prevention

Reducing pro-inflammatory and other nephrotoxins together with maintaining tubular oxygen supply greater than tubular oxygen demand should minimize perioperative renal complications (Box 8.12).

The early restoration of renal perfusion in pure volume-responsive AKI (pre-renal failure) should restore renal function. The correction of hypovolaemia is central to the prevention and progression of AKI in critically ill patients and should be undertaken before instituting any pharmacological intervention.

Renal perfusion pressure is the difference between the MAP and the IVC pressure. The use of vasopressors to increase the MAP is controversial. Although

Box 8.11 Risk factors for renal dysfunction and renal failure following cardiac surgery

Patient factors

Increasing age

Diabetes mellitus

Arterial hypertension/aortic atheroma

Preoperative MI/low CO states

Preoperative creatinine > 130 μmol l^{-1} (> 1.4 mg dl^{-1})

Renal tract obstruction/raised intra-abdominal pressure

Bladder outflow obstruction

Operative factors

Use of CPB and CPB duration/AXC time

Redo and emergency procedures

Valve and combined surgical procedures

Hyperglycaemia

Haemorrhage

Haemodilution/anaemia

Infection/sepsis

Drug-related factors

Contrast media

Loop diuretics

NSAIDs

Antimicrobials (aminoglycosides, amphotericin)

Ciclosporin

Box 8.12 Preventing perioperative renal dysfunction

Reducing inflammatory or other toxins

Withhold nephrotoxic drugs

Maintain glycaemic control in diabetic patients

Avoid radiocontrast-induced nephropathy

Treat sepsis

Reduce CPB time as this will reduce CPB-related inflammatory mediators

Recognize and treat rhabdomyolysis

Retransfuse with washed mediastinal blood

Maintenance of tubular O_2 supply demand balance

Optimize volume status, CO, and systemic arterial pressure

Maintain adequate flow and mean systemic arterial pressure during CPB

Avoid excessive haemodilution

norepinephrine undoubtedly raises the MAP, a simultaneous increase in renal vascular resistance may actually reduce the renal blood flow.

The evidence for pharmacological interventions to protect renal function is weak and no pharmacological renoprotective intervention in cardiac surgery has significantly reduced mortality. Loop diuretics are administered with the aim of converting oliguric AKI into non-oliguric AKI, which has a better prognosis. Without adequate fluid resuscitation, loop diuretics are ineffective in the prevention of AKI and may worsen tubular function.

Mannitol – an alcohol – is an osmotic agent that is freely filtered at the glomerulus and not reabsorbed by the renal tubules. Mannitol has a high diuretic potential and can markedly increase fluid flow rate in all nephron segments, including the proximal tubule. When administered early in the course of AKI, mannitol may flush out cellular debris and prevent tubular cast formation, which in turn may convert oliguric AKI into non-oliguric AKI. Combining mannitol with a loop diuretic prevents compensatory increases in ion reabsorption in the loop of Henle. Mannitol is contraindicated in anuric patients.

Dopamine at low doses (i.e. <3 μg kg^{-1} min^{-1}) increases the CO and the renal blood flow. The authors of a meta-analysis, published in 2001, concluded: 'low-dose dopamine . . . should be eliminated from routine . . . use'.

Diagnosis

A seemingly adequate urine output (i.e. >0.5 ml kg^{-1} h^{-1}) and normal biochemical indices do not preclude renal dysfunction. Serum creatinine concentration tends to remain normal until over 50% of renal tubular function is lost, and doubles with every subsequent halving of renal function. Despite their popularity, these traditional indices are not sensitive enough to detect the early stages of renal dysfunction. This has led to a search for more sensitive biomarkers such as cystatin C, human neutrophil gelatinase-associated lipocalin, alpha-1-microalbumin and N-acetyl-beta-glucosaminidase, glutathione S-transferases and kidney injury molecule 1.

Pre-existing Renal Impairment

Pre-existing renal dysfunction significantly increases operative risk – a creatinine concentration of >200 μmol l^{-1} (>2.3 mg dl^{-1}) adds two points to the

European System for Cardiac Operative Risk Evaluation (EuroSCORE). A number of issues are of importance to the anaesthetist. It is essential that preoperative RRT does not remove excessive solute and render the patient hypovolaemic. For this reason, RRT is avoided in the 12 hours before surgery. Unless the patient is truly anuric, a urethral catheter should be inserted.

The presence of a forearm arteriovenous fistula created for haemodialysis, interferes with pulse oximetry and reduces the number of sites available for arterial and peripheral venous access. In addition, a fistula may represent a significant arteriovenous shunt, which may be worsened following the administration of vasoconstrictors. Occasionally, a large fistula must be excluded from the circulation by ligation or the application of a proximal tourniquet.

Intraoperative 'neutral balance' haemofiltration during CPB may delay the requirement for the reinstitution of RRT in the early postoperative period when anticoagulation may be undesirable. Although peritoneal dialysis avoids many of the potential complications of haemofiltration, diaphragmatic splinting may lead to respiratory impairment.

Uraemia-induced platelet dysfunction may lead to excessive perioperative bleeding. Platelet transfusion and desmopressin (DDAVP) may be of use in this group of patients.

Management

The treatment of patients with AKI after cardiac surgery is largely supportive. In most centres, management is expectant unless there is an indication for intervention or RRT. General measures are shown in Box 8.13.

Indications for RRT include: hyperkalaemia, severe metabolic acidosis, fluid overload, symptomatic uraemia (encephalopathy, neuropathy or pericarditis), to facilitate enteral or parenteral feeding, to facilitate blood-product administration, severe hyponatraemia or hypernatraemia and, rarely, hyperthermia.

RRT can be considered in three broad categories: peritoneal dialysis, intermittent haemodialysis and continuous veno-venous haemofiltration (CVVHF). Most adult patients developing renal failure after cardiac surgery are initially supported with CVVHF, whereas patients with pre-existing renal failure on established peritoneal dialysis may have this therapy reinstituted. Continuous haemodiafiltration, which achieves greater urea clearance, may be considered in patients who do not respond to haemofiltration.

> **Box 8.13 Management of AKI after cardiac surgery**
>
> - Exclude post-renal/obstructive aetiology
> - Optimize circulation and renal perfusion pressure
> - Restrict fluid and K^+ intake
> - Discontinue nephrotoxic drugs
> - Reduce doses of drugs that accumulate in renal failure
> - Consider proton pump inhibitor for GI prophylaxis
> - Exclude and aggressively treat any infection
> - Treat life-threatening hyperkalaemia, acidosis and dysrhythmias
> - Slowly correct metabolic acidosis with isotonic bicarbonate
> - Consider early renal specialist advice

CVVHF requires insertion of a large-bore, double-lumen cannula, specifically designed for CVVHF in the subclavian, internal jugular or femoral vein, and a degree of systemic anticoagulation.

Neurological Complications

Neurological injury following cardiac surgery increases mortality, the length of ICU and hospital stay and reduces the likelihood of a return to independent living. Cardiac surgical patients are largely ignorant of this complication.

Manifestations

The clinical spectrum ranges from changes in cognitive function and transient delirium to the fatal cerebral catastrophe. In most cases a neurological injury becomes evident as soon as the patient emerges from anaesthesia. In a small number of patients, however, significant injury may develop several hours or days after surgery.

The clinical manifestations depend on the location and size of the lesion – a small internal capsule or brainstem infarct will result in an obvious neurological deficit, whereas a considerably larger subcortical or hippocampal lesion may alter cognitive function. Many neurological injuries (e.g. visual field defects, tinnitus and ataxia) go unreported, uninvestigated and undocumented.

Mechanisms

Cerebral injury during cardiac surgery is primarily the result of cerebral embolism or hypoperfusion.

Table 8.2 Putative risk factors for adverse neurological outcome after cardiac surgery

Preoperative (patient) factors		Intraoperative factors	Postoperative factors
Demographic	**Medical history**		
Age	Cerebrovascular disease	Surgery type	Early hypotension
Gender	DM	Aortic atheroma	Long ICU stay
Genotype	Cardiac function	Aortic clamp site	Renal dysfunction
Educational level	IABP use	Microemboli	AF
	Alcohol consumption	Arterial pressure	
	Pulmonary disease	Pump flow	
	Hypertension	Temperature	
	Dysrhythmia	Haematocrit	
	Dyslipidaemia	Use of DHCA	
	Diuretic use		

DHCA, deep hypothermic circulatory arrest.

The two mechanisms are not mutually exclusive, and ischaemia/reperfusion may exacerbate the injury.

Embolic phenomena are thought to account for over half of all perioperative strokes. Cerebral microemboli can be detected in all patients subjected to CPB. There is an association between cognitive decline and intraoperative cerebral microembolic load.

Risk Factors

Patient factors, intraoperative factors and postoperative factors all contribute to the risk of perioperative neurological injury (Table 8.2).

Age is probably the most robust predictor of morbidity and mortality after cardiac surgery. The relationship between age and risk is more a function of age-related co-morbidities than age *per se*.

Higher risk profiles – rather than increased gender susceptibility – is the likely reason why women are at greater risk of complications following cardiac surgery.

DM is an independent risk factor for neurological injury. Although hyperglycaemia is known to worsen outcome from stroke, the greater incidence of hypertension, vascular disease and renal impairment in diabetics may partly explain this phenomenon.

In patients with a history of stroke, the risk does not appear to decline over time. Patients undergoing cardiac surgery within 3 months of a focal event are more likely to extend the area of injury whereas patients with a remote stroke (i.e. >6 months) are more likely to have a stroke in a different vascular territory.

The prevalence and severity of aortic atheroma increases with age, and there is a strong association between proximal aortic atheroma and stroke following cardiac surgery. Surgical manipulation, cannulation and perfusion of the diseased aorta can liberate atheroemboli. Evidence suggests that a change in surgical procedure, prompted by ultrasound detection of proximal aortic atheroma, improves neurological outcome.

Intracardiac and major vascular procedures carry the greatest risk – particularly when DHCA is employed.

The characteristics of 'optimal' CPB perfusion remain to be defined. These are discussed further in Chapter 26.

Intraoperative Strategies

Reducing the incidence and severity of neurological injury requires the identification of patients at increased risk, avoidance of factors known to cause neurological injury (i.e. hypotension, hypoperfusion and emboli), the detection of neuronal ischaemia and avoidance of factors which exacerbate the established injury. Measures for reducing brain injury are summarized in Box 8.14.

Diagnosis

The diagnosis of neurological injury is made on the basis of symptoms and physical signs. The degree of disability should be documented in a systematic and reproducible manner.

The National Institutes of Health Stoke Index provides a simple means of recording level of consciousness, orientation, response to commands, gaze, visual fields, facial movement, limb motor function,

Box 8.14 Measures for reducing brain injury during cardiac surgery*

Class I recommendations

A membrane oxygenator and an arterial line filter ($\leq$40 μm) should be used for CPB

Epiaortic ultrasound for detection of atherosclerosis of the ascending aorta

Avoid hyperthermia during and after CPB

Class IIa recommendations

A single AXC technique should be used for patients at risk for atheroembolism

During CPB in adults α-stat pH management should be considered

NIRS monitoring should be considered in high-risk patients

Class IIb recommendations

Arterial BP should be kept >70 mmHg during CPB in high-risk patients

IV insulin infusion should be given to keep serum glucose <8 mmol l^{-1} (<140 mg dl^{-1})

RBC transfusion should be considered in high-risk patients with Hb $\leq$7 g dl^{-1} or at higher Hb if there is evidence of organ ischaemia

Cardiotomy suction aspirate should be processed with a cell-saver device before returning the blood to the CPB circuit (blood aspirated from open cardiac chamber can be returned directly to the CPB circuit)

*Hogue CW Jr, *et al. Anesth Analg* 2006; 103: 21–37.

Box 8.15 Treatment goals in established brain injury after cardiac surgery

Prevent secondary brain injury

Maintain CO and cerebral oxygenation

Consider therapeutic hypothermia

Avoid hyperthermia and hyperglycaemia

Reduce brain swelling/raised intracranial pressure

Surgery

Evacuation of subdural or intracranial haematoma

Carotid or cerebral artery angioplasty

Intracranial aneurysm coiling/clipping

Ventriculostomy

General supportive measures

Hydration and nutrition

Prevention of pressure sores/contractures

Antimicrobial therapy/thromboprophylaxis

Rehabilitation, speech and language therapy

Specific drug therapy

Seizures – phenytoin, valproic acid

Muscle spasm – baclofen, tizanitidine, Botox

Myoclonus – clonazepam, piracetam, levetiracetam

Agitation – haloperidol, clonidine, olanzepine

Depression – citalopram, fluoxetine, paroxetine

Chronic pain – amitriptylline, gabapentin, pregabalin

limb ataxia, sensory loss, aphasia, dysarthria and inattention.

Conventional CT in the first 24 hours may reveal an undiagnosed extracerebral haemorrhage, but often reveals little or no evidence of intracerebral injury. By contrast, diffusion-weighted MRI can be used to detect cerebral oedema several days before it becomes apparent on CT or conversional MRI.

Assessment of cognitive dysfunction requires formal testing as a patient's subjective opinions are usually inaccurate. It is important to realize that the patient's spouse or other close relatives may be better arbiters of cognitive change.

A number of bedside clinical screening tools (e.g. Confusion Assessment Model ICU) are available for the documentation of delirium.

Postoperative Management

Areas of irreversible brain ischaemia are invariably surrounded by tissue, the so-called ischaemic penumbra, which is viable but vulnerable to further injury. Limiting the extent of brain injury is directed at limiting propagation of the initial ischaemic insult. Depolarization of ischaemic neurones leads to excitatory neurotransmitter release and the activation of cytotoxic pathways. These processes, which ultimately determine the eventual extent of neuronal injury, take place over 36–72 hours. An understanding of the mechanisms of cerebral injury has revealed numerous potential therapeutic targets for cerebral protection.

Treatment goals include recognition of pathology that may be amenable to early neurosurgical intervention, general supportive measures and the prevention of secondary complications. These are summarized in Box 8.15.

Prognosis

One in four patients sustaining a stroke after cardiac surgery will have a long-term disability. Prolonged depression of consciousness, coma and persistent vegetative state are associated with significant (>90%) mortality. The majority of patients with major brain injury succumb to the complications of extended ICU care or aspiration pneumonia. The pattern of neurological recovery within the first 24–72 hours is often an indicator of the eventual extent of recovery. Transient agitation and delirium – once thought to be a 'benign nuisance' – is now recognized as a significant risk factor for short- and long-term morbidity and mortality after cardiac surgery. Longitudinal studies have demonstrated that early postoperative cognitive dysfunction is an independent predictor of longer-term cognitive function, general health and employment status.

Key Points

- A PAWP of >15 mmHg may be required following CPB.
- Tamponade may be difficult to diagnose clinically and should be considered in all cases of hypotension/low CO following cardiac surgery.
- Respiratory failure is common after cardiac surgery.
- Treatment of ARDS is supportive and aims to avoid further organ dysfunction.
- Patients with ARDS tend to die from multiple organ failure.
- A high index of suspicion and a low threshold for an early laparotomy is the most important factor in reducing mortality from GI complications.
- Acute renal hypoxia induces vasoconstriction that may be maintained for several hours after restoration of normoxia.
- No pharmacological renoprotective intervention in cardiac surgery has been shown to significantly reduce mortality.
- Neurological complications are common and often go undiagnosed.
- Neurological complications increase mortality and length of hospital stay.
- Physical interventions such as arterial line filtration, cautious rewarming and α-stat blood-gas management appear to improve neurological outcome.

Further Reading

ARDS Definition Task Force. Acute respiratory distress syndrome: the Berlin Definition. *JAMA* 2012; 307: 2526–33.

Bellomo R, Ronco C, Kellum JA, Mehta RL, Palevsky P. Acute renal failure – definition, outcome measures, animal models, fluid therapy and information technology needs: the Second International Consensus Conference of the Acute Dialysis Quality Initiative (ADQI) Group. *Crit Care* 2004; 8: R204–12.

Bernard GR, Artigas A, Brigham KL, *et al.* The American–European Consensus Conference on ARDS. Definitions, mechanisms, relevant outcomes, and clinical trial coordination. *Am J Respir Crit Care Med* 1994; 149: 818–24.

Buczacki SJA, Davies J. The acute abdomen in the cardiac intensive care unit. In Valchanov K, Jones N, Hogue CW (eds.), *Core Topics in Cardiothoracic Critical Care*, 2nd edn. Cambridge: Cambridge University Press; 2018, pp. 294–300.

Damian MS. Neurological aspects of cardiac surgery. In Valchanov K, Jones N, Hogue CW (eds.), *Core Topics in Cardiothoracic Critical Care*, 2nd edn. Cambridge: Cambridge University Press; 2018, pp. 380–91.

Ely EW, Margolin R, Francis J, *et al.* Evaluation of delirium in critically ill patients: validation of the confusion assessment method for the intensive care unit (CAM-ICU) *Crit Care Med* 2001; 29: 1370–79.

Ercole A, Prisco L. Seizures. In Valchanov K, Jones N, Hogue CW (eds.), *Core Topics in Cardiothoracic Critical Care*, 2nd edn. Cambridge: Cambridge University Press; 2018, pp. 285–93.

Hogue CW Jr, Palin CA, Arrowsmith JE. Cardiopulmonary bypass management and neurologic outcomes: an evidence-based appraisal of current practices. *Anesth Analg* 2006; 103: 21–37.

Koyi MB, Hobelmann JG, Neufeld KJ. Postoperative delirium. In Valchanov K, Jones N, Hogue CW (eds.), *Core Topics in Cardiothoracic Critical Care*, 2nd edn. Cambridge: Cambridge University Press; 2018, pp. 392-401.

Kydd A, Parameshwar J. Cardiovascular disorders: the heart failure patient in the intensive care unit. In Valchanov K, Jones N, Hogue CW (eds.), *Core Topics in Cardiothoracic Critical Care*, 2nd edn. Cambridge: Cambridge University Press; 2018, pp. 256–62.

Mangano CM, Diamondstone LS, Ramsay JG, *et al.* Renal dysfunction after myocardial revascularisation:

risk factors, adverse outcomes and hospital resource utilisation. *Ann Intern Med* 1998; 128: 194–203.

Powell-Tuck J, Varrier M, Osrermann M. Renal replacement therapy. In Valchanov K, Jones N, Hogue CW (eds.), *Core Topics in Cardiothoracic Critical Care*, 2nd edn. Cambridge: Cambridge University Press; 2018, pp. 149–156.

Proudfoot A, Summers C. Respiratory disorders: acute respiratory distress syndrome. In Valchanov K, Jones N, Hogue CW (eds.), *Core Topics in Cardiothoracic Critical Care*, 2nd edn. Cambridge: Cambridge University Press; 2018, pp. 356–71.

Rodriguez R, Robich MP, Plate JF, Trooskin SZ, Sellke FW. Gastrointestinal complications following cardiac surgery: a comprehensive review. *J Card Surg* 2010; 25: 188–97.

Slogoff S, Keats AS. Does perioperative myocardial ischemia lead to postoperative MI? *Anesthesiology* 1985; 62: 107–14.

Aortic Valve Surgery

Pedro Catarino and Joseph E. Arrowsmith

The AV is composed of three semilunar cusps left (posterior), right (anterior) and non-coronary cusp, which are related to the three sinuses of Valsalva. The main functions of the AV are to permit unimpeded LV systolic ejection and to prevent regurgitation of the LV stroke volume during diastole. The normal adult AV orifice area is 2-4 cm^2.

Aortic Stenosis

AS is defined as a fixed obstruction to systolic LV outflow.

Clinical Features

Patients may be asymptomatic for many years, although normally present with one or more of the classic triad of symptoms; angina, syncope or breathlessness. Less fortunate patients may present with sudden death. Fifty per cent survival rates from onset of symptoms are as shown in Table 9.1.

Pathology

In most cases, AS is an acquired disease. Degenerative calcification causes thickening and stiffness of the leaflets. It is associated with advanced age (>70 years) and often with MV annular calcification. Chronic rheumatic AV disease causes commissural fusion and AR is more common.

Bicuspid AV, with a prevalence of 2%, is one of the commonest congenital heart lesions. Patients with a bicuspid AV have a shorter latency period to

Table 9.1 Survival rates from onset of symptoms in AS

Presenting symptom	50% Survival rate
Angina	5 years
Syncope	3 years
Breathlessness	2 years

symptom onset due to earlier degeneration and calcification.

More rarely, AS may be at a supra- or subvalvular level. Similar principles of anaesthetic management apply.

Pathophysiology

The fixed obstruction to LV ejection causes chronic LV pressure overload and increased wall tension (wall tension = LV pressure × LV end-diastolic radius/(2 × LV wall thickness) – Laplace's law). This increase in wall tension is offset by the development of concentric LVH at the price of diastolic dysfunction secondary to impaired relaxation and reduced compliance, manifest as elevated LVEDP (Figure 9.1). LV end-diastolic dimensions are usually preserved in early AS.

Angina Pectoris

An imbalance between myocardial DO_2 and VO_2 may occur even in the absence of significant coronary artery disease. The combination of LVH and wall tension increases the systolic myocardial VO_2, while a reduction in coronary perfusion pressure decreases the myocardial DO_2.

Syncope

Syncope typically occurs on exertion. The SV is limited in moderate or severe AS, giving a 'fixed' or 'limited' CO. An inability to compensate for exercise-induced peripheral arterial vasodilatation is the most common explanation for syncope. Ventricular dysrhythmia is another potential cause.

Dyspnoea

Breathlessness, particularly orthopnoea, is the most sinister of the triad of symptoms and may herald the onset of LV decompensation/dilatation. An increased LVEDP necessitates higher left-sided filling pressures, which leads to pulmonary congestion (Figure 9.2).

69

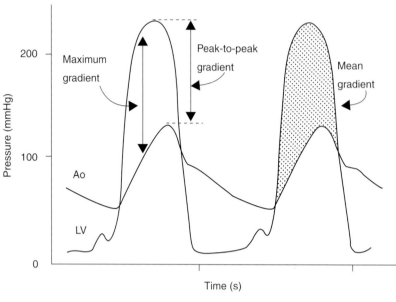

Figure 9.1 Pressure waveforms obtained simultaneously from the LV cavity and the aortic root (Ao) in AS. The peak-to-peak gradient is measured in the catheter laboratory and is the difference between the peak systolic pressures in the LV cavity and aortic root. Note that peak aortic root pressure is reached later than peak ventricular pressure. The maximum or instantaneous gradient is usually measured by CWD ultrasound.

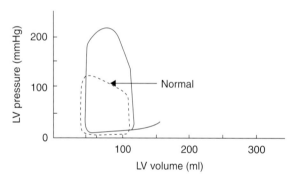

Figure 9.2 LV pressure–volume loop in AS. Note elevated end-diastolic pressure, elevated systolic pressure and preservation of SV.

Decompensation arises when the LV wall tension can no longer be maintained by systolic wall thickening and the LV dilates. LV dilatation is associated with increased wall tension (Laplace's law).

Peripheral Oedema

The presence of peripheral oedema typically indicates advanced or end-stage AS and is invariably associated with biventricular dysfunction, MR, TR and PHT.

Investigations

ECG: Increased R- and S-wave amplitude, T-wave inversion (strain pattern) in anterior chest leads.

2D echocardiography: AV anatomy and function, LV function, aortic root size. Typical features are:

leaflet thickening, calcification, reduced opening. Planimetric measurement of the AV orifice area (AVA) is unreliable in the presence of calcification.

CFD: Turbulence across valve. Does not permit assessment of severity. May demonstrate associated regurgitation.

CWD: Because alignment of the ultrasound beam with blood flow through the AV is easier, TTE provides a more accurate assessment of the AV gradient than TOE using the deep transgastric view (Chapter 34). Peak AV gradient = 4 × peak velocity^2 (modified Bernoulli equation). The AVA can be measured using the continuity equation (Chapter 34).

Coronary angiography: To exclude coronary disease. Mandatory in males >40 years or females >50 years.

Ventriculography: LV function, peak-to-peak AV gradient.

Multidetector row CT (MDCT): To define valvular anatomy and AVA in poor TTE subjects unable to undergo TOE (Figure 9.3).

Anaesthetic Goals

Sinus rhythm and the late diastolic 'atrial kick' are very important in these poorly compliant hearts. Atrial contraction can account for 30–40% diastolic filling in these patients (cf. 15–20% in normal patients).

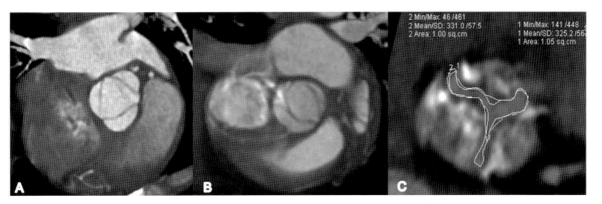

Figure 9.3 64-slice MDCT axial view of AVs. (A) Normal valve. (B) Bicuspid valve. (C) Measurement of AVA by planimetry in a stenotic calcified valve.

Box 9.1	**Anaesthetic considerations in AS**
Preload	'Better full than empty'
HR	60–80 bpm is ideal
Rhythm*	Preserve sinus rhythm
Contractility	Maintain (but most patients tolerate mild depression)
SVR	Maintain (or slight ↑) to maintain coronary perfusion pressure

*Following AVR, the placement of ventricular pacing wires is considered mandatory because of the high incidence of atrioventricular (A-V) block.

AF and nodal rhythms result in the failure to maintain preload and are poorly tolerated (Box 9.1).

TOE provides a better direct objective measure of the LV filling (i.e. LV end-diastolic area) than the PAFC (i.e. the PAWP), but the former is not available during the critical period of induction of anaesthesia.

Tachycardia may cause myocardial ischaemia by reducing diastolic coronary perfusion and should be avoided. Bradycardia should also be avoided due to the 'limited' CO. The systolic function is usually well preserved in the early stages of AS. Maintaining contractility is usually only a problem in end-stage AS associated with LV decompensation. Attempts to improve the SV by reducing afterload are misguided and dangerous in AS, as afterload is effectively fixed at the AV level. The anaesthetic technique must, therefore, preserve the SVR.

In the post-CPB period following AVR for stenosis (i.e. when the fixed obstruction to LV outflow has been removed) the anaesthetist should anticipate significant rebound arterial hypertension. Untreated hypertension may increase bleeding and the risk of aortic dissection during decannulation. The conventional management of hypertension in this setting includes vasodilators, posture-induced preload reduction and volatile anaesthetic agents. Deliberate 'nodal' A-V pacing (i.e. A-V delay <15 ms) can be used in extreme circumstances to effectively remove the contribution of late diastolic LV filling.

Treatment of Hypotension

Hypotension is common following induction of anaesthesia and must be anticipated. Initial treatment is usually IV fluid and a vasoconstrictor to maintain preload and afterload respectively. Early intervention is required to prevent an inexorable downward spiral of hypotension, leading to myocardial ischaemia and cardiac arrest. If cardiac arrest does occur, external cardiac massage is generally ineffective. Survival after prolonged arrest is unusual without the facility for rapid institution of CPB.

Aortic Regurgitation

AR is defined as diastolic leakage across the AV, which causes LV volume overload.

Clinical Features

Presenting features are highly dependent on whether the aetiology is acute or chronic.

Table 9.2 The aetiology of AR

Aortic root dilatation	*Congenital*	Marfan syndrome
	Acquired	Long-standing hypertension, aortic dissection, atheromatous aortic disease, syphilitic aortitis, connective tissue disorders
Leaflet abnormality or damage	*Congenital*	Bicuspid AV (frequently become incompetent after fourth decade and have well-recognized association with coarctation of the aorta)
	Acquired	Aortic dissection, chronic rheumatic heart disease, infective endocarditis, connective tissue disease (e.g. systemic lupus erythematosus, rheumatoid arthritis, ankylosing spondylitis), balloon valvuloplasty

Chronic AR: Compensatory LV changes allow many patients with chronic AR to be asymptomatic for >20 years. Symptoms, typically breathlessness on exertion, accompany LV decompensation. Angina is less common in AR than AS because the increase in myocardial VO$_2$ with volume overload is smaller than that with pressure overload.

Acute AR: This typically presents with acute pulmonary oedema, tachycardia and poor peripheral perfusion.

Pathology

AR may be secondary to dilatation of the aortic root, abnormalities of the valve leaflets or a combination of both (Table 9.2). Both aortic dissection (Chapter 13) and infectious endocarditis cause acute AR. Endocarditis causes leaflet perforation and vegetations may impede diastolic leaflet closure.

Pathophysiology

Factors affecting the severity of AR include: the size of the orifice area, the diastolic pressure gradient across the AV and the length of diastole (inversely related to HR).

In both chronic and acute AR, the primary problem is LV volume overload. In chronic AR, the increase in the diastolic filling volume induces adaptive changes in the LV. Muscle elongation results in an increased LV radius and eccentric LVH. Unlike MR, where the LV offloads into the LA during the early part of ejection, there is no reduction in LV pressure during systole. The LV wall thickness increases to match the increased radius and reduce wall tension (Laplace's law). True compliance is changed only slightly but the ventricle operates much further to the right on the pressure–volume curve (Figure 9.4).

Hearts in chronic AR, so-called 'bovine' hearts, can develop the largest LV end-diastolic volume (LVEDV)

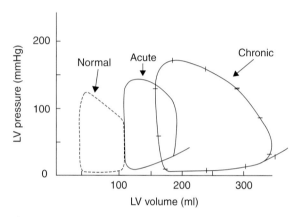

Figure 9.4 Pressure–volume loops for acute and chronic AR. In chronic AR, the LVEDV and SV are greatly increased. In acute AR, where there has been no adaptive increase in LV compliance, the increases in the LVEDV and SV are smaller.

of all the valvular heart lesions. The systolic SV is increased (the LVEDV increases by more than the LV end-systolic volume (LVESV)) in order to compensate for diastolic regurgitant volume and maintain an 'effective' SV. Although Starling mechanisms initially maintain LV systolic function, increasing the LVEDV eventually leads to decompensation, evidenced by a decrease in the slope of end-systolic pressure–volume relationship. The rise in LVESV is accompanied by a fall in LV ejection fraction (LVEF).

Acute AR causes diastolic volume and pressure overload in a normal-sized, non-compliant LV. The acute rise in the LVEDP reduces the coronary perfusion pressure, causes early closure of the MV and the requirement for higher LA filling pressures.

Investigations

2D echocardiography: AV leaflet pathology, aortic root dimensions, LV function. LV end-systolic dimension >5.5 cm and LVEF <50 % are signs of systolic dysfunction and are indications for surgery.

Box 9.2 Anaesthetic considerations in AR

	Acute AR	Chronic AR
Preload	Increase ++	Increase
HR	Fast	Medium to fast
Rhythm*	Sinus	Sinus
Contractility	Inotropic support	Maintain/ support
SVR	Low – maintain	Low

* Following AVR the placement of ventricular pacing wires is considered mandatory because of the high incidence of A-V block.

CFD: To assess the width of the regurgitant jet at origin in relationship to width of the LVOT. Diastolic flow reversal in the descending aorta suggests severe AR. The presence and severity of any associated MR needs to be established.

CWD: Calculation of the regurgitant valve orifice size using the pressure half-time method. The diastolic regurgitant blood flow velocity decreases more rapidly in severe AR.

Coronary angiography: To exclude coronary disease.

Anaesthetic Goals

Preload needs to be greater in acute AR to overcome the higher LVEDP. A modest tachycardia shortens diastole and reduces regurgitant flow. It also reduces the time for anterograde filling through the MV, which reduces LV distention, lowers the LVEDP and improves coronary perfusion. In acute AR and the latter stages of chronic AR, sinus rhythm is particularly beneficial because it facilitates anterograde LV filling.

Contractility must be maintained, inotropic support is often required in acute AR.

Afterload reduction lowers the diastolic AV gradient and, therefore, the regurgitant volume. Vasodilator therapy is commonly used to delay the development of systolic dysfunction. Afterload

reduction may not be tolerated in the presence of a low diastolic BP, particularly in the emergency setting (Box 9.2).

Treatment of Hypotension

Strategies are based on inotropes and vasodilators. Preoperative use of the IABP is contraindicated due to its tendency to worsen regurgitation and cause LV dilatation.

Surgical Approach

In recent years, the use of a J-shaped upper partial ('mini') sternotomy has been advocated in patients requiring AV or aortic root surgery. Proponents of the technique claim improved wound healing, reduced hospital stay and faster postoperative recovery when compared to conventional ('full') sternotomy.

Anaesthetic considerations, most of which arise from limited surgical access, include the need for external defibrillation equipment, a greater reliance on TOE, being prepared for rapid conversion to full sternotomy and the risk of incomplete intracardiac de-airing prior to separation from CPB.

Key Points

- AS produces both systolic and diastolic LV dysfunction.
- Tachycardia, *severe* bradycardia and vasodilatation are poorly tolerated in AS.
- Hypotension should be treated early in AS to prevent haemodynamic collapse.
- Deliberate 'nodal' A-V pacing can be used in extreme circumstances to treat hypertension following AVR for AS.
- Volume overload in chronic AR results in the largest LVEDV of all the valvular heart lesions.
- A-V conduction abnormalities are common after AV replacement. Epicardial pacing and close monitoring after ICU discharge are considered mandatory.

Further Reading

Bonow RO, Brown AS, Gillam LD, *et al.* Appropriate use criteria for the treatment of patients with severe aortic stenosis: a report of the American College of Cardiology Appropriate Use Criteria Task Force, American Association for Thoracic Surgery, American Heart Association, American Society of Echocardiography, European Association for Cardio-Thoracic Surgery, Heart Valve Society, Society of Cardiovascular Anesthesiologists, Society for Cardiovascular Angiography and Interventions, Society of

Cardiovascular Computed Tomography, Society for Cardiovascular Magnetic Resonance, and Society of Thoracic Surgeons. *J Am Soc Echocardiogr* 2018; 31: 117–47.

Nair SK, Sudarshan CD, Thorpe BS, *et al.* Mini-Stern trial: a randomized trial comparing mini-sternotomy to full median sternotomy for aortic valve replacement. *J Thorac Cardiovasc Surg* 2018; 156: 2124–32.

Nishimura RA, Otto CM, Bonow RO, *et al.* 2014 AHA/ACC guideline for the management of patients with valvular heart disease: executive summary. A report of the American College of Cardiology/American Heart Association task force on practice guidelines. *J Am Coll Cardiol* 2014; 63: 2438–88.

Chapter 10

Mitral Valve Surgery

Jonathan H. Mackay and Francis C. Wells

The normal adult MV area is 4–6 cm^2. Unlike other heart valves, the MV consists of two asymmetric leaflets. The *aortic* (anterior) leaflet makes up 65% of the valve area but its base forms only 35% of the circumference. The *mural* (posterior) leaflet usually consists of three main scallops, although there may be up to five. The leaflets are joined at the anterolateral and posteromedial ends of the commissure. The aortic MV leaflet shares the same fibrous attachment as the non-coronary cusp of the AV.

The complete valve apparatus consists of the leaflets, which arise from the A-V junction and the chordae tendinae. The chordae connect the leaflets to the papillary muscles, muscular projections from the non-compacted layer of the LV (Figure 10.1). There are two principal fibrous condensations that form the trigones; posterosuperior and antero-inferior. They are placed approximately equidistant within the sector of the valve between the two lateral ends of the commissure. This fibrous condensation extends for up to a third of the circumference of the orifice. It is commonly misstated that there is a complete annulus of circumferential fibrous tissue.

During diastole, MV leaflet opening should permit unimpeded flow from LA to LV. During systole, coaptation of the MV leaflets protects the pulmonary circulation from high LV pressures. The tensor apparatus, consisting of the chordae tendinae and papillary muscles, makes significant contributions to the LV function and ejection fraction.

MV surgery is still most often undertaken through a sternotomy though right thoracotomy may be used particularly for redo MV surgery. Minimal access surgery, which entails peripheral cannulation and a right mini-thoracotomy, is becoming more widespread. Its benefits await substantiation by a prospective randomized study (see Chapter 12).

Mitral Stenosis

MS in adults is defined as a valve area of less than 2 cm^2 and is classified as severe or critical when the valve area is less than 1 cm^2. The vast majority of cases are secondary to rheumatic fever, although a history of an earlier acute febrile illness is often absent. Leaflet thickening and commissural fusion occurs secondary to the inflammatory process. Other valve diseases, particularly involving aortic and tricuspid valves, are common. Pure MS is less common than mixed stenosis and regurgitation, as a result of the fixed orifice.

Clinical Features

Exertional dyspnoea is the commonest presentation and the onset is usually insidious. Other presentations include haemoptysis, new-onset AF or peripheral embolic events.

Pathophysiology

Fixed obstruction to blood flow between the LA and the LV creates a pressure gradient across the MV. The left atrial pressure (LAP) increases to maintain the CO.

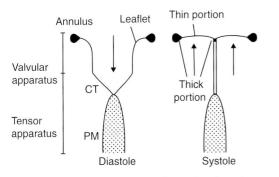

Figure 10.1 Mitral leaflet opening during diastole, and coaptation (central overlap) and apposition (relative height of leaflets) during systole. CT, chordae tendinae; PM, papillary muscle.

$$\text{Pressure gradient} = [\text{ Flow Rate}/(\, K \times \text{valve area} \,) \,]^2$$

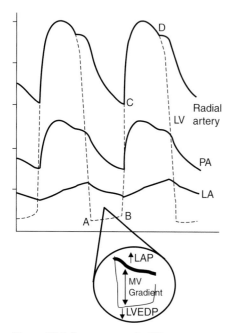

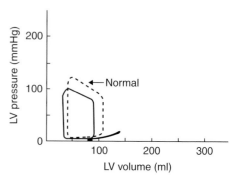

Figure 10.3 LV pressure–volume loop in MS

Figure 10.2 Pressure waves for MS

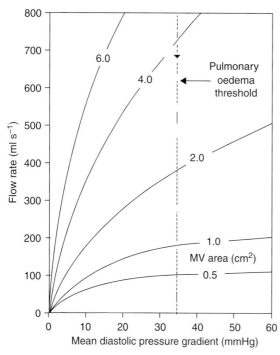

Figure 10.4 Rate of transmitral diastolic blood flow versus mean diastolic MV gradient for normal (4–6 cm^2) and stenotic MVs (0.5–2 cm^2)

where K is the hydraulic constant. An elevated LAP and the presence of a low LVEDP results in an increased MV gradient (Figure 10.2). The consequences of an elevated LAP include:

- LA hypertrophy and, later, dilatation
- AF
- Reduced pulmonary compliance
- PHT and eventually RV 'stress' and TR

AF reduces the LV filling particularly when associated with fast ventricular rates. PHT is initially reversible but becomes irreversible following sustained chronic elevation of PVR.

The LV pressure–volume loop in MS is small and shifted to the left due to a reduction in LV pressure and volume loading (Figure 10.3).

The LV systolic function may be depressed due to myocardial fibrosis and chronic underloading. Figure 10.4 illustrates the effect of reducing the valve orifice area on the relationship between transmitral flow rate and pressure gradient. Decreasing the MV area has a dramatic effect on the flow rate required to generate the diastolic pressure gradient at which pulmonary oedema develops.

Investigations

2D echocardiography: Leaflets thickened, possibly calcified, doming and reduced opening.

PWD gradient (pressure half-time; PH-T): MV inflow is quantified with PWD or CWD (Figure 10.5). The rate of fall of blood flow velocity of the E (early diastolic filling) wave is attenuated in MS. The PH-T method uses the slope of E-wave deceleration to calculate the MV

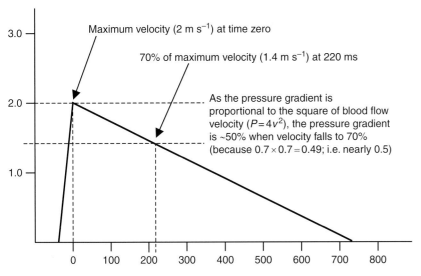

Maximum velocity (2 m s^{-1}) at time zero

70% of maximum velocity (1.4 m s^{-1}) at 220 ms

As the pressure gradient is proportional to the square of blood flow velocity ($P=4v^2$), the pressure gradient is ~50% when velocity falls to 70% (because $0.7 \times 0.7 = 0.49$; i.e. nearly 0.5)

Figure 10.5 Estimation of the MV orifice area using diastolic transmitral blood flow velocity to calculate the PH-T. The latter is defined as the time required for the magnitude of the instantaneous transmitral pressure gradient to fall by half. From the modified Bernouilli equation $P = 4 \times v^2$ (where P = pressure and v = velocity) it can be deduced that for pressure to halve, velocity must fall by 30%. In the example above, the PH-T is 220 ms, which gives an MV area of 220/220 = 1.0 cm^2.

area. Calculation of the latter by the PH-T method is unreliable in the presence of an incompetent AV. AR contributes to LV diastolic filling, causing transmitral blood flow velocity to decline more rapidly. The net result is an underestimation of the severity of MS.

CFD: The proximal isovelocity surface area (PISA) method can be used to estimate the MV orifice area.

$$\text{MV orifice area (cm}^2) = 220/\text{Pressure half-time (ms)}$$

Anaesthetic Goals

A high LAP is required to overcome the resistance to LV filling. Excessive preload may cause LA distension and AF. Control of HR is paramount. Tachycardia does not allow sufficient time for LV filling and results in a reduced LVEDV. Bradycardia is poorly tolerated due to the relatively fixed SV. Loss of sinus rhythm can decrease the CO by 20%. Consider synchronized DC shock in acute onset AF - if no LA thrombus is present.

The SVR needs to be maintained particularly in patients with tight stenosis and an active sympathetic nervous system. LV contractility is rarely a problem in pure MS where greater emphasis should be placed on protecting the RV from increases in PVR and PHT (Box 10.1).

Box 10.1	Anaesthetic considerations in MS
Preload	High
HR	Avoid tachycardia
Rhythm	Sinus rhythm better than AF
SVR	Maintain
Contractility	Maintain
PVR	Avoid increase

Treatment of Hypotension

Hypotension is usually associated with tachycardia. Consider DC cardioversion if tachycardia is due to acute-onset AF. Sinus tachycardia is generally best treated initially with IV fluid and phenylephrine. Esmolol is useful if these measures fail to improve the haemodynamics.

External CPR is unlikely to be successful in patients with severe MS. In the event of full-blown cardiac arrest, the emphasis should be on institution of internal cardiac massage and emergency CPB.

Surgery

Percutaneous transeptal balloon valvotomy is an alternative to surgery in patients with favourable valve morphology (non-calcified, pliable leaflets and absence of commissural calcification) in the absence of significant MR or LA thrombus. Valvotomy is a palliative procedure and recurrence is common. Patients with valvular calcification, thickened fibrotic leaflets and subvalvular fusion have higher incidences of complications and recurrence, and tend to fair better with open surgery.

Mitral Regurgitation

Mild MR is a common finding in patients with IHD undergoing cardiac surgery. Most of these patients do not require surgical intervention to the valve. Lesions that are typically amenable to repair include myxomatous degeneration, mural (posterior) leaflet prolapse and chordal rupture. Cardiac anaesthetists can assist the surgical decision-making process using TOE by providing information on likely aetiology, severity and the natural history of the regurgitant lesion.

Pathology

Acute MR is usually due to rupture or ischaemia of a papillary muscle or rupture of the chordae tendinae. Posterior papillary muscle dysfunction is more common than anterior papillary dysfunction, because the former is supplied by a single coronary artery whereas the latter is supplied by two coronary arteries.

- *Myxomatous degeneration of valve leaflets* most commonly affects the mural (posterior) more than the aortic (anterior) leaflet. The chordae are thin and prone to rupture. Leaflets appear redundant and thickened. A size disproportion between mitral leaflets and the LV cavity causes prolapse.
- *Chronic rheumatic heart disease* leads to scarring and contraction of chordae and leaflets, which become thickened and often calcified.
- *Ischaemic MR* papillary muscle dysfunction with reduced contractility and consequent prolapse, mitral annular dilatation, papillary muscle rupture.
- *Endocarditic* leaflet perforation, chordal rupture, vegetations, abscess formation or scarring may interfere with coaptation.
- *Congenital* cleft or fenestrated mitral leaflets, double orifice MV and endocardial cushion defects.

Clinical Features

Chronic MR commonly presents with exertional dyspnoea and fatigue. Symptoms frequently worsen following the onset of AF. Patients with acute MR do not have time to develop LA enlargement and may present with acute LV failure and pulmonary oedema.

Pathophysiology

The effect of systolic ejection of blood into the low-pressure LA is largely dependent on whether the onset of MR is acute or chronic.

- *Acute MR* results in a sudden increase in the LAP. The LA and LV are not accustomed to increased volume load. An increased LVEDP and increased LAP result in acute pulmonary oedema. The SVR increases to maintain BP. The balance between myocardial oxygen supply and demand is adversely affected by a reduced CO and an increased HR. There is a particularly high risk of subendocardial ischaemia when acute MR is secondary to ischaemic papillary muscle dysfunction or rupture.
- *Chronic MR* results in LV volume overload, LV dilatation and a rightward shift of the LV pressure–volume loop (Figure 10.6). An increased LVEDV occurs without any increase in the LVEDP early in the course of the disease process.

Anaesthetic Goals

Patients with chronic MR are frequently in AF. Sinus rhythm is useful, but less critical than for other valve lesions, as the blood entering the LV in late diastole is

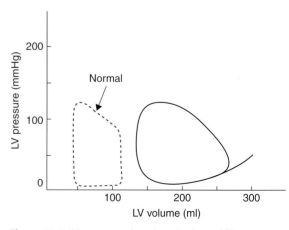

Figure 10.6 LV pressure–volume loop in chronic MR

immediately returned to the LA in early systole. Reduced afterload is generally desirable because of improved forward flow. Patients with non-ischaemic MR tolerate a lower MAP than patients with AR because the coronary perfusion pressure (i.e. aortic root pressure) is maintained during diastole (Box 10.2).

Treatment of Hypotension

The risk of downwardly spiralling hypotension, resistant to medical treatment, is less than in stenotic valvular lesions. Hypotension therefore rarely interferes with the important and interesting task of acquiring good TOE images of the valve. Nevertheless, profound hypotension may occur, particularly in MR secondary to acute ischaemia. Patients with a competent AV usually respond to small doses of phenylephrine, otherwise inotropes are the first-line treatment.

Investigations

The LA provides an excellent acoustic window for examination of the MV. TOE is superior to TTE for examining posterior cardiac structures. MV repair and endocarditis surgery are both high-level indications for intraoperative TOE. A thorough 2D examination using oesophageal and transgastric views provides the cornerstone of MV evaluation. Figure 10.7 illustrates the scanning planes through the MV for mid-oesophageal views at 0, 60, 90 and 150 degrees. TOE assessment of MV function is discussed in Chapter 34.

Surgery

In comparison to MV replacement with complete valve excision, MV repair is associated with better preservation of LV function. Moreover, MV repair is associated with a lower risk of bacterial endocarditis, reduced need for postoperative anticoagulation, lower operative mortality and better long-term survival. Virtually all Carpentier type I, and the majority of type II lesions,

Box 10.2 Anaesthetic considerations in acute and chronic MR

	Acute MR	Chronic MR
Preload	Maintain	Maintain
HR	Maintain	Control ventricular rate
Rhythm	Sinus preferable	Generally in AF
SVR	Maintain coronary perfusion	Slight decrease normally tolerated
Contractility	Support	Maintain
PVR	Maintain	Maintain

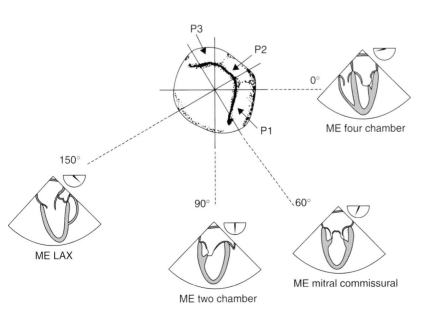

Figure 10.7 Mid-oesophageal (ME) TOE scanning planes perpendicular to the MV demonstrating the effect of ultrasound plane rotation. P1, anterior scallop of mural (posterior) leaflet; P2, middle scallop of mural leaflet; P3, posterior scallop of mural leaflet. All three scallops of the mural leaflet can usually be visualized with the mid-oesophageal 60° (commissural) and 150° views.

79

are amenable to satisfactory repair. Common problems and their solutions are shown in Table 10.1.

Emergency surgery in the setting of acute MR carries greater morbidity and mortality. LA enlargement, which typically accompanies chronic lesions and facilitates surgical access, is normally absent in MR of acute onset.

Surgical repair of rheumatic and ischaemic (Carpentier type III) lesions is challenging. Extensive rheumatic leaflet calcification often leaves little pliable leaflet tissue remaining. Partial or complete homograft replacement or the use of pericardial extension has yet to demonstrate long-term stability and durability.

Myocardial ischaemia may result in type I (annular dilatation), type II (papillary muscle rupture) or type III (fibrosis of subvalvular apparatus) lesions. The mechanisms of MR are often complex – having more to do with LV function than a structural valve abnormality. Type III lesions caused by fibrotic distortion of the ventricular wall following infarction are particularly difficult to repair. Ischaemic rupture of the head of a papillary muscle is best treated with valve replacement as reattachment of the papillary muscle head all too frequently

breaks down. Patients with mild MR will often improve with coronary revascularization alone. More severe regurgitation may be better treated with valve replacement, with preservation of the subvalvular apparatus.

The mechanical complications of MV repair include persistent regurgitation, iatrogenic stenosis and LVOT obstruction (Table 10.2).

High-velocity regurgitant jets may produce severe haemolysis. Anaemia and haematuria may necessitate repeat surgery. Obstruction of the LVOT secondary to SAM (Figure 10.8) is a rare complication, ranging from severe (failure to wean from CPB) to mild/transient (exertional symptoms). The aetiology of SAM is presented in Table 10.3.

Postoperative management specific to the MV repair patient includes anticoagulation, treatment of dysrhythmias and prevention of secondary infection.

- *Anticoagulation*

  If in sinus rhythm after surgery:

  Long-term anticoagulation not necessary

  Evidence for use of antiplatelet therapy weak

Table 10.1 Surgical solutions for MR

Carpentier type	Mechanism	Solution
Type I	Annular dilatation	Annuloplasty ring
	Leaflet perforation	Pericardial patch
Type II	Posterior leaflet prolapse (cord rupture/elongation)	Quadrangular resection + simple/sliding annuloplasty
	Anterior leaflet prolapse	Posterior leaflet flip over; Gortex® cords; edge-to-edge (Alfieri) apposition
	Commissural prolapse	Resection/plicaton; edge-to-edge; partial homograft
Type III	Restricted leaflet motion	Challenging – difficult to repair

Table 10.2 Mechanical complications of MV repair

Problem	Mechanism	Discussion
Regurgitation	Leaflet distortion	Badly positioned or ill-sized annuloplasty ring
	Paravalvular leak	Gaps between the sutures or annuloplasty sutures cutting out through the annulus creating a hole between the ventricle and the LA
Stenosis	Severe reduction of the MV orifice	May be trivial – all degrees possible
		Repeat surgery may be indicated
LVOT obstruction	Systolic anterior motion (SAM) of the anterior MV leaflet	Anterior leaflet moves into the LVOT during systole

Table 10.3 Aetiology of SAM of the aortic (anterior) mitral leaflet

Aetiology	Mechanism	Prevention/treatment
Excessive height of the posterior leaflet	Pushes anterior leaflet into the LVOT in early systole. As systole progresses the leaflet is carried further and further into the LVOT, producing potentially complete obstruction	Ensure that the posterior leaflet is not left too tall when being reconstructed
Small/rigid annuloplasty ring		Use of appropriate ring size
Septal hypertrophy	Reduces the LVOT diameter	
LV cavity size	Reduces the LVOT diameter	Avoidance of hypovolaemia Cautious use of inotropes

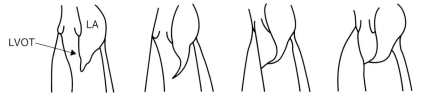

Figure 10.8 The mechanism of LVOT obstruction due to SAM

If in AF after surgery:

Anticoagulation indicated at the level determined by AF as the primary indication

- *Dysrhythmias*

AF is the most common dysrhythmia – particularly in the elderly

Onset is often accompanied by hypokalaemia/hypomagnesaemia

Amiodarone has replaced digoxin as first-line therapy

Amiodarone continued until at least the first outpatient clinic visit

- *Infection*

The risk of bacterial endocarditis is lower following MV repair than MV replacement.

Changes in international guidelines since the last edition mean that antibiotic prophylaxis is *no longer recommended* before dental, genitourinary and GI surgery.

Consult local or national formulary for latest details.

Up to 50% of patients in AF before surgery will revert to sinus rhythm when the atrial stretching effect of MR has been corrected. The likelihood and durability of reversion to sinus rhythm is determined by the duration of AF prior to surgery.

Key Points

- The mitral subvalvular apparatus is important for normal LV function.
- Tachycardia and *severe* bradycardia are poorly tolerated in MS.
- The assessment of LV function is difficult in severe MR.
- Relative hypovolaemia and reduced SVR during anaesthesia may lead to an underestimation of the severity of MR.

Further Reading

Anderson RH, Spencer DE, Hlavecek AM, Cook AC, Backer CL. *Surgical Anatomy of the Heart*, 4th edn. Cambridge: Cambridge University Press; 2013.

Nishimura RA, Otto CM, Bonow RO *et al.* 2017 AHA/ACC focussed update of the 2014 AHA/ACC guidelines for the management of patients with valvular heart disease: a report of the American College of Cardiology/American Heart Association task force on practice guidelines. *J Am Coll Cardiol* 2017; 70: 252–89.

Tricuspid and Pulmonary Valve Surgery

Joanne Irons and Yasir Abu-Omar

The Tricuspid Valve

The TV complex lies between the RA and RV in a slightly more apical position than the MV on the left side. Anatomy of the TV apparatus consists of:

- Three unequal membranous leaflets – anterior (usually largest), septal and posterior
- A saddle-shaped annulus
- The chordae tendinae
- The papillary muscles

Tricuspid Stenosis

TS is defined as a fixed obstruction to RV filling due to TV orifice narrowing. It is most commonly of rheumatic origin, and often combined with regurgitation. Rheumatic TS is invariably associated with left-sided valvular disease.

Non-rheumatic TS is rare. Causes include congenital atresia or stenosis, right heart tumours (e.g. RA myxoma), systemic lupus erythematosus, endomyocardial fibroelastosis, carcinoid syndrome, prosthetic-valve endocarditis and pacemaker lead infection or adhesions.

Clinical Presentation

Clinical features are often overshadowed by left-sided (particularly mitral) valve disease. The normal TV area is 7–9 cm^2, making it the largest cardiac valve. Clinically significant TS only develops when the TV area reaches less than 2 cm^2 and, hence, there can be a long asymptomatic period as stenosis develops.

Isolated TS presents with features of systemic venous hypertension and RV failure (dyspnoea, fatigue, peripheral oedema, hepatomegaly and ascites). An opening snap and high-pitched, mid-diastolic murmur are best heard at the left lower sternal edge, and a dominant a-wave and a slow y-descent can be seen on the CVP (Figure 11.1). A pansystolic murmur may indicate concomitant TR (Chapter 2).

Investigations

ECG: This may show tall peaked P-waves in leads II, III and aVF indicative of RA enlargement. AF or flutter may be present.

Echocardiography: This is the most useful investigation and can be used to assess the anatomy, measure the severity and diagnose concomitant TR in addition to left-sided valve lesions. 2D and 3D assessment of the TV may reveal thickening or calcification of the leaflets, with restricted movement. Diastolic doming of the leaflets may be seen and RA and IVC enlargement is common. Quantification of the orifice area by 2D and 3D planimetry is difficult and currently not validated or recommended.

CWD: This technique may be of limited use for assessing the severity of TS. Tricuspid inflow velocities are affected by respiration, HR and rhythm and the presence of TR. The pressure

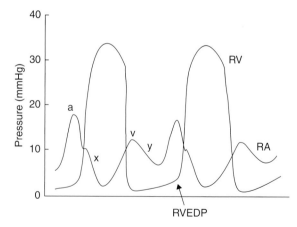

Figure 11.1 RA and RV pressure waveforms in TS. The RA pressure tracing shows the prominent a-wave and a slow y-descent. At end diastole, there is a significant pressure gradient between the RA and RV due to the elevated RA pressure and a drop in RV end-diastolic pressure (RVEDP).

half-time is less valid than in MS and the continuity equation (the SV can be derived from the LV or RV outflow) is unreliable in the presence of more than mild TR. Mean pressure gradients in a normal TV are usually less than 1 mmHg. Features indicative of significant TS are listed in Box 34.1.

Right heart catheterization: This is rarely used but may be useful in determining the contribution of TS to the patient's symptoms. The relative changes in RA pressure and RV end-diastolic pressure mirror left heart pressure changes in MS (Figure 11.1).

Surgery

TV surgery is usually performed with other valve procedures. The need for isolated tricuspid surgery is determined by both the severity of symptoms and the degree of stenosis. Surgery is preferred to percutaneous balloon valvotomy due to the high incidence of concomitant TR, the risk of creating or worsening the TR and the lack of long-term outcome data.

Surgical options include repair by open commissurotomy and valve replacement. If the valve is replaced, biological prosthesis is preferred due to the higher risk of thrombosis with mechanical valves and the durability of bioprosthetic valves in the tricuspid position.

Anaesthetic Goals

These are summarized in Box 11.1.

Tricuspid Regurgitation

TR is defined as retrograde blood flow from the RV into the RA during systole. Mild or 'physiological' TR is present in as many as 70% of asymptomatic, normal individuals. Clinically significant TR is usually functional in origin – occurring secondary to RV enlargement and dilatation of the tricuspid annulus. This is often seen in association with other cardiac disorders such as left-sided mitral and AV disease, PHT, congenital heart disease and cardiomyopathies.

Secondary TR carries a poor prognosis with a vicious cycle of disease whereby progressive dilatation and remodelling of the RV causes TV annular dilatation, papillary muscle displacement and leaflet tethering. This causes worsened TR with a further increase in RV and RA size and a further increase in the dimensions and flattening of the TV annulus. Furthermore, the increase in RV pressure can cause a leftwards shift of the interventricular septum with a decrease in the LV size, an increase in the LV diastolic pressures, an increase in PAPs and further worsening of RV function and TR.

Primary TR is rare; causes include Ebstein's anomaly, infective endocarditis, rheumatic heart disease, carcinoid syndrome and iatrogenic damage from surgery, endocardial biopsies, catheter placements and pacemaker leads.

Clinical Presentation

Isolated TR may be tolerated for many years without symptoms. Like TS, patients with significant TR present with fatigue, dyspnoea, exercise intolerance and features of systemic venous hypertension. A pansystolic murmur is best heard at the left lower sternal edge and the CVP is characterized by a prominent cv-wave, an absent x-descent, and a sharp y-descent (Figure 11.2).

Box 11.1 Anaesthetic considerations in TS

- Preoperative medical management – includes diuretics for heart failure and hepatic congestion and treatment of atrial arrhythmias.
- Attention to left-sided valvular disease.
- RV filling – the need for adequate preload, to maintain forward flow, has to be balanced against the risk of worsening venous congestion.
- Heart rate – AF and other SVTs may cause rapid cardiovascular collapse and should be treated promptly. Conversely, bradycardia can also be harmful and a sinus rhythm of 70–80 bpm should be targeted.
- RV contractility – a sudden drop in RV contractility can cause a severe decrease in CO and increase in RA pressure. Adequate perfusion pressure and RV coronary blood flow should be maintained, and arterial hypotension avoided.
- PA catheters – may be almost impossible to place and will have to be removed during surgery. Surgical assistance in placement is advised if required following CPB.

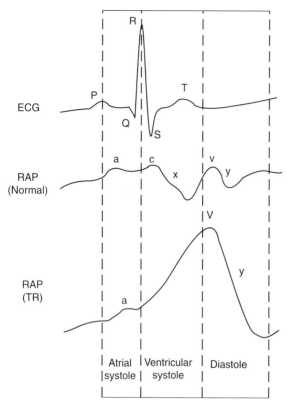

Figure 11.2 The RA pressure (RAP) waveform in TR shows a large cv-wave caused by the regurgitant jet, disappearance of the x-descent and a steep y-descent. The jugular vein pressure may feel pulsatile with a systolic thrill in patients with severe TR, and may be confused with the carotid pulse.

Investigations

ECG: This may reveal RV dysfunction, right-axis deviation, tall P-waves, RBBB and AF.

Echocardiography: An assessment of the TV can be difficult as it is challenging to visualize all three cusps simultaneously, and measurements are less robust than for the MV. Assessment should consider the 2D and 3D anatomy of the valve, right heart chambers, IVC and Doppler measures of severity. Endocarditis, catheter and pacemaker trauma can be well seen on TOE. Significant TR is identified on 2D echocardiography by significant leaflet tethering and annular dilatation. Tethering can be assessed by measuring the systolic tenting area (the area between the annulus and leaflet body in mid systole in the apical four-chamber view) or the tethering distance (the distance between the coaptation point and the annular plane). A tenting area of over 1 cm^2 or tethering distance of over

0.8 cm indicates severe TR. The tricuspid annulus can be measured in diastole in the four-chamber view. The normal diameter is 28 ± 5 mm. A diameter of over 40 mm is considered dilated and an indication for surgery (it corresponds to intraoperative measurement from anterior–septal commissure to anterior–posterior commissure of over 70 mm).

CWD: An assessment of severity is less robust than for MR and has significant limitations due to eccentric jets, haemodynamics and equipment settings.

CFD: This Doppler technique, however, is commonly used and detection of a large eccentric jet extending to the posterior wall of the RA lies in favour of severe TR while thin central jets usually are mild. Although the geometry of the TV is complex and CFD measurements can be difficult, a vena contracta greater than 7 mm, an effective regurgitant orifice area of more than 75 mm^2 and a proximal isovelocity surface area (PISA) of 9 mm at a Nyquist limit of 28 cm s^{-1} usually indicates severe TR. PA systolic pressure can be estimated using the modified Bernoulli equation.

Estimated PA systolic pressure = 4 × (peak TR jet velocity)^2 + RA pressure.

PWD: This can be used to look at the TV inflow and, in the absence of TS, a peak E-wave of greater than 1 m s^{-1} indicates severe TR, while the density of the CWD TR jet can also indicate severity. This is summarized in Table 34.5.

Other findings on TOE indicative of severe TR include PWD systolic flow reversal in the hepatic veins (specific to severe TR), a dilated and pulsatile IVC, a dilated coronary sinus, an enlarged RA with bowing of the interatrial septum towards the LA and RV dysfunction.

Surgery

Tricuspid surgery is indicated for severe TR and is usually undertaken at the time of surgery for left-sided valves. It should also be considered in patients with moderate primary TR and mild–moderate secondary TR with dilatation of the annulus greater than 40 mm. Isolated TV surgery should be considered in patients with severe primary TR who are symptomatic and those with progressive RV dilatation or early dysfunction.

Ring annuloplasty is usually all that is required for isolated annular dilatation, although repair may

---

Box 11.2   Anaesthetic considerations in TR

- As TR is usually secondary, the anaesthetic management is generally dictated by the primary pathology.
- RV preload – adequate filling must be achieved to maintain forward flow and limit TR. A drop in CVP can severely reduce CO. Airway pressures during mechanical ventilation should be minimized to avoid reduced RV filling.
- HR – most patients are in chronic AF and are impossible to convert to NSR. A normal to high HR is preferred to maintain forward flow.
- RV contractility – RV failure is usually the cause of severe clinical deterioration in these patients and inotropic support is often required.
- PVR – hypercarbia, hypoxia, acidosis and other factors that increase PVR should be avoided and consideration given to the use of pulmonary vasodilators such as inhaled NO. If inotropic support is necessary, inodilators such as enoximone or dobutamine should be considered.
- Immediately post TV surgery, the RV will be compromised as the entire SV is ejected forward without the pressure relief of blood into the RA through a leaking TV. This may require inotropic support to prevent RV failure.

---

be indicated when the leaflets are deformed. Some utilize suture (DeVega) annuloplasty with excellent outcomes. If TV replacement is necessary, large bioprosthetic valves are generally preferred to mechanical valves as they are associated with a lower risk of thromboembolic complications.

Anaesthetic Goals

These are summaraized in Box 11.2.

The Pulmonary Valve

The PV separates the RVOT from the main PA. Its structure mimics that of the AV, comprising three cusps, each with its own sinus of Valsalva and a sinotubular junction. The annulus has ventricular muscular attachments, making it susceptible to the effects of RV preload and afterload. The normal adult PV has an orifice area of 2 cm^2.

Pulmonary Stenosis

PS may be subvalvular, valvular, supravalvular or proximal pulmonary arterial. In the majority of cases PS is congenital and valvular in nature; this may be trileaflet, bicuspid, unicuspid or dysplastic (e.g. Noonan's syndrome), and is characterized by commissural fusion, leaflet thickening and doming. Supravalvular stenosis may be found in congenital rubella and Williams syndromes, while subvalvular or infundibular stenosis is often associated with a VSD (e.g. tetralogy of Fallot, double-chamber RV). Physiological proximal arterial PS is frequently seen in neonates. Acquired PS is rare, and causes include carcinoid syndrome and rheumatic heart disease.

External compression by a tumour or sinus of Valsalva aneurysm may also lead to PV narrowing.

Clinical Presentation

Adults with PS usually present with an asymptomatic systolic murmur, detected during routine examination. Children with moderate to severe PS may develop exertional dyspnoea that should prompt early intervention. The features of severe PS are those of systemic venous congestion and RV failure. A right-to-left shunt across a PFO or ASD may produce cyanosis. A prominent venous a-wave, a precordial thrill and a parasternal heave indicate severe PS (Chapter 2).

Diastolic RV dysfunction, secondary to RVH, occurs at an early stage. RV pressure overload causes RV systolic dysfunction, RV dilatation, TR and systemic venous congestion.

Investigations

ECG: This may show evidence of RVH and right-axis deviation.

Echocardiography: Evaluation of the anatomy is important to determine the level of stenosis. Leaflets may be thickened, calcified or dysplastic depending on aetiology. Other findings may include systolic doming, post-stenotic PA dilatation and RVH (>5 mm). Muscular subvalvular stenosis and an associated VSD should be excluded when adult PS is suspected.

Doppler: Assessment of stenosis is based on the transpulmonary pressure gradient using CWD (Figure 11.3 and Table 34.6). Care is required to identify the level of stenosis using this technique

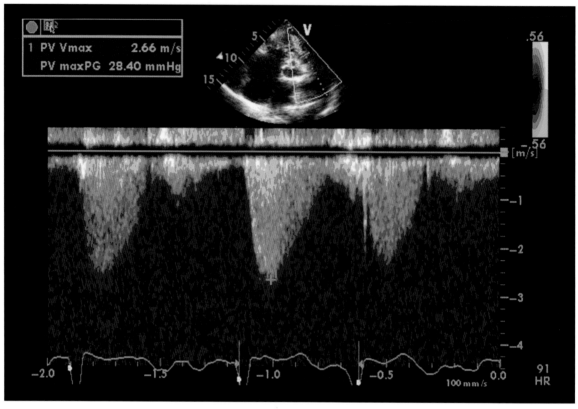

Figure 11.3 CWD applied across a stenotic PV. The peak velocity is 2.66 m s^{-1}, which corresponds to a peak gradient of 28.4 mmHg, indicating mild PS.

and 2D anatomy and PWD may help. Valve area by planimetry is not possible and the continuity equation is rarely used for the PV.

Anaesthetic Goals

These are summaraized in Box 11.3.

Pulmonary Regurgitation

PR is defined as retrograde blood flow from the PA into the RV during diastole. Like TR, mild 'physiologic' PR is a frequent echocardiographic finding in normal hearts.

In adults, pathological PR is most commonly due to annular dilatation secondary to PHT. PR is also a common finding after surgical intervention for PS, and a frequent complication of surgery for tetralogy of Fallot. Consequently, a significant number of patients with severe PR presenting for valve replacement will have already undergone some form of cardiac surgery.

Box 11.3   Anaesthetic considerations in PS

- Patients with PS often have other structural cardiac abnormalities, which need to be considered in the perioperative period.
- HR - bradycardia should be avoided. Modest elevation of HR (80–100 bpm) is generally better tolerated than in AS.
- SVR - Subendocardial blood flow falls as the RV hypertrophies. Aortic root pressure should be maintained to ensure adequate coronary perfusion and prevent RV subendocardial ischaemia.
- PVR - In contrast to AS, there is no absolute requirement to maintain 'post-stenotic' afterload.

Other causes include infective endocarditis, carcinoid syndrome, rheumatic heart disease, PA catheter trauma and connective-tissue disorders (e.g. Marfan syndrome). Congenital causes, such as absent pulmonary valve syndrome, are extremely rare.

Clinical Presentation

PR is well tolerated, with the majority of patients remaining asymptomatic for many years. As the disease progresses, exercise intolerance and clinical features of right heart failure may arise as a result of RV dilatation. Patients present late, often with irreversible RV dysfunction, which places them at an increased risk of ventricular arrhythmias and sudden cardiac death.

Clinical examination may reveal a parasternal heave, a soft diastolic murmur at the left upper sternal edge and a loud P2. In the presence of PHT, a high-pitched early diastolic (Graham Steel) murmur may be audible (see Chapter 2).

Investigations

ECG: This may show evidence of RVH, RBBB, right axis deviation and arrhythmias.

2D and 3D echocardiography: This is useful to identify cusp number, motion (doming or prolapse) and structure. RV dilatation, a flattening of IVS in diastole (volume overload) and TR may also be seen.

Doppler: The severity of PR can be determined by assessing jet width and extent of penetration into the RVOT on CFD. A jet width that occupies more than 50% RVOT width suggests severe PR. The vena contracta width can also be used but lacks validation. CWD of the PR jet can also be used to assess the severity, although this lacks validation also. A faint jet with slow deceleration indicates mild PR, while a dense, steep jet with early termination indicates severe PR. A pressure half-time less than 100 ms may also indicate severe PR. Flow reversal on CWD or CFD in the pulmonary arteries is a very specific sign of severe PR (Table 34.7).

Cardiac magnetic resonance imaging: This remains the gold-standard imaging modality in the assessment and follow-up of patients with PR. RV function and severity of PR can be accurately assessed to aid timely intervention in patients with chronic PR.

Surgery

Surgery is considered when PR is severe with symptoms or signs of RV dysfunction.

Anaesthetic Goals

These are summaraized in Box 11.4

> **Box 11.4 Anaesthetic considerations in PR**
>
> - RV preload – needs to be maintained to promote forward flow.
> - HR – a modest tachycardia shortens diastole and reduces regurgitant flow.
> - PVR – afterload reduction lowers the regurgitant flow. Hypercarbia, hypoxia, acidosis and other factors that increase PVR should be avoided and consideration given to the use of pulmonary vasodilators such as inhaled NO.
> - Contractility – RV function must be maintained and optimized. If inotropic support is necessary, inodilators such as enoximone or dobutamine should be considered.
> - SVR – higher systemic arterial pressures are both desirable and well tolerated.

Carcinoid Heart Disease

Carcinoid tumours are rare neuroendocrine neoplasms of amine precursor uptake decarboxylation cells. Around 70% of carcinoid tumours are found in the GI tract, although in a small proportion of cases carcinoid may arise in a bronchopulmonary system or other endocrine glands and organs. When these tumours invade and metastasize (usually to the liver) they may produce carcinoid syndrome.

Carcinoid syndrome refers to a constellation of symptoms and signs caused by the release of vasoactive substances (e.g. serotonin, prostaglandins, histamine), which bypass hepatic inactivation and enter the systemic circulation. The syndrome is characterized by episodic bronchospasm, flushing, GI hypermotility and cardiovascular symptoms.

Pathophysiology

Carcinoid heart disease is found in about 50% of patients with carcinoid syndrome, which typically causes abnormalities in the right side of the heart. Characteristic pearly white fibrous plaques may be deposited anywhere on the endocardium and may cause restrictive diastolic dysfunction. Subvalvular involvement causes restriction and distortion of valve anatomy.

One in five patients with a carcinoid tumour present with symptoms and signs of right heart failure secondary to TV and PV disease. TR is found in practically all patients, followed by PR, and less commonly TS and PS. Left-sided valvular disease is

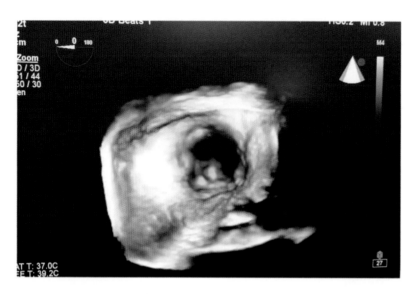

Figure 11.4 3D TOE image of a TV in carcinoid disease from the RA during systole. Note the closure of the anterior leaflet but complete retraction and restriction of the septal and posterior leaflets, leaving a large defect for severe TR.

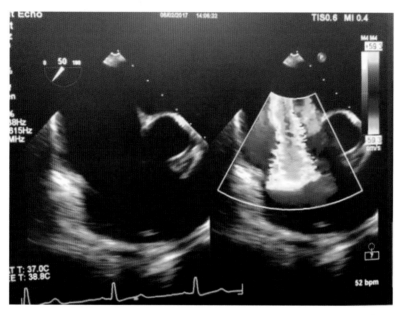

Figure 11.5 2D TOE image of a TV in carcinoid disease with simultaneous CFD during systole. There is severe restriction and retraction of the septal and posterior leaflets with a large defect and severe TR.

uncommon, due to inactivation of vasoactive substances by the lung, and is usually associated with an interatrial shunt or bronchial carcinoid. A significant number of patients with symptoms of heart failure die within a year.

Investigations

Echocardiography: The TV and PV leaflets appear thickened, retracted and sometimes fixed in a semi-open position. Thickening and shortening of the subvalvular apparatus is commonly seen (Figure 11.4). Any right-sided valvular abnormality may be present, but TR is almost universal (Figure 11.5). Other findings include RA and RV dilatation with evidence of RV volume overload and reduced ejection fraction. CWD of the TR jet shows a characteristic 'dagger-shaped' signal.

Biochemical screening: Serotonin is the major vasoactive amine secreted by carcinoid tumours and is metabolized to 5-hydroxyindoleacetic acid (5-HIAA) and excreted in the urine. A 24-hour urinary concentration of 5-HIAA is key to

Box 11.5 Anaesthetic considerations in carcinoid heart disease

- Medical therapy – cardiac and carcinoid symptoms should be stabilized on medical therapy prior to surgery. Somatostatin analogues, such as octreotide, which bind to somatostatin receptors, have become the mainstay of medical therapy.
- Haemodynamic goals – largely dictated by the primary cardiac lesion and RV function.
- Preventing carcinoid crisis.

establishing the diagnosis as well as assessing disease progression and response to treatment. Patients with carcinoid heart disease have characteristically much higher levels of urinary 5-HIAA and serum serotonin than those without cardiac involvement.

Anaesthetic Goals

These are summaraized in Box 11.5.

Preventing Carcinoid Crisis

Factors which can precipitate a crisis include hypothermia, hypotension, hypercarbia, emotional stress and drugs (e.g. thiopental, atracurium, succinylcholine and morphine). Benzodiazepines, propofol, etomidate, steroidal muscle relaxants (e.g. vecuronium, rocuronium, pancuronium) and synthetic opioids (e.g. fentanyl and sufentanil) have all been shown to be safe.

A multidisciplinary approach is essential in managing these complex patients. A pre-emptive infusion of octreotide (50–200 µg h^{-1}) should be started before induction of anaesthesia and continued into the postoperative period. Additional doses may be given during surgery as necessary. Since the introduction of octreotide, previous concerns about catecholamine-induced carcinoid crisis have proven unfounded. Serum glucose concentration should be monitored closely as octreotide suppresses insulin production and elevates blood glucose levels. Antihistamines may also be used perioperatively to prevent flushing and bronchospasm, whereas corticosteroids can be used to reduce bradykinin production.

Hypotension

Hypotension may be caused by RV dysfunction, carcinoid crisis, blood loss and post-CPB vasodilatation. Intraoperative TOE, in addition to invasive CVP and PAP monitoring, can assist in diagnosis.

Hypovolaemia should be treated with fluid replacement. If a carcinoid crisis is suspected, a bolus of octreotide should be administered. Poor ventricular function can be managed safely with exogenous catecholamines, calcium and phenylephrine.

Surgery

Valve replacement is the treatment of choice for carcinoid heart disease and should be considered in symptomatic patients with worsening RV function. Traditionally, this was with mechanical valves on the grounds that they are more resistant to carcinoid plaque deposition. However, the use of bioprosthetic valves is an alternative, as these patients, with hepatic metastases, are at a high risk of bleeding associated with warfarin therapy. The choice is challenging and should be tailored to the individual patient. Furthermore, the median survival following valve replacement is around 6–11 years and it is likely that the durability of the modern generation of bioprosthetic valves is greater than life expectancy.

Key Points

- TS is rare and often rheumatic in origin. Symptoms and signs are often overshadowed by left-sided valvular disease.
- TR is usually functional in origin, occurring secondary to RV enlargement and dilatation of the tricuspid annulus. Surgery is usually undertaken at the time of surgery for left-sided valves.
- Echocardiographic assessment of right-sided valves is essential to grade severity and guide timing of surgical intervention.
- Factors increasing PVR should be avoided during surgery for right-sided valve lesions.
- A multidisciplinary approach is essential when dealing with patients with carcinoid disease. The main anaesthetic challenges are prevention of RV failure and carcinoid crisis.

Further Reading

Baumgartner H, Hung J, Bermejo J, *et al.* Echocardiographic assessment of valve stenosis: EAE/ASE recommendations for clinical practice. *Eur J Echocardiogr* 2009; 10: 1-25.

Castillo JG, Filsoufi F, Adams DH, *et al.* Management of patients undergoing multivalvular surgery for carcinoid heart disease: the role of the anaesthetist. *Br J Anaesth* 2008; 101: 618-26.

Kaltsas G, Caplin M, Davies P, *et al.* ENETS consensus guidelines for the standards of care in neuroendocrine tumors: pre- and perioperative therapy in patients with neuroendocrine tumors. *Neuroendocrinology* 2017; 105: 245–54.

Lancellotti P, Tribouilloy C, Hagendorff A, *et al.* Recommendations for the echocardiographic assessment of native valvular regurgitation: an executive summary from the European Association of Cardiovascular Imaging. *Eur Heart J Cardiovasc Imaging* 2013; 14: 611–44.

Nishimura RA, Otto CM, Bonow RO, *et al.* 2017 AHA/ACC focused update of the 2014 AHA/ACC guideline for the management of patients with valvular heart disease: a report of the American College of Cardiology/American Heart Association task force on clinical practice guidelines. *Circulation* 2017; 135: e1159–95.

Vahanian A, Alfieri O, Andreotti F, *et al.* Guidelines on the management of valvular heart disease (version 2012): the Joint Task Force on the Management of Valvular Heart Disease of the European Society of Cardiology (ESC) and the European Association for Cardio-Thoracic Surgery (EACTS). *Eur J Cardiothorac Surg* 2012; 42: S1–44.

12 Minimally Invasive and Off-Pump Cardiac Surgery

Ben Gibbison

Cardiac surgery is a major insult to homeostasis. Attempts have been made to reduce the inflammatory response to cardiac surgery by limiting the stimulus. The two biggest stimuli to this inflammation are thought to be surgical tissue destruction and the interaction with the extracorporeal circuit. Therefore, techniques have been developed to reduce these stimuli – either by minimizing them (minimally invasive surgery) or eliminating them completely (off-pump surgery).

Off-Pump Surgery

Off-pump coronary artery bypass (OPCAB) surgery describes coronary revascularization without the use of CPB. This should not to be confused with 'beating heart surgery', involving the use of CPB without arresting the heart.

History

Coronary artery bypass in humans was developed in the 1950s. Techniques evolved and improved facilitating cardiac surgery on a massive scale in the 1960s onwards with CPB and cardioplegic arrest, transforming both the safety and scope of cardiac surgery. It was rapidly apparent that there were considerable side effects associated with cardiac surgery, many of which were attributed to the use of CPB. The evolution of surgical techniques and the development of cardiac stabilization devices, retractors and intra-coronary shunts led to a resurgence of interest in OPCAB.

OPCAB had been performed for many years, particularly in territories where cost was a limiting factor, enabling surgery without using expensive disposables. The absence of a significant reduction in major morbidity and mortality, coupled with technical challenges, have limited the uptake of OPCAB in the developed world.

Rationale

Resurgence in interest and wider utilization of OPCAB were motivated by the desire to limit morbidity and mortality – much of which was attributed to CPB. Advances in surgical equipment were supported by commercial interest in providing new equipment and devices to facilitate OPCAB. As the profile of the procedure rose, demand from cardiologists and patients rose, although this has now fallen – mainly because the rise in percutaneous intervention has changed the profile of those referred for surgery. Patients are now older, have more complex coronary disease and a greater number of co-morbidities. They also have pathology that is less amenable to OPCAB, including those with deep intramuscular coronary arteries, a need for endarterectomy and poor LV function.

Surgical Approach

The usual approach for multi-vessel revascularization is median sternotomy. The heart will need to be displaced to position it suitably for surgical anastomosis. LAD artery grafts require minimal repositioning of the heart and, if isolated, can be amenable to minimal access surgery via a small left anterior thoracotomy. Bypass grafts to the inferior and right sides of the heart require extensive elevation or rotation of the heart.

Positioning is often achieved using a swab attached to the posterior pericardium or a bespoke suction cup to manipulate the heart. A stabilization device is used to keep the anastomotic site still. Stabilizer devices can be thought of like a 'sewing-machine foot', and indeed initial equipment was based on this principle. Equipment has now evolved to include tiny suction cups on the stabilizer and bespoke sternal retractors.

In the initial development of OPCAB, blood flow to the anastomotic site would be interrupted by surgical sutures. Modern practice utilizes flexible olive-ended silicone shunts, which maintain both a relatively bloodless field and arterial flow throughout the process of grafting. Tiny amounts of blood still contaminate the field, which are too small for standard suction equipment. Therefore, CO_2 is used to 'blow' this away.

The proximal anastomoses on the ascending aorta require the use of a 'side-biting' aortic clamp. It is the continued use of an aortic clamp that contributes most to morbidity and it is for this reason that 'off-pump' isolated left internal mammary artery (LIMA) to the LAD artery grafting (i.e. the aortic clamp is not needed) has a clear outcome benefit (Table 12.1).

Anaesthetic Management

Off-pump CABG requires a greater degree of communication between anaesthetist and surgeon than 'on-pump' surgery. The anaesthetic technique has a much greater impact on the ease of surgery – it is much easier to perform 'off-pump' surgery on a 'soft heart' with a slow HR.

Manipulation of the heart leads to cardiac chamber compression, valvular distortion, valvular regurgitation (notably the MV), reduced venous return, RV outflow obstruction, myocardial ischaemia and arrhythmias. The resultant decrease in the CO and MAP has consequences for end-organ perfusion. Most haemodynamic disturbances can be resolved by returning the heart to

its normal anatomical position or by reducing retraction on the heart. If this does not happen rapidly, myocardial function is likely to be impaired. The rate of return to normal haemodynamics when the heart is returned to its usual position is more predictive of the heart tolerating the surgery than absolute haemodynamic values.

General Considerations

Patients scheduled for OPCAB surgery require the same preoperative assessment and management as those scheduled for conventional surgery. The goals of anaesthetic management are:

- Prevention of intraoperative cardiac ischaemia
- Tight haemodynamic control
- Minimization of cardiovascular depression
- Maximization of surgical access – a double-lumen endotracheal tube may be required

Multiple anaesthetic techniques have been utilized; none has been shown to be superior.

Monitoring

Standard cardiac anaesthetic monitoring is required in all cases (Chapter 4). Although CO monitoring (e.g. PA catheter, oesophageal Doppler, pulse contour analysis) is advocated in many centres, it is not routinely required.

TOE is routinely used to assess regional wall motion although cardiac displacement and swabs placed behind the heart may obscure images. Nevertheless, TOE may be used to guide fluid management and exclude other cardiac pathology. Neurological monitoring (e.g. TCD, EEG and near-infrared spectroscopy) have all been used, but with little evidence of alteration in the clinical outcome.

Heat Conservation

Convective, evaporative and radiated heat loss during surgery may cause significant cooling and should be anticipated as rewarming using CPB is not available. Measures to reduce hypothermia include:

- Maintaining high ambient temperature (approximately 25 °C) – although this is likely to be resisted by the surgical team
- Use of underbody heating, e.g. heated mattresses
- Use of a sterile lower-body forced air blanket following saphenous vein harvest

Table 12.1 Advantages and disadvantages of off-pump surgery

Advantages	Disadvantages
No cardioplegia (K+ load/ fluid load)	Technically more challenging
No aortic or atrial cannulation (fewer sites for bleeding/dissection)	Incomplete revascularization – not all arteries well reached by technique (fewer grafts per patient)
No AXC (isolated LIMA → LAD grafts)	Higher rates of early graft failure
Less inflammatory mediator release	
Less bleeding/transfusion	
More time-efficient	

- Use of fluid warming devices for all IV fluids
- Insulation of the head and neck to decrease cranial heat loss

Haemodynamic Management

Physical

Fluid administration: Avoid hypovolaemia and remember that there is no fluid input from CPB prime. Maintain preload, but do not over fill during grafting as over distension of the heart makes the surgery more difficult.

Maintain the cerebral perfusion pressure: Maintain the MAP and avoid gross/prolonged CVP elevation.

Posture: Use of Trendelenburg position ± lateral tilt ameliorates a decrease in CO from decreased venous return.

Opening the right pleural cavity reduces the impact of cardiac rotation.

IABP placement pre-grafting in high-risk cases has been described.

Pharmacological

HR: Aim for 60–80 bpm. Use IV β-blocker (e.g. esmolol) if required.

Contractility: Avoid inotropes during grafting if possible – tachycardia may cause ischaemia. Low-dose dobutamine or a phosphodiesterase inhibitor may be used if absolutely necessary.

Vasoconstriction: Metaraminol provides vasoconstriction with reflex cardiac slowing. A noradrenaline infusion is generally not useful during grafting as it is not rapidly titratable.

Vasodilatation: GTN, sodium nitroprusside or phentolamine drugs may be useful if there is cardiac distension.

Cardiac rhythm: K^+ and Mg^{2+} supplementation to reduce myocardial irritability.

Electrical

Epicardial pacing: Increasing the HR with fixed-rated atrial (AOO) pacing maintains CO and may decrease the risk of cardiac distension. Ventricular pacing may be required during RCA grafting if transient heart block arises.

Anticoagulation

The interruption of normal blood flow and the pro-thrombotic effect of breaching the vascular endothelium mandates a degree of anticoagulation, although there is no consensus on the ideal strategy. Unfractionated heparin remains the drug of choice as it can be titrated to a measurable effect and is rapidly reversible. The degree of anticoagulation varies by centre and operator – some surgeons prefer full anticoagulation (i.e. ACT >400 s). Alternatively, a heparin dose of ~150 IU kg^{-1} of heparin – sufficient to double the baseline ACT or achieve an ACT >300 s – may be used. Heparin reversal also varies between centres; ranging from complete to no reversal at all. Variations in anticoagulation practice may well be the reason for the blood-conserving potential benefit of off-pump surgery.

Postoperative Management

Principles of postoperative management are no different from those of conventional surgery.

Avoiding CPB and using partial anticoagulation typically results in less bleeding and reduced transfusion requirements.

Although the postoperative temperature 'after drop' often seen after CPB is avoided, patients may still be hypothermic at the time of ICU admission.

Avoiding CPB spares the patient from the effects of the pump prime and cardioplegia. Obsessive intraoperative fluid management may, however, render a patient hypovolaemic.

Conversion to On-Pump Surgery

CPB may be required during OPCAB. In some cases, the institution of CPB constitutes an emergency. Full anticoagulation will be required with an ACT >400 s. Common indications are:

- Inadequate surgical access
- Gross haemodynamic instability
- Refractory dysrhythmia
- Newly diagnosed valvular pathology requiring surgical correction

Table 12.2 Advantages and disadvantages of MICS

Advantages	Disadvantages
Reduced postoperative pain	Challenging in the very obese, previous thoracic surgery and in those with pectus excavatum
Increased early mobility and faster return to normal activity	Increased risk of peripheral vascular complications due to large-vessel cannulation for CPB
Lower incidence of wound infections	Technically more challenging
Improved cosmetic outcome	Multiple procedures (e.g. AVR and MVR) more difficult
Can reduce trauma and difficult dissection in redo procedures (e.g. mini thoracotomy approach)	Retrograde arterial perfusion (i.e. aortic cannula placed via the femoral artery) may increase the risk of stroke
Better visualization of pathology with high-definition screen and fibreoptic cameras	Rapid institution of CPB in the unstable patient may be technically difficult

Outcome

The many putative benefits of OPCAB surgery have failed to be realised. While the range of complications seen differs from conventional surgery, there appears to be little difference in mortality. Recent studies suggest that patients undergoing OPCAB have fewer grafts (twice the rate of incomplete revascularization), have reduced intermediate-term graft patency and have a greater risk of repeat surgery.

Minimally Invasive Cardiac Surgery

Proponents of minimally invasive cardiac surgery (MICS) claim that reducing the size of the surgical incision reduces tissue damage and improves outcomes by reducing the inflammatory response to surgery. Although the acronym MICS is widely used – a better description of this type of surgery is 'minimal access surgery'. Surgery still involves gaining access to the chest, instituting CPB, arresting the heart and performing the same reparative techniques, albeit through smaller incisions. The limited view of the heart and mediastinum means that there is a heavy reliance on TOE to guide the surgery. In expert hands, surgical outcomes are non-inferior to standard procedures in terms of repair of the pathology. The benefits are thought to come from the preservation of the structural integrity of the chest wall, leading to reduced pain, fewer respiratory complications and a more rapid return to normal function. The cosmetic outcome is also better – while this may not very important to anaesthetists, it is to patients! The advantages and disadvantages of MICS are outlined in Table 12.2.

> **Box 12.1 Types of cardiac surgery amenable to a minimally invasive approach**
> - MV repair/replacement
> - TV repair/replacement
> - Removal of atrial mass
> - Repair of ASD/PFO
> - AV repair/replacement (mini-sternotomy)
> - CABG surgery (LIMA → LAD - minimally invasive direct coronary artery bypass (MIDCAB))

Types of MICS

MICS encompasses a range of surgical procedures and approaches. At its most basic, this can be near 'standard', using a smaller incision such as a mini-sternotomy for AVR (Chapter 9) or mini-thoracotomy for single-vessel OPCAB to the anterior surface of the heart. At the other end of the spectrum, robotic port-access MV surgery represents MICS at its most developed. The types of surgery achievable with MICS are shown in Box 12.1.

Preoperative Assessment

Preoperative assessment for MICS should follow the same principles as any other cardiac surgical procedure. This means that the severity of the lesion should be established, and its consequent symptoms and end-organ effects elucidated. These are then placed on the background of the patient's other co-morbidities and a risk/benefit decision taken. Particular points relevant to MICS are:

Cardiovascular:

- Cardiac pathology and ventricular performance
- Other cardiac pathologies (venous drainage anomalies, coexistent valve disease) should be excluded
- Significant extracardiac atheromatous disease should be excluded and the adequacy of femoral vessels for cannulation should be confirmed (CT angiography)

Respiratory:

- Airway assessment and pulmonary function tests to ensure suitability for one-lung ventilation in those undergoing a thoracotomy approach
- Previous cardiac surgery, lung conditions and chest wall deformity/irradiation all lead to increased adhesions that may make surgical access difficult

Gastrointestinal:

- TOE is essential for MICS – a contraindication for TOE (e.g. oesophageal varices, strictures, pouches, oesophagectomy) is a contraindication for MICS

Conduct of Anaesthesia

The conduct of anaesthesia is dictated by the planned operative procedure. Thoracotomy approaches typically require one-lung ventilation and the use of either a double-lumen tracheal tube or bronchial blocker.

Use of an endo-aortic balloon clamp means that bilateral radial arterial lines are useful – right radial pressure monitoring can detect innominate artery occlusion by migration of the balloon. TCD and cerebral oximetry are also useful in this situation to monitor the cerebral circulation. Access for internal defibrillation may also be limited; therefore, external defibrillation pads should be affixed to the patient prior to surgery, taking care to place them away from the surgical field.

Cardiopulmonary Bypass

The use of conventional CPB cannulae within a reduced surgical field may be technically challenging and may reduce surgical access to such an extent that surgery is rendered impossible. A 'flattened' low-profile venous cannula may improve mini-sternotomy access (Figure 12.1). In port-access MICS, CPB cannulae are usually sited away from the operative site. Venous cannulae may be placed in the internal jugular or femoral veins using the Seldinger technique (Figure 12.2). The use of ultrasound and TOE is advocated to ensure correct placement (Figure 12.3).

Other CPB equipment that can be placed peripherally includes the retrograde cardioplegia cannula and the PA vent. Both of these may be inserted via the internal jugular vein. The retrograde cardioplegia cannula is inserted into the coronary sinus via the RA and guided into position using TOE. It is critical that the operator is certain that the tip is 1 cm into the coronary sinus as misplacement risks inadequate myocardial protection or coronary sinus perforation. The PA vent is useful if there is only one venous

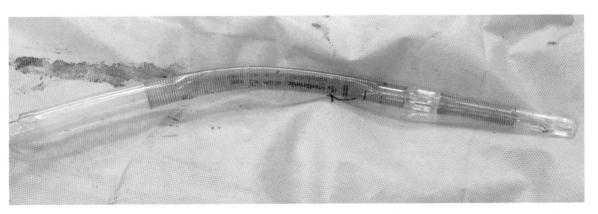

Figure 12.1 Medtronic low-profile, two-stage venous cannula. The flattened mid-section of the cannula is reinforced with metal coil.

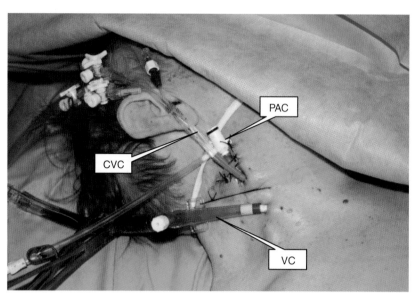

Figure 12.2 Jugular venous cannulation for port-access surgery. A multi-lumen central venous catheter (CVC), pulmonary artery catheter (PAC) introducer sheath and CPB venous cannula (VC) have been inserted.

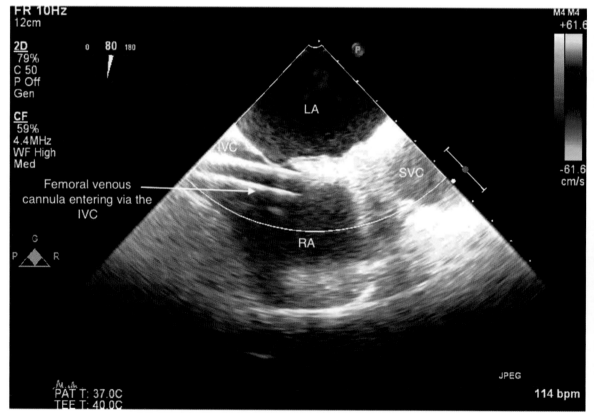

Figure 12.3 Mid-oesophageal bicaval TOE view of femoral venous cannula entering the RA

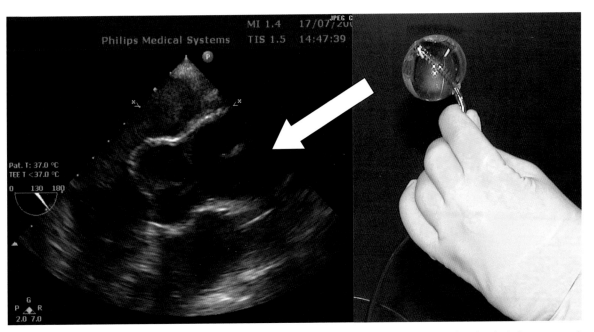

Figure 12.4 The endo-aortic balloon clamp (right). The mid-oesophageal long-axis TOE view is used to confirm that the balloon is correctly positioned in the proximal ascending aorta (left).

cannula in the RA. Its passage can be followed through the right side of the heart using TOE and should be placed at the bifurcation of the main PA.

Aortic Clamping

Aortic cross-clamping is either achieved in a conventional manner by a long external clamp (introduced via either the operative site or a separate incision) or via an endo-aortic balloon clamp introduced via the femoral or subclavian artery. The endo-aortic balloon clamp is inflated in the proximal ascending aorta under TOE guidance (Figure 12.4). Anterograde cardioplegia can then be delivered via the distal port of the balloon clamp or via a separate aortic root cannula.

Postoperative Care

Postoperative care for patients undergoing MICS should follow the same principles as those having cardiac surgery via a conventional approach. The gains of MICS in terms of hospital efficiency and shorter ICU and hospital stay cannot be realized without a systematic approach to the perioperative clinical pathway. Pain is often greater compared to median sternotomy in the first 48 hours. Beyond this point, however, return to normal function is faster and pain scores are lower. Many centres use a multimodal approach comprising IV opiates, local anaesthetic infiltration and peripheral nerve blocks. NSAIDs are excellent, but generally are not used until more than 48 hours after the operation due to the risk of renal failure.

Key Points

- Off-pump surgery requires a greater degree of understanding and communication between the surgeon and anaesthetist than on-pump surgery.
- Off-pump coronary artery surgery is associated with lower blood loss and fewer transfusions, but a greater risk of incomplete revascularization and early reoperation.
- In minimal access cardiac surgery, reduction in surgical access leads to a greater reliance on TOE.
- Non-sternotomy approaches to cardiac surgery require modifications to anaesthetic technique and mandates equipment changes.

Chapter 13

Thoracic Aortic Surgery

Seema Agarwal and Andrew C. Knowles

Thoracic aortic disease is often difficult to detect and may remain asymptomatic until presenting acutely, which in turn is associated with high rates of complications, morbidity and mortality. This chapter provides an overview of anaesthesia for both elective and emergency thoracic aortic surgery.

Pathology

Surgical disease of the thoracic aorta includes aneurysm and dissection. These may occur separately or together and may be congenital or acquired. Acquired disease is usually the result of arterial hypertension and atherosclerosis although, historically, syphilis was an important cause. Congenital causes include connective tissue diseases, such as Marfan, Ehlers–Danlos, Turner and Loeys–Dietz syndromes, and polycystic kidney disease.

Aneurysm

A true aneurysm of the aorta is a permanent dilatation that is at least 50% greater than its original diameter, involving all layers of the aorta. A pseudoaneurysm is a rupture through the layers of the aorta, held together by blood, thrombus and surrounding tissues. A dissection is a disruption of the aortic intima with bleeding into the media.

Untreated aneurysms of the descending and thoracoabdominal aorta that are greater than 6 cm in diameter have a 14.1% annual risk of rupture, dissection or death and the 5-year survival in conservatively managed patients is only 10–20%. Indications for surgery are based on individual patient assessment when the predicted operative risk is less than the risk of optimal medical management and include:

- A rupture or an acute dissection
- Symptomatic enlargement of the aorta – pain or compression of adjacent structures

- Aneurysm enlargement of >1 cm per year or a rapid increase in size
- An absolute diameter of >6.5 cm, or >6.0 cm in patients with connective tissue disease

Aortic Dissection

Dissection of the aorta is often associated with acute arterial hypertension following physical activity or stress. An intimal tear occurs, usually in the presence of a weakened aortic wall and predominantly involving the middle and outer layers of the media. In this area of weakening, the aortic wall is more susceptible to shear forces produced by pulsatile blood flow in the aorta. The most frequent locations of intimal tears are the areas subjected to the greatest mechanical shear forces; the ascending and isthmic (just distal to the left subclavian artery) segments of the aorta are relatively fixed and thus subject the aortic wall to the greatest amount of mechanical shear stress (Figure 13.1).

Classification of Dissection

The DeBakey classification (Figure 13.2) comprises three types, depending on where the intimal tear is located and which section of the aorta is involved:

Type I: The intimal tear is located in the ascending portion, but the dissection involves all portions (ascending, arch and descending) of the thoracic aorta.

Type II: The intimal tear is in the ascending aorta, but the dissection involves the ascending aorta only, stopping before the origin of the innominate artery.

Type III: The intimal tear is located in the descending segment, and the dissection almost always involves the descending portion of the thoracic aorta only, starting just distal to the origin of the left subclavian artery; type III dissections can propagate proximally into the arch, but this is rare.

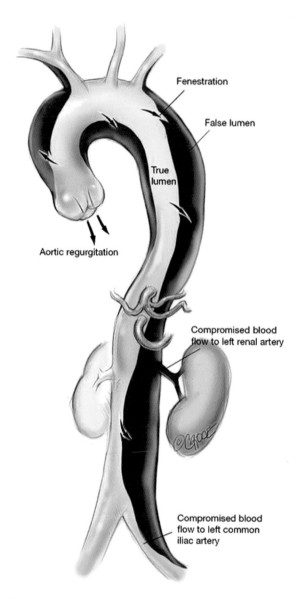

Figure 13.1 A dissection of the aorta (reproduced with kind permission from the Annals of Cardiothoracic Surgery: www.annalscts.com)

The Stanford (Daily) classification (Figure 13.2) comprises two types:

Type A: Dissections that involve the ascending aorta, regardless of where the intimal tear is located and regardless of how far the dissection propagates; clinically, type A dissections run a more virulent course.

Type B: Dissections that involve the aorta distal to the origin of the left subclavian artery.

Classification of aortic dissection

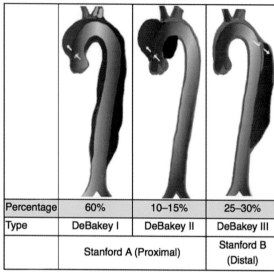

Percentage	60%	10–15%	25–30%
Type	DeBakey I	DeBakey II	DeBakey III
	Stanford A (Proximal)		Stanford B (Distal)

Figure 13.2 The DeBakey and Stanford classifications of an aortic dissection

The survival rate of untreated patients with an aortic dissection is poor, with a 2-day mortality of up to 50% and a 6-month mortality approaching 90%. The usual cause of death is the rupture of the false lumen and a fatal haemorrhage. The overall surgical mortality is approximately 30%, but surgical therapy is often the only viable option for most patients.

Preoperative Assessment

A thorough preoperative assessment should take place, as time allows (Figure 13.3). Specific items to bear in mind include:

- Assessment of premorbid functional capacity
- Examination for evidence of compression of adjacent structures:
  - Stridor or dyspnoea are associated with encroachment onto the trachea or left main bronchus
  - Dysphagia may suggest oesophageal compression
  - Hoarseness may indicate stretching of the recurrent laryngeal nerve
- Baseline neurological examination to document any neurological deficit
- Enquiry into any history of angina, MI, CVA or renal dysfunction

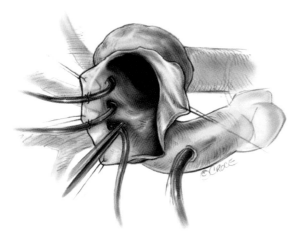

Box 13.1 Investigations prior to major aortic surgery

- Bloods: FBC, urea and electrolyte, liver function tests, clotting screen, glucose, cross-match
- ECG
- Plain posteroanterior and lateral CXR
- Pulmonary function tests: basic spirometry and transfer factor
- CT aorta
- TTE
- Coronary angiography
- Cardiopulmonary exercise testing to determine maximum VO_2 and anaerobic threshold

Figure 13.3 Anterior cerebral cannulation utilized in aortic arch surgery. The aorta is opened under DHCA and arterial cannulae placed directly into the ostia of the innominate, left carotid and left subclavian arteries (reproduced with kind permission from the Annals of Cardiothoracic Surgery: www.annalscts.com).

Baseline investigations are summarized in Box 13.1. They should be performed where possible according to the urgency of surgery and the stability of the patient. Where possible, coronary angiography should be performed to assess the need for concomitant coronary artery bypass surgery. In aneurysmal disease, CT angiography of the aorta allows 3D reconstruction and surgical planning, specifically the presence of thrombus at clamping sites and the patency of key vessels. Imaging may also indicate the presence of trachea or left main bronchus compression that may make insertion of a double-lumen endotracheal tube challenging. Some centres advocate identification of the greater radicular or Adamkiewicz artery, a large segmental artery usually found between vertebral levels T5 and L2, through which the anterior spinal artery may receive a significant proportion of its blood supply.

Anaesthesia for Aortic Surgery

Regardless of the extent of the intended surgery, routine cardiac anaesthetic management should be employed – large-bore IV access, invasive arterial pressure monitoring and central venous access. The need for additional monitoring or vascular access is discussed below. Monitoring of Hb concentration, glucose, electrolytes, ACT, ABG and acid–base status must be undertaken at regular intervals throughout the case.

Surgery Involving the Aortic Root and Ascending Aorta

In situations where an AXC can be applied proximal to the innominate artery, management is similar to that of AV surgery. Where root replacement is performed with reimplantation of the coronary arteries, TOE is indicated before CPB to assess the anatomy of the aorta and after CPB to assess valvular and ventricular function.

Surgery Involving the Aortic Arch

This inevitably involves a period of interruption to the cerebral blood supply, necessitating the use of full CPB and deep hypothermic circulatory arrest (DHCA). The venous cannula is commonly placed in either the RA or a femoral vein. The arterial cannula is usually placed in a femoral or right axillary artery, either directly or via a vascular graft to prevent distal limb ischaemia.

The use of DHCA undoubtedly provides cerebral protection, although opinions on the degree of hypothermia required vary. DHCA at 14–20 °C typically provides 20–30 minutes of safe circulatory arrest (without additional cerebral perfusion) whereas moderate hypothermia (20–28 °C) permits only 10–20 minutes of safe arrest. Surrounding the head with ice or using a cold-water jacket may supplement brain cooling and provide an additional margin of safety, although there is no objective evidence of outcome benefit.

In an attempt to reduce the time required for cooling and rewarming on CPB, some centres combine modest hypothermia with either selective antegrade cerebral perfusion or retrograde cerebral perfusion. These perfusion techniques undoubtedly increase the complexity of the surgical procedure and may provide a false sense of security.

Anaesthetic Management

The right radial artery is preferred for uninterrupted BP monitoring, should the AXC be applied proximal to the left subclavian artery. Following induction of anaesthesia, the trachea is intubated using a double-lumen endotracheal tube when access to the descending aorta is required. Additional vascular access includes a femoral arterial line and large-bore femoral venous access (often a haemofiltration catheter) to allow monitoring of the distal arterial pressure and the rapid infusion of fluids.

Monitoring of the brain and core temperature is required during cooling and rewarming, to ensure that excessive thermal gradients are not created. The nasopharynx temperature correlates closely with the cerebral temperature, whereas the rectal or bladder temperature is a reasonable reflection of the core temperature.

Cerebral Oxygenation Monitoring

Near-infrared spectroscopy (NIRS) is increasingly used during aortic surgery, to provide continuous, real-time, non-invasive monitoring of anterior cerebral circulation (see Chapter 31).

A baseline measurement should be obtained as soon as possible, ideally prior to the induction of anaesthesia. The regional cerebral oxygen saturation (rSO2) should be maintained within 25% of the baseline level and a fall below this level should be investigated and addressed promptly. It has been suggested that the use of NIRS is associated with a lower incidence of postoperative neurological dysfunction. Increasing the CPB flow rate, the Hb concentration and the depth of anaesthesia, and decreasing temperature may be effective in increasing the rSO2. An abrupt decrease in rSO2 should prompt exclusion of CPB cannula displacement or cerebrovenous obstruction.

Surgery Involving the Descending Aorta

Positioning

Access to the entire thoracoabdominal aorta is achieved via a thoracolaparotomy. The patient is positioned with support from a vacuum bean bag in the left helical or semi-lateral position, with the torso and shoulders rotated approximately 60° and the hips, 30° (Figure 13.4).

Surgical Approach

The surgical approach will vary according to the extent of the aneurysm, and clear communication between the surgical and anaesthetic teams is essential. The surgical team must decide between

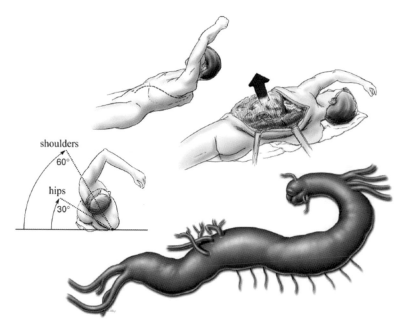

Figure 13.4 Positioning for thoracoabdominal aortic surgery. The patient is positioned such that the upper body is at 60° from horizontal and the hips at 30° from horizontal. A sigmoid-shaped skin incision is made from behind the left scapula, along the 7th rib, across the costal margin, and toward the left periumbilical region. The chest is entered through the 6th intercostal space. (reproduced with kind permission from the Annals of Cardiothoracic Surgery: www.annalscts.com.)

shoulders
60°

hips
30°

approaches requiring left heart bypass (LHB) or conventional CPB with DHCA. Where there is involvement of the aortic arch, or it is otherwise impossible to place a clamp distal to the left subclavian artery, full CPB must be used. Where there is to be no interruption to the cerebral blood supply, the use of LHB is practicable. Figure 13.5 shows a typical LHB system.

The prolonged CPB and hypothermia, with an extensive, adherent aneurysm, is associated with a significant inflammatory response and marked coagulopathy. Although this can also develop following LHB, the response is usually of a lesser magnitude. A final approach, which may be used when the patient is unable to tolerate one lung ventilation and has suitable clamp zones, is to use CPB with cannulae in the ascending/arch of the aorta and in the femoral artery with distal and proximal clamps, respectively.

Anaesthetic Management

A standard anaesthetic induction is performed using a short-acting, non-depolarizing muscle relaxant to facilitate neurophysiological monitoring. To allow exposure of the thoracic aorta (and deflation of the left lung) a double-lumen endotracheal tube is inserted. An arterial catheter is sited in a femoral artery to allow monitoring of the distal perfusion pressure. Large-bore IV access is gained using a haemofiltration catheter in a femoral vein, allowing rapid infusion at rates of up to 750 ml min^{-1} when

required. A central venous catheter and percutaneous introducer sheath are inserted into the *left* internal jugular vein (IJV); insertion into the right IJV may lead to problems with kinking once the patient is positioned. Anaesthesia is maintained with propofol and opiate infusions to allow effective and more reliable neurophysiological monitoring, as described later. TOE is often used to assess cardiac and valvular function, and to confirm positioning of any cannulae inserted peripherally.

LHB

Whilst replacement of the abdominal aorta can be performed with use of an AXC, application of this to the descending thoracic aorta may precipitate marked haemodynamic compromise and organ ischaemia. Cross-clamping of the descending thoracic aorta leads to an abrupt increase in LV afterload and proximal BP. There is a consequent rise in myocardial contractility and oxygen demand, which may outstrip supply, potentially precipitating acute myocardial ischaemia. All organs distal to the proximal AXC will suffer from a lack of perfusion, which may last for hours.

Partial LHB provides perfusion of the distal aorta by pumping blood directly from the left heart whilst maintaining perfusion of the heart and brain via their native circulations. The spinal cord and organs distal to the AXC are afforded some protection with relief of proximal arterial hypertension and LV afterload. LHB can be achieved between the LA or a pulmonary

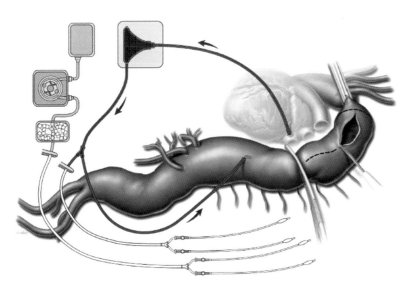

Figure 13.5 LHB. The inflow cannula is placed in the LA via the left inferior pulmonary vein. The outflow cannula is placed in the descending thoracic aorta. (reproduced with kind permission from the Annals of Cardiothoracic Surgery: www.annalscts.com)

vein and either a common femoral artery or the aorta distal to the AXC. The relatively small-volume extra-corporeal circuit and the absence of an oxygenator necessitates only partial heparinization – ACT 200–300 s. Maintaining cerebral perfusion through-out the procedure obviates the need for anything more than passive cooling, with mild hypothermia at around 34 °C.

LHB is typically instituted prior to application of the AXC. Whilst the presence of the LHB circulation reduces the rise in afterload associated with cross-clamping, this is still a time of potential instability and close attention to proximal and distal BPs is required. Unacceptable proximal hypertension may be alleviated by increasing distal bypass flow or by vasodilators or a volatile anaesthetic agent.

Following application of the AXC, the aorta is opened, at which point there may be a significant blood loss and haemodynamic compromise. Cell sal-vage together with rapid infusion devices are often used to allow rapid return of circulating volume to the patient. It is vital that the perfusionist and anaesthetist work in harmony to preserve adequate cerebral per-fusion – this may require a reduction or even cessa-tion of distal LHB flow.

Removal of the AXC in the latter stages of surgery may also be associated with haemodynamic com-promise. The resumption of flow through the des-cending aorta precipitates a fall in LV afterload and BP. Where there has been tissue hypoperfusion, the release of vasoactive mediators may lead to myocar-dial depression and a further fall in the SVR. Pre-emptive vasoconstriction, fluid administration and a gradual removal of the AXC may reduce the magni-tude of this phenomenon.

Maintenance of Spinal Cord Perfusion

Paraplegia following thoracic aortic surgery is a dev-astating and life-limiting complication that occurs in 4–16% of cases. Application of the AXC leads to a reduced distal arterial blood flow and a rise in CVP, which compromises spinal cord perfusion. The replacement of diseased sections of the aorta requires temporary or permanent interruption of arterial col-laterals, leading to spinal cord ischaemia and subse-quent reperfusion injury. Ischaemia causes spinal oedema, hyperaemia and inflammation, thus raising the intra-spinal fluid pressure and compromising spinal cord perfusion further. Risk factors for spinal

cord ischaemia include the extent of the aneurysm, the longer duration of AXC application, emergency surgery, previous surgery to the distal aorta, severe atherosclerotic disease, perioperative hypotension, advanced age and DM.

Interventions thought to reduce the risk of spinal cord injury include sequential clamping of the aorta with reimplantation of intercostal and lumbar seg-mental vessels, neurophysiological monitoring and drainage of the CSF.

CSF Drainage

The spinal cord perfusion pressure (SCPP) is equal to the MAP minus the intrathecal pressure (ITP), thus the insertion of a CSF drainage catheter is performed to reduce the ITP and increase spinal cord perfusion. In most centres, the drain is placed at either L_{34} or L_{45} after induction of general anaesthesia and placement of all invasive lines. Although some centres advocate inserting the drain *before* the induction of anaesthesia, the risk of direct spinal cord or nerve root damage is small.

The ITP is maintained at 10–15 mmHg by draining the CSF – typically at rates up to 20 ml h^{-1}. In most centres, a target SCPP of 70 mmHg is used. This typically requires that ITP >15 mmHg and MAP ≥80 mmHg, a target that may require infusion of a vasopressor such as noradrenaline. Where it is not possible to maintain the ITP at <15 mmHg through CSF drainage, the MAP must be increased further. Where there is evidence of spinal cord ischaemia, the SCPP and MAP target can be increased in 5 mmHg increments, until the level suitable to improve perfu-sion is achieved.

Neurophysiological Monitoring

Neurological function can be assessed using motor evoked potentials (MEPs) or somatosensory evoked potentials (SSEPs). Assessment is performed throughout the perioperative period to allow early identification of spinal cord ischaemia and timely intervention. The use of neurophysiological moni-toring with sequential clamping of the aorta identi-fies key vessels for spinal cord perfusion that must be reimplanted, and helps to ascertain the min-imum acceptable MAP for adequate spinal cord perfusion.

MEPs monitor activity in the descending motor pathways on the anterior spinal cord. Subdermal elec-trodes are used to stimulate the motor cortex, and recordings of the consequent muscle contractions are monitored peripherally. MEPs disappear in the presence of neuromuscular blocking agents, hence the need for short-acting muscle relaxants.

SSEPs, although less frequently used, allow monitoring of the posterior ascending sensory columns and involve stimulation of large mixed sensory and motor nerves. As well as information about spinal cord function, SSEPs can give an indication of the adequacy of perfusion to areas of the cerebral cortex that are supplied by the middle and anterior cerebral arteries.

A fall in amplitude of the electrophysiological signal of more than 50% should prompt reinsertion of intercostal arteries into the graft, along with measures to improve spinal cord perfusion. These involve the maintenance of spinal cord perfusion with a MAP >80 mmHg and distal aortic pressure >60 mmHg. The Hb concentration should be maintained at or above 100 g l^{-1}, and the CSF may be drained at 20 ml h^{-1}. The decision for surgical intervention is usually made within 3–5 minutes of the change in the neurophysiological parameters.

Maintaining Spinal Cord Perfusion in the ICU

Neurophysiological monitoring, ITP monitoring and CSF drainage continue for up to 72 hours after surgery. Once sedation is reduced and the patient is able to cooperate with clinical examination, assessment should focus on the strength of both the proximal and distal leg muscles.

Where there is evidence of neurological impairment, the so-called COPS protocol, as described by Estrera, is initiated, to optimize spinal cord perfusion. COPS is an acronym for **C**SF drain status, optimizing **O**xygen Delivery and assessing the **P**atient **S**tatus (MAP, cerebral perfusion pressure and cognitive status). Where the spinal catheter is patent the patient should be positioned flat and the ITP ideally maintained at <5 mmHg. Oxygen delivery should be optimized through administration of supplemental oxygen or intubation and ventilation to ensure that SpO$_2$ >95%. The Hb concentration is maintained at >120 g l^{-1} and the CI at >2.5 l min^{-1} m^{-2}. The SCPP should be >80mmHg and the MAP >90mmHg. In situations where a drain was not sited perioperatively, for example prior to emergency surgery, the development of delayed neurological symptoms has been successfully treated with postoperative drain insertion.

Fluid Management and Haemostasis

Peri- and postoperative bleeding is a common occurrence. Platelet dysfunction, thrombin activation, disruption of coagulation factor function, hypothermia, fibrinolysis and use of systemic anticoagulant drugs all contribute. Fibrinolysis generally serves to limit coagulation to the site of injury but can become excessive in situations of major blood loss or surgery. Various drugs can be used to counteract this including tranexamic acid, ε-aminocaproic acid and aprotinin.

Cell salvage should be considered as a routine practice. Prior to separation from CPB, point-of-care coagulation tests are performed to assess the extent of coagulopathy. On separation from CPB, protamine is administered to reverse residual heparinization and blood products given as indicated by thromboelastography and laboratory tests of coagulation. These may be FFP, cryoprecipitate and platelets or, more recently, factor concentrates such as prothrombin complex and fibrinogen concentrate. Further transfusions are guided by repeat tests. In cases of ongoing bleeding refractory to administration of clotting products, the use of recombinant factor VIIa has been advocated.

Postoperative Management

Sedation and Analgesia

Sedation is maintained in the postoperative period using IV agents such as propofol, alfentanil and dexmedetomidine. Minimal sedation should be used to allow assessment of neurological function. In surgery where there has been disruption to cerebral blood flow, there is an increased incidence of neurocognitive dysfunction.

The extensive surgical incision required for thoracoabdominal aortic surgery leads to significant pain, which can impede weaning from sedation and mechanical ventilation. The presence of the spinal catheter provides a route for administration of intrathecal diamorphine, providing excellent analgesia.

Complications

Whilst surgery for an aortic aneurysm is potentially lifesaving, there is significant morbidity and mortality. The reported incidence of an adverse outcome (e.g. renal failure requiring dialysis at hospital discharge, stroke or permanent paraplegia or paraparesis) is 16% with an overall operative mortality of 8–10%.

Key Points

- An acute type A aortic dissection is a surgical emergency associated with high mortality.

- Aortic arch surgery is likely to involve circulatory arrest and may involve selective cerebral perfusion techniques.
- Paraplegia following descending thoracic aortic surgery may occur despite all precaustion.

Further Reading

Bavaria J (ed.). Aortic arch surgery (I). *Ann Cardiothorac Surg*: 2013; 2: 147–244.

Bavaria J (ed.). Aortic arch surgery (II). *Ann Cardiothorac Surg*: 2013; 2: 247–386.

Cameron D, Price J (eds.). Type A aortic dissection (I). *Ann Cardiothorac Surg*: 2016; 5: 155–255.

Cameron D, Price J (eds.). Type A aortic dissection (II). *Ann Cardiothorac Surg*: 2016; 5: 257–406.

Catarino P, Iyer S. Aortic surgical patients in the intensive care unit. In Valchanov K, Jones N, Hogue CW (eds), *Core Topics in Cardiothoracic Critical Care*, 2nd edn. Cambridge: Cambridge University Press; 2018, pp. 347–55.

Coselli J, LeMaire S (eds.). Thoracoabdominal aortic aneurysm repair. *Ann Cardiothorac Surg* 2012; 1: 264–425.

Estrera AL, Sheinbaum R, Miller CC, *et al.* Cerebrospinal fluid drainage during thoracic aortic repair: safety

and current management. *Ann Thorac Surg* 2009; 88: 9–15.

O'Neill B, Bilal H, Mahmood S, Waterworth P. Is it worth packing the head with ice in patients undergoing deep hypothermic circulatory arrest? *Interact Cardiovasc Thorac Surg* 2012; 15: 696–701.

Subramaniam K, Park KW, Subramaniam B (eds.). *Anesthesia and Perioperative Care for Aortic Surgery*. New York: Springer-Verlag; 2011.

Chapter

14

Surgery for Cardiomyopathy and Pericardial Disease

Jonathan Brand and Florian Falter

Cardiomyopathy is a disease spectrum that alters the shape, function and conduction of cardiac muscle. Affecting 1 in 500 people it is often incurable; however, symptom control can improve life quality and expectancy.

Hypertrophic Obstructive Cardiomyopathy

Hypertrophic obstructive cardiomyopathy (HOCM) is a progressive disease, caused by a mutation in one of the nine sarcomeric genes. Its inheritance is autosomal-dominant with some heterogeneous phenotypes. The incidence is 0.2–0.5%.

Pathophysiology

Ventricular septal hypertrophy causes LVOT narrowing with thinning of the LV free wall. The narrowing of the LVOT during systole leads to increased systolic ejection velocity, creating a Venturi effect, drawing the anterior mitral valve leaflet (AMVL) toward the hypertrophied septum. Simultaneously, systolic anterior motion (SAM) brings the AMVL into contact with the septum, leading to LVOT obstruction and MR secondary to distortion of the MV in mid to late systole (Figure 14.1). Factors influencing this physiology are summarized in Table 14.1. Decreased compliance and diastolic dysfunction occur through increased muscle mass, decreased LV volume, increased myoplasmic $[Ca^{2+}]$ and myocardial fibrosis.

Clinical Features

The most common presentation is sudden death in previously asymptomatic and athletic individuals. A small number of patients develop exertional symptoms similar to those of AS. Atrial and ventricular dysrhythmias are common.

Investigations

Imaging is the basis of investigation in HOCM, although genetic testing should be undertaken when there is a family history of unexplained sudden death. Common modalities include: echocardiography, cardiac catheterization and cardiac MRI.

Echocardiography characterises the septal thickness and LVOT diameter alongside real-time visualization of pathophysiology. CWD reveals a characteristic 'shark tooth' velocity contour that is different from AS (Figure 14.2), corresponding to velocity increases from SAM during systole.

Table 14.1 Factors determining LVOT obstruction in HOCM

Factors increasing likelihood	Factors decreasing likelihood
↓ Arterial BP	↑ Arterial BP
↓ Preload	↑ LV volume
↑ Blood flow velocity – inotropes	↓ Blood flow velocity – β-blockers/verapamil
↓ SVR	↑ SVR

Eject ⟶ Obstruct ⟶ Leak

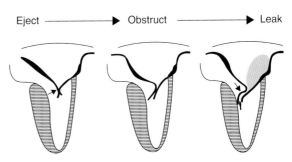

Figure 14.1 SAM of the AMVL dynamic LVOT obstruction and MR in HOCM. Adapted from Grigg LE, Wigle ED, Williams WG, Daniel LB, Rakowski H. *J Am Coll Cardiol* 1992; 20: 42–52.

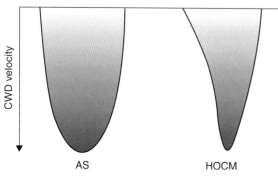

Figure 14.2 CWD findings in AS and HOCM

Box 14.1	Anaesthetic considerations in HOCM
Preload	Better full than empty
HR	Rather 60 than 80 bpm
Rhythm	Preserve NSR
Contractility	Maintain (most patients will tolerate mild depression as long as they are well filled)
SVR	Maintain or slightly increase to preserve coronary perfusion

Management

Medical: β-blockers are the first-line treatment. If the LVOT gradient and symptoms persist, a calcium channel antagonist of the verapamil type should be substituted. Implantation of a dual-chamber pacing device can improve symptoms. High-risk patients can be considered for a combined pacemaker and ICD.

Interventional: Septal myectomy through the AV orifice can relieve LVOT obstruction and is offered to symptomatic patients on maximal medical therapy. In a select group of patients, septal ablation by alcohol injection into LAD septal branches can yield similar results. Complications following intervention include a residual LVOT obstruction, a VSD and conduction abnormalities.

Anaesthetic Goals

Anaesthesia should avoid haemodynamic worsening of any LVOT obstruction and perioperative TOE is always indicated.

Dilated Cardiomyopathy

Dilated cardiomyopathy (DCM) is the most common form of cardiomyopathy, affecting mainly males aged 20–60 years. It causes a third of all cases of congestive heart failure, and although many cases are idiopathic, secondary causes arise due to myocardial damage from toxic, infectious or metabolic insults, which include: sickle cell disease, Duchenne muscular dystrophy, ischaemia, infection (viral, trypanosomal), toxins (ethanol, doxorubicin, cobalt, ionizing radiation), stimulants (amphetamine), thyroid disease (myxoedema), morbid obesity and pregnancy.

Autosomal-dominant inheritance accounts for between 20–40% of patients.

Pathophysiology

DCM is characterized by impaired systolic and diastolic function with progressive ventricular enlargement and reduced compliance, function and increased risk of intracardiac thrombus formation due to low flow. Subsequent atrioventricular valve regurgitation worsens atrial enlargement, increasing the likelihood of AF.

Clinical Features

Patients can be asymptomatic but often develop progressive ventricular failure and declining functional status. Ventricular dysrhythmias are common, as are systemic embolic phenomena in the later stages of disease.

Investigations

DCM is usually diagnosed using echocardiography. 2D echocardiography shows dilatation of all four chambers and poor ventricular contractility. Other investigations such as MRI and cardiac catheterization are rarely of diagnostic value, although the latter may reveal coronary artery and valvular disease that is amenable to surgery.

Management

Patients are treated with standard heart failure therapy, comprising ACE inhibitors, diuretics and possibly digoxin. A pacemaker or ICD should be considered in patients with conduction abnormalities or arrhythmias. Despite medical therapy, a significant number of

Box 14.2	Anaesthetic considerations in DCM
Preload	Already high, avoid overfilling
HR	Avoid tachycardia – impaired ventricular relaxation
Rhythm	NSR preferred – little dependence on late diastolic filling
Contractility	Maintain – inotropic support invariably needed
SVR	Maintain or slight decrease – increase poorly tolerated

Box 14.3	Anaesthetic considerations in restrictive cardiomyopathy
Preload	High
HR	High – in view of fixed SV
Rhythm	NSR preferred – but a little dependent on late diastolic filling
Contractility	Maintain – inotropic support invariably needed
SVR	Maintain – in view of fixed SV

patients die within 3 years of the onset of symptoms. Mechanical ventricular assist devices and cardiac transplantation are of proven prognostic benefit.

Anaesthetic Goals

These are summarized in Box 14.2.

Restrictive Cardiomyopathy

Restrictive or obliterative cardiomyopathy is a rare cause of severe diastolic dysfunction with a high mortality – 70% of patients die within 5 years of symptom onset. Causes are divided into primary, which are often idiopathic; and secondary: to amyloidosis, sarcoidosis, haemochromatosis, carcinoid disease, glycogen-storage diseases, post-radiation and tropical endomyocardial fibrosis.

Pathophysiology

The condition is characterized by increasing ventricular stiffness and endocardial thrombosis, leading to poor ventricular compliance with rapid early diastolic filling. The myocardium is not normally thickened and there are similarities to constrictive pericarditis.

Clinical Features

Patients usually present with signs and symptoms of biventricular failure, although signs of right heart failure predominate. Chest pain and syncope are less common.

Investigations

This include echocardiography, endomyocardial biopsy, CT and cardiac MRI. The key features on echocardiography include biatrial dilatation, normal

systolic function with restricted diastolic relaxation and restrictive filling patterns.

Management

The aim of management is to reduce filling pressures without reducing the CO. Standard heart failure treatment is not helpful as is reduces venous return and systemic BP. On occasion, diuretics are indicated to relieve oedema.

Anaesthetic Goals

These are summarized in Box 14.3.

Constrictive Pericarditis

Constrictive pericarditis causes diastolic dysfunction. Previously a common cause, TB now accounts for 2% of cases. Frequently the aetiology is unknown; however, suspected causes include: infection, chest radiotherapy, connective tissue disease, chest trauma, cardiac surgery and chronic renal failure.

Pathophysiology

Chronic pericardial inflammation causes fibrosis and calcification, encasing the heart in a non-compliant sac, which prevents diastolic filling. This causes rapid early diastolic filling, which ceases when ventricular expansion limits are reached (Figures 14.3 and 14.4). Intracardiac volumes are fixed, leading to exaggerated ventricular interdependence with dissociation of intrathoracic and intracardiac pressures.

Clinical Features

Signs of impaired RV filling predominate, although hepatomegaly and ascites are more common than oedema. In the latter stages of the disease patients often appear malnourished and jaundiced. Although

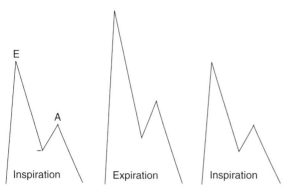

Figure 14.3 PWD transmitral diastolic flow pattern in constrictive pericarditis. Note the high velocity E-wave and short deceleration time.

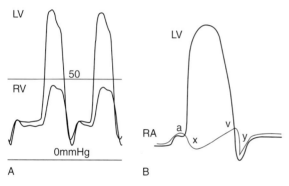

Figure 14.4 Typical pressure waveforms in constrictive pericarditis. (A) The pathognomonic 'square-root sign' can be seen in both the LV and RV pressure traces. (B) Rapid, unimpeded early diastolic filling gives rise to a deep y-descent in the RA pressure trace. The short duration of the y-descent is due to abrupt cessation of early diastolic filling.

it may be difficult to distinguish constrictive pericarditis from restrictive cardiomyopathy, the treatments are different (Table 14.2).

Investigations

Diagnosis is often difficult and requires a high index of suspicion.

Management

Mild pericardial constriction may be amenable to diuretic therapy that is aimed at lowering venous filling pressure. Definitive treatment requires a pericardiectomy. This heralds a significant risk with an associated mortality of 6%. Patients are often in poor physiological condition, and are prone to major haemorrhage and haemodynamic instability during dissection. Pressure-controlled ventilation with no PEEP should be used to maximize LV filling.

Anaesthetic Goals

Anaesthetic considerations are similar to cardiac tamponade, although in constrictive pericarditis ventricular filling occurs in early diastole, in tamponade it occurs in late diastole (Box 14.4).

Ventricular Aneurysms

LV aneurysms can either be false or true. A false ventricular aneurysm (pseudoaneurysm) is a rupture of the ventricular free wall contained by the surrounding pericardium (Figure 14.5). These aneurysms occur following MI, MV, AV and congenital heart surgery. Surgical repair is indicated because of the risk of further rupture and tamponade.

A true ventricular aneurysm is where stretched scar tissue replaces muscle. This appears during diastole as a protruding ventricular wall beyond the expected outline of the cavity, during systole it appears either akinetic or dyskinetic (Figure 14.6).

The majority of LV aneurysms affect the anterior or apical walls and are associated with coronary disease or infarction (often the LAD artery). Functional MR is often present, whilst ventricular arrhythmias and LV failure are the commonest causes of death. A risk of mural thrombus exists in patients with low flow states.

Indications for Surgery

Asymptomatic patients often have a good prognosis without surgery. Surgical repair is often performed with concomitant CABG to reduce ventricular size, wall stress and the risk of subsequent rupture.

Non-Compaction Cardiomyopathy

Non-compaction cardiomyopathy (NCC) or spongiform cardiomyopathy is a rare congenital myocardial abnormality diagnosed by echocardiography and MRI when the trabeculations are more than twice the thickness of the underlying ventricular wall. NCC may be completely asymptomatic, it may present acutely with ventricular tachyarrhythmia or thromboembolism, or with symptoms of progressive cardiac failure.

Takotsubo Cardiomyopathy

Takotsubo cardiomyopathy is a non-ischaemic reversible 'stress' cardiomyopathy, defined by a sudden weakening of cardiac muscle in relation to severe physical or emotional stress. The condition is more common in postmenopausal women and its

Table 14.2 Differential diagnosis of constrictive pericarditis and restrictive cardiomyopathy

	Constrictive pericarditis	Restrictive cardiomyopathy
CXR	Diffuse calcification of pericardium	Normal heart size
CVP	Prominent y- >> x-descents	Elevated. Prominent cv-wave in the presence of TR
PA catheter	PA systolic pressure normally <40 mmHg	PA systolic pressure ≥50 mmHg
LV catheter	'Square-root sign', RVEDP = LVEDP RV systolic pressure ≤50 mmHg	LVEDP – RVEDP >5 mmHg RV systolic pressure ≥50 mmHg
2D echocardiography	Pericardial thickening and effusion	Normal pericardium
Doppler echocardiography	Restrictive pattern Respiratory swing >25% variation in peak mitral velocities during inspiration	Little respiratory swing in velocities
CT and MRI	Pericardial thickness >4 mm	Pericardial thickness <4 mm

Box 14.4 Anaesthetic considerations in pericardial constriction

Preload	Increased
HR	High – in view of fixed SV
Rhythm	NSR preferred – little dependence on late diastolic filling
Contractility	Maintain – inotropic support may be needed
SVR	Maintain

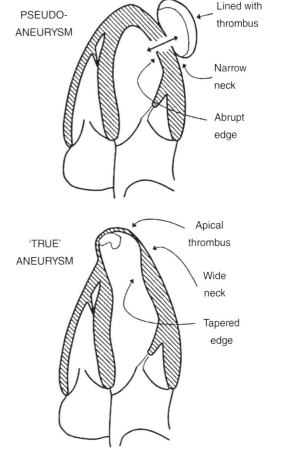

Figure 14.5 False and true aneurysm of the LV (from Otto CM. *Textbook of Clinical Echocardiography*, 2nd edn. WB Saunders, Philadelphia 2000: 221)

presentation often mimics an anterior MI with ECG changes. The pathognonomic systolic LV apical ballooning and basal hyperkinesis are seen during investigation, often in the absence of coronary disease to explain the wall motion abnormalities. The name comes from the Japanese word for octopus trap, which the LV cavity resembles in systole. Treatment is supportive, although avoidance of catecholamine-inducing medications is advised. The prognosis is excellent and LV function normalizes within weeks to months.

Arrhythmogenic Right Ventricular Cardiomyopathy

Since its first report by Marcus *et al.* in 1982, arrhythmogenic right ventricular cardiomyopathy (ARVC) has been identified as one of the leading causes of

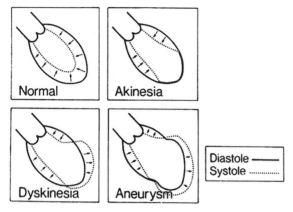

Figure 14.6 The natural history of a true LV aneurysm (from Grondin P, Kretz JG, Bical O, *et al*. Natural history of saccular aneurysms of the LV. *J Thorac Cardiovasc Surg* 1979; 77: 57–64).

arrhythmic cardiac arrest in young people and athletes. This predominanty autosomal-dominant hereditary disease is characterized by progressive replacement of the RV myocardium with fibrofatty tissue. Biopsy samples show abnormalities or loss of desmosomes, leading to disrupted cell junctions, myocyte detachment and cell death. The fatty tissue replacing the myocardium is thought to contribute to the development of ventricular arrhythmias through scar-related macro re-entry mechanisms, similar to those seen following MI. The prevalence of ARVC has long been underestimated. It is now thought to be 1:5,000 in the general population and 1:2,000 in some European countries such as Italy and Germany. It tends to be more malignant in men, which is either due to the direct influence of sex hormones or the gender-specific difference in exercise intensity.

ARVC typically becomes clinically apparent between the ages of 20 and 40 years, with exercise-induced palpitations or syncope. ECG signs include T-wave inversion in the right precordial leads and ventricular arrhythmias with LBBB. However, sudden cardiac death may be the first clinical manifestation of the disease. The diagnosis is difficult due to the low specificity of ECG signs, the array of different causes for ventricular arrhythmias and the often-inconclusive results of genetic testing. To help standardize the diagnosis and to make family screening more accurate a task force produced guidelines on quantitative diagnostic and genetic molecular criteria in 2010.

The aim of any therapeutic approach is palliative. Medical therapy with β-blockers, often together with amiodarone, ICD implantation or catheter ablation is aimed at reducing the risk of sudden cardiac death and increasing the quality of life but to not change the progression of the disease. Mechanical biventricular support or transplantation are the ultimate treatment options for ARVC in cases of untreatable arrhythmias or end-stage heart failure refractory to other therapies.

Fortunately, drugs used for general anaesthesia do not appear to increase arrhythmogenicity. In fact, the opposite appears to be true; by decreasing sympathetic drive they are thought to decrease the incidence of arrhythmias.

Key Points

- Strategies to reduce LVOT obstruction in HOCM include increasing preload and afterload, and reducing myocardial contractility.
- DCM is the most commonly seen cardiomyopathy, resulting in systolic and diastolic heart failure.
- The differentiation between constrictive pericarditis and restrictive cardiomyopathy can be difficult.
- A false ventricular aneurysm is a ventricular free rupture wall contained by the pericardium.
- The first manifestation of ARVC can be sudden cardiac arrest in previously fit and healthy individuals.

Further Reading

Corrado D, Link MS, Calkins H. Arrhythmogenic right ventricular cardiomyopathy. *N Engl J Med* 2017; 376: 61–72.

Irpachi K, Kumar KA, Kapoor PM. Echocardiography for hypertrophic obstructive cardiomyopathy. *Ann Card Anaesth* 2017; 20: 279.

Marcus FI, Fontaine GH, Guiraudon G, *et al*. Right ventricular dysplasia: a report of 24 adult cases. *Circulation* 1982; 65: 384–98.

Pick JM, Batra AS. Implantable cardioverter–defibrillator implantation for primary and secondary prevention: indications and outcomes. *Cardiol Young* 2017; 27: S126–S131.

Varian K, Tang WHW. Therapeutic strategies targeting inherited cardiomyopathies. *Curr Heart Fail Rep* 2017; 14: 321–30.

Weintraub RG, Semsarian C, Macdonald P. Dilated cardiomyopathy. *Lancet* 2017; 390: 400–14.

Zhang L, Piña IL. Stress-induced cardiomyopathy. *Heart Fail Clin* 2019; 15: 41–53.

Chapter 15

Surgery for Pulmonary Vascular Disease

Choo Y. Ng and Andrew Roscoe

Pulmonary vascular surgery comprises emergency procedures such as pulmonary embolectomy and post-traumatic repair, and elective procedures such as palliation of PHT, pulmonary thromboendarterectomy (PTE), tumour resection and the Ross procedure. The focus of this chapter will be PHT and the management of patients undergoing PTE.

Pulmonary Hypertension

PHT is defined as a mean PAP (mPAP) greater than 20 mmHg at rest and can be graded as mild (mPAP 20–30 mmHg), moderate (mPAP 30–40 mmHg) and severe (mPAP > 40 mmHg). It is divided according to PAWP into pre-capillary PHT (PAWP < 15 mmHg) and post-capillary PHT (PAWP > 15 mmHg). The classification of PHT is based on pathophysiology (Box 15.1).

The PVR (in Wood units) is derived from the CO and mPAP:

$$PVR = \frac{mPAP}{CO}$$

A normal PVR is under 3 Wood units (3 mmHg min l^{-1}, i.e. 240 dyne s cm^{-5}).

Management

The treatment of PHT is based on the underlying aetiology.

Class 1 PHT is characterized by medial hypertrophy intimal proliferation of the distal pulmonary arteries. Treatment comprises anticoagulation and pharmacological therapy with pulmonary vasodilators (Table 15.1). Patients whose disease progresses despite maximal medical therapy, with evidence of RV failure, can be considered for lung transplantation.

Class 1' PHT (pulmonary veno-occlusive disease) involves fibrotic occlusion of pulmonary venules. There is no established therapy and early referral for lung transplantation is recommended.

Class 2 PHT is post-capillary in nature and typically presents with pulmonary vein engorgement, capillary dilatation and interstitial oedema. Treatment is aimed at relieving the underlying left-heart pathology. The use of pulmonary vasodilators is not recommended and may be detrimental to outcome.

Class 3 PHT involves intimal obstructive proliferation of distal pulmonary arteries. There is no specific therapy other than oxygen supplementation.

Class 4 PHT is due to CTEPH, with formation of organized thrombi, webs and bands replacing the normal intima, occluding the PAs. In addition, smooth-muscle cell proliferation results in medial thickening and pulmonary vascular remodelling. The mainstay of treatment is surgery, in the form of PTE.

Class 5 PHT is a heterogeneous group of conditions with varying pathology and management is dependent upon aetiology.

Atrial Septostomy

Patients with class 1 PHT have a survival benefit if they have a concurrent PFO. Patients who are refractory to optimal pulmonary vasodilator therapy can be considered for balloon atrial septostomy (BAS) as a palliative or bridging procedure. BAS can decompress the right heart and increase LV preload, enhancing the CO. However, BAS is contraindicated in patients with a baseline SaO_2 below 80%, as the right-to-left shunt will worsen the SaO_2.

RV Pathophysiology

The normal RV is a thin-walled chamber, vulnerable to acute elevations in the PVR, such as PE. The resultant acute increase in RV afterload can precipitate a lethal RV failure. Chronic increases in the PVR lead initially to compensatory RV hypertrophy and, if left untreated, to dilatation and, ultimately, to RV failure. Right coronary artery (RCA) perfusion

Table 15.1 Pulmonary vasodilators

Inhaled	IV	Oral
NO	PDE-5 inhibitors	PDE-5 inhibitors
PGI$_2$ analogues	PGI$_2$ analogues	PGI$_2$ analogues
Milrinone	Milrinone	ET antagonists
	Dobutamine	Riociguat
	Nitroglycerine	Calcium channel blockers

ET, Endothelin; PDE, phosphodiesterase; PGI$_2$ prostaglandin I$_2$.

Box 15.1 Classification of PHT

Class 1 Pulmonary arterial hypertension
   1.1 Idiopathic
   1.2 Inherited
   1.3 Drug-induced
   1.4 Associated with connective tissue disease, HIV infection, portal hypertension, congenital heart disease, schistosomiasis
1' Pulmonary veno-occlusive disease
1" Persistent PHT of the newborn

Class 2 PHT due to left-sided heart disease
   2.1 LV systolic dysfunction
   2.2 LV diastolic dysfunction
   2.3 Valvular disease
   2.4 Congenital/acquired left heart inflow/outflow tract obstruction and congenital cardiomyopathy

Class 3 PHT due to lung disease and/or hypoxia
   3.1 Chronic obstructive pulmonary disease
   3.2 Interstitial lung disease
   3.3 Other pulmonary diseases with mixed restrictive and obstructive pattern
   3.4 Sleep-disordered breathing
   3.5 Alveolar hypoventilation disorders
   3.6 Chronic exposure to high altitude
   3.7 Developmental lung diseases

Class 4 Chronic thromboembolic pulmonary hypertension (CTEPH)

Class 5 PHT with unclear or multifactorial mechanisms
   5.1 Haematological disorders: chronic haemolytic anaemia, myeloproliferative disorders, splenectomy
   5.2 Systemic disorders: sarcoidosis, pulmonary histiocytosis, lymphangioleiomyomatosis
   5.3 Metabolic disorders: glycogen storage disease, Gaucher disease, thyroid disorders
   5.4 Others: tumoural obstruction, fibrosing mediastinitis, chronic renal failure, segmental PHT

From 5th World Symposium on Pulmonary Hypertension, Nice, France.

---

pressure is determined by the aortic root pressure and the RV pressure, and in the normal heart occurs throughout the cardiac cycle. As PHT develops, coronary perfusion becomes predominantly diastolic. When suprasystemic PHT occurs, RV perfusion is confined to diastole, which itself is reduced in duration secondary to the compensatory tachycardia of RV dysfunction (Figure 15.1).

The subsequent imbalance between oxygen supply and demand exposes the RV to ischaemia and dysfunction. This in turn results in an elevated RV end-diastolic pressure (RVEDP), a reduced CO and systemic hypotension, which further reduces the coronary perfusion pressure, producing a downward spiral of a worsening RV function and decreased CO, ultimately culminating in RV failure.

Pulmonary Thromboendarterectomy

CTEPH is an under-recognized disease process, which carries a poor prognosis if not treated. The incidence of CTEPH in patients surviving an acute PE is up to 4%. CTEPH may occur following a single PE and is more likely if the patient is over 70 years old and the initial mPAP is >50 mmHg. PTE is the treatment of choice for the majority of patients with CTEPH, where the disease process is proximal enough to allow surgical excision. Distal disease is managed medically.

Anaesthetic Considerations

Anxiolytic premedication is usually avoided due to the potential worsening of hypoxia or hypercarbia, which may precipitate an increase in the PVR and RV afterload. Preoperative anticoagulation therapy is ubiquitous, although warfarin is now less prevalent following the introduction of newer direct thrombin inhibitors and factor Xa inhibitors. These agents are typically stopped several days prior to surgery and anticoagulation treatment bridged with low-molecular-weight

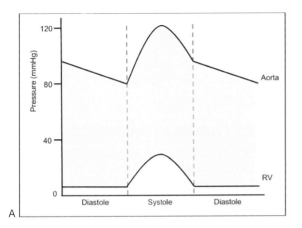

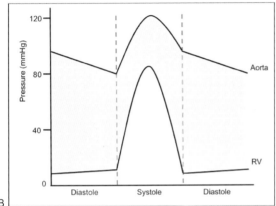

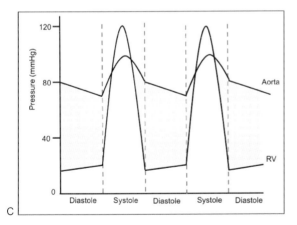

Figure 15.1 RV coronary perfusion (shaded area) in (A) normal heart, (B) moderate PHT, (C) suprasystemic PHT

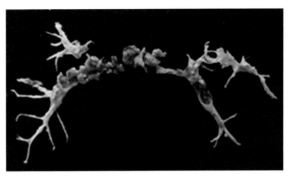

Figure 15.2 Typical surgical specimen excised during PTE surgery

typically determined by institutional guidelines. The anaesthetic goals are:

- Maintain RV perfusion
- Maintain sinus rhythm/avoid bradycardia
- Augment RV contractility
- Avoid increases in RV preload
- Avoid hypoxaemia and hypercarbia

These are achieved by avoiding systemic hypotension during induction with vasopressors, and augmenting RV contractility with positive inotropic agents. Patients are usually anaesthetized in a semi-recumbent position to avoid acute increases in RV preload. Once the trachea is intubated, the patient can be hyperventilated with a high FiO_2 to decrease the risks of hypoxaemia and hypercarbia.

Post-induction monitoring includes CVP, PA catheter, TOE and cerebral oximetry. Maintenance of anaesthesia is achieved by an IV infusion of propofol.

Following sternotomy, CPB is instituted and the patient is cooled to 20 °C. Deep hypothermic circulatory arrest (DHCA) is used to arrest blood flow in the bronchial circulation, which has often developed significant collateral vessels and impedes surgical vision during the endarterectomy dissection. Cerebral protection involves IV administration of methylprednisolone, topical head cooling and cerebral oximetry monitoring to limit the duration of each DHCA. A typical excised endarterectomy specimen is shown in Figure 15.2.

During the rewarming phase other procedures, such as valve surgery or CABG, can be performed if required. Weaning from CPB is attempted when the core body temperature is stable at 36 °C. A low-dose inotrope infusion is commenced and TOE is useful to assess RV function. Successful surgery is reflected by a decrease in the PVR and mPAP.

heparin. Vitamin K is often administered to patients to ensure full warfarin reversal in those with INR >1.3.

Routine monitoring and invasive arterial pressure are standard prior to induction. IV induction can be achieved with any combination of agents and is

Complications

Reperfusion injury: Reperfusion oedema may occur in up to 15% of patients. It typically occurs 24–48 hours after PTE, but may be evident immediately after CPB. In its mildest form it manifests as persistent hypoxaemia and treatment is supportive. At its worst it results in florid pulmonary oedema. In this scenario, veno-venous ECMO is instituted to provide oxygenation until the oedema resolves, usually within 1 week.

PA disruption: Rupture of the pulmonary vessels during surgical dissection is a rare but potentially fatal complication. It presents during weaning from CPB as frank blood in the endotracheal tube. On TOE examination, persistent air is seen in the left side of the heart. Management is to immediately reinstitute CPB to reduce blood flow through the pulmonary circulation. The patient is then weaned from CPB onto central veno-arterial ECMO. Anticoagulation is reversed and the patient can remain on ECMO until bleeding into the airway resolves.

RV failure: The management of PHT and RV failure involves optimizing RV preload, reducing RV afterload and enhancing RV contractility by maintaining the coronary perfusion pressure. Volume loading in RV failure is usually detrimental. The RV has a flatter Starling curve than the LV, so increases in preload result in RV dilatation with little increase in SV. The negative sequelae of RV dilatation include:

- Increase in the RVEDP, reducing the RV perfusion pressure
- Increase in RV free wall tension, increasing oxygen demand
- Tricuspid annulus dilatation, exacerbating TR
- Shift of the interventricular septum to the left, impeding LV diastolic filling

RV afterload can be reduced by avoiding hypoxaemia, hypercarbia and acidaemia, and by administering pulmonary vasodilators (Table 15.1). The RV perfusion pressure is maintained by avoiding systemic hypotension and RV contractility is augmented by positive inotropic agents.

Balloon Pulmonary Angioplasty

In CTEPH patients who are considered inoperable, or patients with residual PHT, post PTE, catheter-based balloon angioplasty dilatation of the PA circulation can be offered. Target vessels are typically subsegmental and can be dilated with a 2 mm angioplasty balloon. The procedure is usually done under local anaesthesia with little or no sedation. Complications include reperfusion oedema and PA perforation, both of which carry a high mortality.

Outcomes

After successful PTE, haemodynamic recovery is often immediate, with a reduced PVR and RV size. RV reverse remodelling occurs over the following months and functional capacity recovers. Reported 1-year survival is approximately 93%.

Key Points

- CTEPH is an under-diagnosed condition.
- PTE is the treatment of choice for the majority of patients with CTEPH.
- Right coronary perfusion pressure must be maintained to avoid RV ischaemia.
- RV failure carries a poor prognosis.
- Balloon pulmonary angioplasty may provide an alternative treatment in inoperable CTEPH patients.

Further Reading

Ashes CM, Roscoe A. Transesophageal echocardiography in thoracic anesthesia: pulmonary hypertension and right ventricular function. *Curr Opin Anesthesiol* 2015; 28: 38–44.

Delcroix M, Lang I, Pepke-Zaba J, et al. Long-term outcome of patients with chronic thromboembolic pulmonary hypertension. *Circulation* 2016; 133: 859–71.

Galie N, Humbert M, Vachiery JL, *et al.* 2015 ESC/ERS Guidelines for the diagnosis and treatment of pulmonary hypertension. *Eur Heart J* 2016; 37: 67–119.

Haddad F, Elmi-Sarabi M, Fadel E, *et al.* Pearls and pitfalls in managing right heart failure in cardiac surgery. *Curr Opin Anesthesiol* 2016; 29: 68–79.

Hosseinian L. Pulmonary hypertension and noncardiac surgery: implications for the anesthesiologist. *J Cardiothorac Vasc Anesth* 2014; 28: 1064–74.

Kanwar MK, Thenappan T, Vachiery JL. Update in treatment options in pulmonary hypertension. *J Heart Lung Transplant* 2016; 35: 695–703.

Ogo T. Balloon pulmonary angioplasty for inoperable chronic thromboembolic pulmonary hypertension. *Curr Opin Pulm Med* 2015; 21: 425–31.

Shenoy V, Anton JM, Collard CD, *et al.* Pulmonary thromboendarterectomy for chronic thromboembolic pulmonary hypertension. *Anesthesiol* 2014; 120: 1255–61.

Simonneau G, Montani D, Celermajer DS, *et al.* Haemodynamic definitions and updated clinical classification of pulmonary hypertension. *Eur Respir J* 2019; 53: 1801913.

Chapter

16

Ventricular Assist Device Implantation

Nicholas J. Lees

Introduction

Mechanical circulatory support (MCS) can be used in a setting of either acute or chronic heart failure in selected patients refractory to medical management, to augment the failing circulation due to pump failure and to avert organ failure. There are a variety of devices available, which may be employed for short- or long-term support. Longer-term support may only be afforded by a ventricular assist device (VAD) or cardiac transplantation. VADs are used most commonly for left ventricular support (LVADs), but may also be used for the RV (RVADs) or for biventricular support (BIVADs).

Over recent years there have been considerable technological advances in the various devices available, making them smaller and less traumatic once implanted, with improved safety profiles and reliability. The principal driver has been the gap between the supply and demand of organs for cardiac transplantation, which remains the 'gold standard' of treatment for eligible patients with non-recoverable heart failure.

VADs may be implanted as destination therapy for those ineligible for transplant (age or co-morbidities) or as either a bridge to recovery of heart function after a period of ventricular unloading; or as a bridge to transplantation (BTT) which represents the bulk (80–90%) of implants. Destination therapy is not currently approved in the UK.

The main aims of LVAD therapy are to improve heart failure symptoms, which are a huge burden to affected patients in terms of quality of life and prognosis. Other than transplantation, LVADs are the only option that can significantly improve the symptoms of advanced NYHA classes 3–4 heart failure. In addition, LVADs allow stabilization and indeed reversal of organ dysfunction (renal and liver in particular), PHT and PVR, which if high may preclude transplantation. Published in 2001, the Randomized

Evaluation of Mechanical Assistance for the Treatment of Congestive Heart Failure (REMATCH) trial showed better survival (more than double at 1 year) and quality of life compared with optimal medical management using a first-generation LVAD (Heart-Mate V). With current devices there is >70% survival at 2 years.

Devices and Design

VADs comprise an inflow cannula, a pump (which may be implantable or extracorporeal), a power supply and an outflow cannula. The pump is connected to a controller unit by a driveline. In the case of an LVAD, blood from the LA or LV is pumped to the aorta, maintaining the circulation and decompressing the LV. In an RVAD, blood from either the RA or RV is pumped to the PA to support the failing RV. For biventricular support, two separate pumps are required; in the case of the Total Artificial Heart this may be a fully implantable system. Devices differ in their flow characteristics (non-pulsatile or pulsatile), implantability and ability to support the left or right heart. Newer devices generate a continuous non-pulsatile flow, so generate no pulse, and are designed to be small, easily implantable and cause minimal damage to the blood. LVAD patients may or may not have a pulse depending on intrinsic LV function and VAD flow.

Indications and Patient Selection

For MCS devices, the Interagency Registry for Mechanically Assisted Circulatory Support (INTERMACS) profile is a useful guide that helps classify patients with heart failure at the time of implantation (Table 16.1). The management strategy and choice of device largely depends on urgency and risk. Other factors involved in decision-making include anatomical barriers to device placement and function, perioperative risk (sepsis, bleeding risk, organ failure, etc.), the likely need for additional temporary or

Table 16.1 INTERMACS® patient profiles

Profile	Description/patient characteristics	Time frame
1	**Critical cardiogenic shock** 'Crashing and burning', life-threatening hypotension and rapidly escalating inotropic and vasopressor support, with critical organ hypoperfusion often manifested by worsening acidosis and lactate levels	Hours
2	**Progressive decline** 'Dependent' on inotropic support but deterioration of nutrition, renal function, fluid retention or other major status indicator	Days
3	**Stable but inotrope-dependent** Clinically stable on, but unable to wean off, mild–moderate doses of IV inotropes (or with a temporary MCS device)	Days–weeks
4	**Symptoms at rest** Patients can be managed at home on oral therapy	Weeks–months
5	**Comfortable at rest but *limited by exertion*** Patients can be managed at home on oral therapy	Months–years
6	**Comfortable at rest but *exertion intolerant*** Patients can be managed at home on oral therapy	
7	**NYHA class 3 equivalent** Patients can be managed at home on oral therapy	

long-term RV support (RVAD or BIVAD) and the estimated time a patient might spend on the transplant waiting list.

Acute Heart Failure and Cardiogenic Shock

In the situation of critical cardiogenic shock refractory to inotropic support, or with progressive organ dysfunction despite the use of inotropes (INTERMACS profile 1), temporary MCS is indicated. The IABP is commonly used as a temporizing measure especially in the setting of cardiogenic shock following acute MI and coronary intervention; however, outcomes have not been shown to be significantly different to standard care. Veno-arterial ECMO is usually the first-line treatment in this setting as it is can be instituted relatively quickly (especially when inserted percutaneously) and provides rapid support of the failing circulation.

There are a variety of other short-term MCS devices that may be used (Table 16.2), some designed for a few days (e.g. Impella); others suitable for longer. The aim is to bridge the patient to recovery, or to the next 'decision' – definitive reparative surgery, additional medical therapy, long-term VAD implantation or transplantation. The most common indications for acute VAD implantation outside of the setting of the cardiac catheter laboratory are post-cardiotomy heart failure (i.e. failure to wean from CPB) and acute myocarditis, where there is potential for recovery. An LVAD has particular advantages over ECMO in that it will unload a failing LV and reduce the LV wall tension, which may better

facilitate recovery. A common indication for a temporary RVAD is RV failure after LVAD implantation. Long-term implantable VADs are very rarely used in the acute setting, particularly when the patient's neurological status is unknown.

A commonly used device in the emergent setting is the CentriMag® system (Figure 16.1). This comprises a high durable magnetically levitated centrifugal (impeller) pump, capable of generating flows of up to 10 l min^{-1} with minimal damage to blood. This system may be used as an LVAD or RVAD, with or without an oxygenator. Tunnelling the inflow and outflow cannulae through the epigastric skin permits chest closure and aids nursing care.

Bridge to Transplant or Destination Therapy

A successful outcome depends very much on appropriate patient selection. In the case of BTT, patients are often those who deteriorate on medical therapy while already waiting for a heart transplant or have potentially reversible contraindications such as organ dysfunction, which may improve once on VAD therapy (INTERMACS profiles 2-4). In this situation it is usual to use a long-term VAD, unless the patient has had an acute, critical deterioration whilst on the 'urgent' transplant list.

Table 16.3 shows some of the commercially available long-term LVADs (Figures 16.2–16.4). Continuous-flow devices have demonstrated better safety profiles compared to older pulsatile devices. Once the LVAD is in place the patient can be

Table 16.2 Short-term VADs

Device	Mechanism	Notes
CentriMag® (Thoratec Corporation, St Jude Medical)	Impeller, centrifugal flow	LVAD, RVAD or BIVAD support An oxygenator may be incorporated into circuit
Thoratec pVAD	Pneumatic, pulsatile flow	Capable of LVAD, RVAD or BIVAD support Bulky Paracorporeal >30 years' clinical experience
Protek Duo catheter (CardiacAssist Inc, USA)	Connect to blood pump such as CentriMag to work as a continuous flow RVAD	Percutaneously placed dual-lumen catheter, diverts blood from RA to PA
Abiomed Impella (Abiomed Inc, USA)	Sits across AV into LV, flow using microaxial blood pump Up to 2.5 and 5 l min^{-1} blood flow capability versions available	Percutaneously placed in catheter laboratory Impella 5.0™ can support blood flow up to 5 l min^{-1}, licensed up to 6 days Can also be placed surgically (Impella LD™)
HeartMate PHP (Thoratec Corporation, St Jude Medical)	Similar to Impella Flows around 4 l min^{-1}	Percutaneous, catheter based

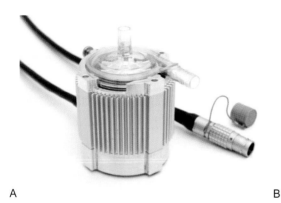

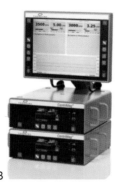

Figure 16.1 CentriMag® VAD. (A) CentriMag® impeller unit sitting on motor unit and (B) drive console. (Images courtesy of St. Jude Medical, Inc.)

A

B

discharged from hospital, followed up as an outpatient and placed on the transplant list once fit. Many patients will not end up being transplanted. In this case the LVAD represents destination therapy because some patients die on the waiting list and some patients never end up meeting criteria for transplantation. VADs for destination therapy will likely become more commonplace as device costs fall and donor organs remain in short supply.

Preoperative Assessment

Patients may be acutely unwell in the case of postcardiotomy heart failure and already in the operating room. In this situation, the inflow cannula required for LVAD support is placed directly into the LA or LV and the outflow cannula into the ascending aorta. Once VAD flow has started, the patient can be weaned from CPB and transferred to intensive care for further management. In the case of long-term VAD implantations, either as BTT or destination therapy, the patient is typically not acutely unwell but has severe heart failure. Assessment should include the likely aetiology, current medication and other co-morbidities. Patients often have cardiac resynchronization therapy devices or ICDs, which should be interrogated, and therapies deactivated immediately prior to surgery. The decision to proceed

Table 16.3 Long-term VADs

Device	Mechanism	Notes
HeartMate II (Thoratec Corporation, St Jude Medical, USA)	Continuous axial flow 6,000–15,000 rpm $\leq$10 l min^{-1} flow	Intraperitoneal placement Over 20,000 implants worldwide
HeartWare HVAD (HeartWare International Inc., USA)	Magnetically suspended impeller, continuous centrifugal flow, 1,800–4,000 rpm $\leq$10 l min^{-1} flow	Intrapericardial placement Over 10,000 implants worldwide Non-inferior to HeartMate II with respect to survival free from disabling stroke
HeartMate 3 (Thoratec Corporation, St Jude Medical, USA)	Magnetically suspended, continuous flow, 4,800-6,500 rpm, $\leq$10 l min^{-1} flow	Intrapericardial placement
ReliantHeart aVAD (ReliantHeart, USA)	Magnetically suspended, axial flow	Intrapericardial (pump placed in ventricle), true flow measured
Syncardia Total Artificial Heart (Syncardia Systems, USA)	Pneumatically driven, pulsatile, four mechanical valves	Intrapericardial Only long-term biventricular support licensed as BTT
HeartMate VE/XVE LVAD (Thoratec Corporation, St Jude Medical, USA)	Pulsatile, older generation	Licensed in USA as destination therapy

to LVAD implantation is usually made by a multidisciplinary team, comprising surgeons, cardiologists, intensivists and other transplant team members – documentation supporting the decision should be examined. Of particular importance is the evaluation of the right heart function, as poor RV function may be a contraindication for LVAD insertion. There are a number of echocardiographic features of RV function that should be noted because preoperative RV dysfunction significantly increases the risk of requiring a temporary RVAD.

Perioperative Management

An arterial cannula and a large-bore venous cannula are placed prior to induction of anaesthesia. Induction is slow and careful. The airway is secured using an endotracheal tube; note that in some circumstances the surgeon may choose a less invasive approach such as thoracotomy, in which case lung isolation using a double-lumen tube is required. Following induction, a central venous catheter, a PA catheter, additional venous access for fluid, a urinary catheter and a TOE probe are placed. External defibrillation pads should be placed on the chest away from

the intended site of operation. One should have available infusions of vasopressors, inotropes (typically milrinone and/or adrenaline) and inhaled NO. The procedure is usually performed on CPB using a midline sternotomy; however, there are various sternum-sparing approaches. The current practice at our institution is femoral cannulation for CPB and bilateral anterior thoracotomies; left-sided to place the device into the apex of the LV and right-sided for the aortic outflow graft.

TOE examination of the heart once the VAD has been implanted is essential to confirm optimal device positioning, cardiac de-airing and competence of the AV (Box 16.1). Following VAD activation, TOE allows visual assessment of the extent of the LV unloading, movement of the interventricular septum and RV function. Close communication between the anaesthetist/TOE operator, surgeon, perfusionist and VAD operator is required at the point of weaning from CPB and increasing the flow on the VAD. Signs of RV failure need to be recognized and promptly addressed. Inotropes are commenced prior to weaning from CPB, inodilators such as milrinone may have benefits in reducing the PVR but it is very likely that vasopressors will be needed. Epinephrine is

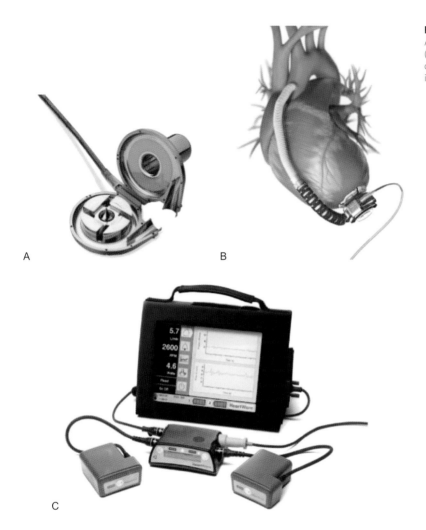

Figure 16.2 HeartWare HVAD. (A) A pump unit opened to show impeller, (B) as implanted and (C) with external controllers (small portable and larger in-hospital devices shown) with batteries.

A

B

C

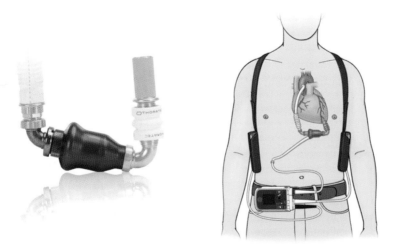

Figure 16.3 HeartMate II LVAD (images provided courtesy of St. Jude Medical, Inc.)

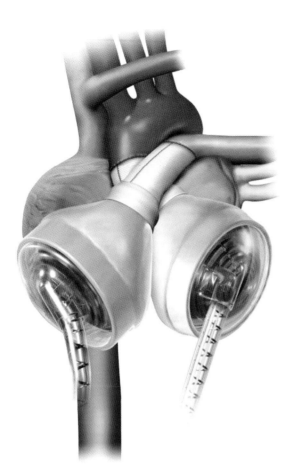

Box 16.1 TOE considerations for VAD implantation

Pre-VAD assessment

RV function

Degree of TR

Presence of shunts (ASD, PFO, small VSD) (need closing at time of surgery)

AR (requires surgical intervention if moderate or severe)

PR (for RVADs)

MS (may require replacement if moderate or severe)

Aortic pathology (aneurysm, dissection, plaque)

Intracardiac thrombus

Post-VAD insertion assessment

De-airing of cardiac chambers

RV function assessment, TR

Cannula alignment and flow (outflow usually not visible in LVADs)

Ventricular septum position

LV unloading

AV movement (may be intermittently or not opening once VAD functioning)

AR

New shunts

Post-surgical collections

Figure 16.4 Syncardia Total Artificial Heart showing prosthetic 'ventricles' attached to the native atria and ascending aorta and PA (courtesy of Syncardia.com)

commonly used, but choice is largely down to institutional preference. Inhaled NO is usually used at the time of separation from CPB, as a potent pulmonary vasodilator to reduce the RV afterload.

Bleeding should be managed before transferring the patient to the ICU, taking care to avoid volume overload. Many of the patients will have been on antiplatelets or anticoagulants pre-op. Prothrombin complex concentrates are often used; one of the benefits is the lower volume of administration required. Excessive bleeding and transfusion are risk factors for RV dysfunction and the need for RVAD support.

Postoperative Care

Patients are transferred to the ICU sedated and mechanically ventilated, with full monitoring and typically inhaled NO still running. Early management of the

LVAD patient in ICU is mainly focused on preserving the RV function. CO monitoring is continued using the PA catheter, with a low threshold for further TOE. Signs of RV failure will be a rise in the CVP and PAP with hypotension, a fall in the CO/index and falling VAD flows. In these situations inotropic support can be increased to augment the RV function. Signs of RV failure, worsening metabolic acidosis, rising serum lactate concentration and oliguria in the face of escalating support should prompt early consideration of an RVAD. In some circumstances, VA ECMO can be used as a bridge to RV recovery. This is less invasive than RVAD implantation and can be instituted at the bedside. Recently, a percutaneous RVAD has been developed (Protek Duo cannula), which can be placed with imaging guidance via the internal jugular vein. Arrhythmias should be controlled (DC cardioversion is not contraindicated) so as not to worsen RV function. Renal replacement therapy is often used to manage volume status as well as acute kidney injury, which occurs in more than 10% of patients.

Once surgical bleeding is controlled and there is no concern about RV function, the inhaled NO is weaned off and the patient woken and the trachea extubated. In some situations, the inhaled NO can be changed to IV or oral sildenafil if there is an ongoing concern about PHT and RV function. A heparin infusion is then usually commenced. Once stable and discharged to the ward, patients will be established on antiplatelet and anticoagulant therapy, heart failure medication and daily symptom surveillance. VAD malfunction is very rare, but complications related to the VAD include the risks of anticoagulation, stroke, pump thrombosis and driveline infections.

Key Points

- VADs may be used as a bridge to cardiac recovery or as a bridge to cardiac transplantation.
- VADs may be used as destination therapy in some territories but this indication is currently unlicensed in the UK.
- The commonest indications for acute LVAD support are post-cardiotomy shock and acute myocarditis.
- Maintenance of the RV function is essential during and after LVAD implantation.
- Patients with an LVAD may have no palpable pulse, making conventional NIBP measurement difficult if not impossible.

Further Reading

Desai SR, Hwang NC. Advances in left ventricular assist devices and mechanical circulatory support. *J Cardiothorac Vasc Anesth* 2018; 32: 1193–213.

Feldman D, Pamboukian SV, Teuteberg JJ, *et al.* The 2013 International Society for Heart and Lung Transplantation guidelines for mechanical circulatory support: executive summary. *J Heart Lung Transplant* 2013; 32: 157–87.

Lampert BC. Perioperative management of the right and left ventricles. *Cardiol Clin* 2018; 36: 495–506.

Rogers JG, Pagani FD, Tatooles AJ, *et al.* Intrapericardial left ventricular assist device for advanced heart failure. *N Engl J Med* 2017; 376: 451–60.

Rose EA, Gelijns AC, Moskowitz AJ, *et al.* Long-term use of a left ventricular assist device for end-stage heart failure. *N Engl J Med* 2001; 345: 1435-43.

Heart Transplantation

Lenore F. van der Merwe and Alan D. Ashworth

The first successful human-to-human heart transplant was performed by Christiaan Barnard in 1967 but the initial outcomes were poor. The introduction of ciclosporin resulted in a significant improvement in survival, leading to an increase in heart transplantation through the 1980s. A total of 5,149 heart transplants, including 4,547 adult transplants, were performed at 302 transplant centres worldwide in the year to July 2017, with 86% 1-year survival, just over 50% survival at 10 years and a median survival of 11 years.

In the last few years, transplantation after donation after circulatory-determined death (DCD) has been investigated as an additive alternative to donation after brain death (DBD). Adoption of this technique may increase the number of donor organs by more than 20%. Initial studies suggest that 2-year survival after DCD transplantation is the same as DBD transplantation.

Indications

Heart transplantation remains the definitive treatment for end-stage heart failure with impaired LV systolic function and NYHA class 3–4 symptoms despite optimal medical, device and surgical treatment. The aetiology of end-stage heart failure leading to heart transplantation are summarized in Box 17.1.

Contraindications

The timing of patient evaluation for heart transplantation is of key importance. Patients should be referred before irreversible complications occur, as these may complicate or contraindicate transplantation (Box 17.2).

Contraindications to heart transplantation include conditions that would significantly increase morbidity or mortality after transplantation, shorten life-expectancy, complicate postoperative recovery or

> **Box 17.1** Aetiology of heart failure in adult heart transplant recipients
>
> - Cardiomyopathy – predominantly dilated cardiomyopathy (56%)
> - IHD (35%)
> - Valvular heart disease (3%)
> - Adult congenital heart disease (3%)
> - Re-transplant for graft failure (3%)
> - Other less common indications for transplantation include:
>
> Persistent ventricular arrhythmias, refractory to standard therapies
>
> Refractory debilitating angina, unresponsive to conventional therapy
>
> Restrictive cardiomyopathy
>
> Hypertrophic cardiomyopathy
>
> Arrhythmogenic right ventricular cardiomyopathy
>
> Peripartum cardiomyopathy
>
> Acute myocarditis

preclude long-term compliance with immunosuppression (Box 17.3).

Organ dysfunction may occur as a result of severe heart failure and may be potentially reversible with medical therapy or the use of mechanical circulatory support (MCS) as a bridge to transplantation. PHT secondary to pulmonary venous congestion is common in heart-transplant recipients and is associated with RV dysfunction and increased mortality. A TPG above 15 mmHg and a PVR above 5 Wood units (400 dyne s cm^{-5}) is associated with a significant increase in mortality and is therefore a contraindication to heart transplantation.

TPG = mean PAP − PAWP
PVR = TPG/CO

Box 17.2 Indications for referral for heart transplantation evaluation

- RV failure or increasing PAP on optimal treatment
- Deteriorating renal function attributable to heart failure
- Persistent heart failure and/or increasing brain natriuretic peptide on optimal medical treatment
- Two or more admissions within 12 months for treatment of decompensated heart failure
- Significant ventricular arrhythmias despite optimal medical, electrophysiology and device therapy
- Seattle Heart Failure Model (SHFM*) score indicating $\geq$20% 1-year mortality
- Liver dysfunction, hyponatraemia, anaemia or involuntary weight loss attributable to heart failure

Indications for urgent inpatient referral:

- Requirement for continuous inotrope infusion and/or IABP
- Persisting coronary ischaemia
- Persistent circulatory shock as a result of a primary cardiac disorder

*Data from *Circulation* 2006; 113: 1424–33.

Box 17.3 Contraindications to heart transplantation

- Allosensitization – anti-human leucocyte antigen antibodies
- Severe irreversible PHT
- Age >70 years (transplant unlikely >65 years in UK)
- Obesity: BMI >35 kg m^{-2}
- DM with end-organ damage or poor glycaemic control
- Severe renal dysfunction (estimated GFR <30 ml min^{-1} per 1.73 m^2)
- Active malignancy or a history of malignancy with probability of recurrence
- Severe cerebrovascular disease
- Severe peripheral vascular disease
- Advanced liver or lung disease
- Recent PE
- Infection (sepsis and active infections)
- Frailty
- Active substance abuse
- Severe cognitive-behavioural disabilities, dementia, insufficient social supports or other demonstrated inability to comply with instructions and drug therapy
- Mechanical ventilation
- Autoimmune disorders
- Infiltrative cardiac diseases
- Severe skeletal myopathies

Anaesthesia for Heart Transplantation

Heart transplantation presents significant anaesthetic challenges. Patients in end-stage heart failure typically have both systolic and diastolic dysfunction manifested by a low CO (SV), elevated ventricular end-diastolic volume and pressure, and pulmonary and hepatic venous congestion. Levels of circulating catecholamines are elevated, leading to down-regulation of adrenergic receptors, diminished myocardial catecholamine stores and reduced sensitivity to inotropes. The failing heart is preload-dependent and afterload-sensitive – minor changes in the SVR, CVP, HR, heart rhythm and cardiac contractility are poorly tolerated. In addition, heart failure alters the pharmacodynamics and pharmacokinetics of many anaesthetic drugs. The anaesthetist should anticipate these changes to avoid excessive myocardial depression and changes in vascular resistance.

The functional status of patients ranges from the ambulatory outpatient to the obtunded critically ill patient on multiple IV inotropes, an IABP and MCS. As a consequence of the shortage of donor organs, around half of recipients are bridged with MCS.

Heart transplantation is generally considered to be an urgent or emergent procedure, as delays to organ implantation increase the ischaemic time and the risk of ischaemia-reperfusion injury. Minimizing the delay requires close communication between the donor harvest and implantation teams.

With the exception of the most urgent cases, the majority of recipients will have already undergone extensive assessment, investigation and preparation. Nevertheless, a rapid yet thorough preoperative assessment should be undertaken; focusing on current symptoms and functional status, current medication (including anticoagulation and antiplatelet therapy), the current level of cardiovascular support, fasting status and airway evaluation. Recent laboratory investigations, imaging, pulmonary function tests and right heart catheter studies should be reviewed to exclude any recent deterioration.

The timing of implant surgery and organ procurement will have to take into account any factors that might prolong recipient preparation, for example previous cardiac surgery. A modified rapid sequence induction may be indicated as patients are often inadequately fasted.

Recipients often have an implanted rhythm management device that will be removed at the end of surgery. These should be interrogated, and therapies deactivated prior to the induction of anaesthesia.

A suitable quantity of cross-matched blood and blood products should be immediately available. These should be leucocyte-depleted and should be cytomegalovirus (CMV) negative if both the donor and recipient are CMV negative.

Vascular Access and Monitoring

Standard AAGBI-recommended monitoring should be used along with core temperature and urine output. These patients will also require invasive pressure monitoring (MAP, CVP, PAP), a means of measuring the CO and TOE to monitor cardiac function. Depth of anaesthesia monitoring and cerebral oximetry may be useful.

Large-bore peripheral IV access and invasive arterial monitoring is the minimum requirement prior to the induction of anaesthesia. Depending on the preoperative condition of the patient, central venous access may also be considered prior to induction. All patients undergoing heart transplantation require the insertion of a multi-lumen central venous catheter and a central venous sheath for rapid infusion of fluid and insertion of the PA catheter. It is important to withdraw the PA catheter from the right heart prior to CPB. Central venous access can be challenging in these patients as insertion sites may have been used repeatedly and there may be a degree of anticoagulation. Strict adherence to sterile technique is critical, due to immunosuppression therapy and increased infection risk.

Induction and Maintenance of Anaesthesia

The goal is maintenance of haemodynamic stability and vital organ perfusion until the institution of CPB.

Induction may be challenging, as anaesthetic drug-induced suppression of sympathetic tone produces vasodilatation and myocardial depression, which untreated may rapidly progress to haemodynamic decompensation and cardiovascular collapse. The choice of anaesthetic drugs is far less important than the manner in which they are administed. Pre-emptive inotropic and vasoconstrictor support (or an escalation of the existing therapy) may be required to offset the deleterious effects of anaesthesia and positive pressure ventilation.

In addition to providing information about cardiac anatomy and function, TOE allows the assessment of cardiac filling, the severity of PHT and the presence of intracardiac thrombus, significant aortic atheroma and pleural effusions.

Reperfusion and Separation from CPB

The donor heart is denervated and, in the absence of vagal stimulation, has an intrinsic rate of 80–110 bpm. Bradycardia and junctional rhythms may indicate surgical or ischaemic injury to sinoatrial and atrioventricular nodal tissue. Temporary epicardial pacing is used in all patients to maintain the HR in the range of 90–110 bpm. Up to 12% of patients will eventually require a permanent pacemaker. Normal neurohumoral mechanisms that control inotropy and chronotropy are absent, so that the modulation of the HR and contractility will be depend on circulating catecholamines. Infusions of inotropes and vasoactive drugs are usually commenced in the reperfusion period to assist with separation from CPB.

TOE is crucial at separation from CPB, to assess the adequacy of the de-airing of the cardiac chambers, to monitor ventricular function and filling and to evaluate flow across surgical anastomoses.

Following satisfactory weaning from CPB and the reversal of anticoagulation, scrupulous attention to haemostasis is required. A degree of coagulopathy is to be expected and the anaesthetist should be prepared to deal with ongoing haemorrhage. Factors contributing to the development of coagulopathy include:

- Preoperative anticoagulation or antiplatelet therapy
- Impairment of hepatic synthetic function secondary to liver congestion
- CPB-induced coagulopathy secondary to platelet degradation, haemodilution, hypothermia and the activation of coagulation, fibrinolytic and inflammatory pathways
- Surgical bleeding due to multiple suture lines and (in some cases) re-sternotomy

Patients on preoperative MCS and those who have previously undergone complex cardiac surgery are at a particularly high risk of significant intraoperative

127

> **Box 17.4** Factors contributing to primary graft dysfunction
>
> **Recipient factors**
>
> Increasing age
>
> PHT parameters (even within acceptable limits for transplantation)
>
> Congenital heart disease as aetiology of heart failure
>
> Increasing severity of pre-transplant condition, including dependence on IV inotropes, mechanical ventilation and mechanical circulatory support
>
> **Donor factors**
>
> Increasing age
>
> Gender mismatching
>
> Brain death
>
> Cardiac dysfunction
>
> High inotropic requirements
>
> Concomitant lung retrieval
>
> **Procedural factors**
>
> Ischaemic time
>
> Donor-to-recipient weight mismatch

bleeding. A multi-modal approach to the management of coagulopathy is advisable – meticulous surgical haemostasis, prophylactic antifibrinolytic therapy and the targeted use of blood products and coagulation factor concentrates. Laboratory measures of coagulation and point-of-care tests of platelet function, coagulation and fibrinolysis may be useful to guide blood product administration.

Early Complications

Significant early complications following heart transplantation include graft dysfunction, infection, renal impairment, pulmonary dysfunction, multi-organ failure and acute rejection.

Early graft dysfunction, manifested as univentricular or biventricular failure, is common and the incidence appears to be increasing. Primary graft dysfunction (Box 17.4) and subsequent multi-organ failure may account for two-thirds of deaths in the early postoperative period. Secondary graft dysfunction occurs as a result of discernible causes such as pre-existing PHT, hyper-acute rejection or surgical complications.

Early graft failure is defined as death or re-transplantation within 30 days post-transplantation.

While it occurs in only 4% of recipients, it accounts for 40% of deaths within this period. Medical management of graft dysfunction comprises inotropic support, vasodilators, vasopressors and an IABP. Levosimendan may have a role as an adjuvant therapy in milder cases. Phosphodiesterase inhibitors and inhaled NO are particularly helpful in RV dysfunction with PHT. MCS may be used as a bridge to recovery (or re-transplantation in select patients) if medical management is ineffective.

Antimicrobial Therapy

Antibiotic prophylaxis should be administered perioperatively in accordance with local protocols to cover usual skin flora; however, if a chronically infected MCS or rhythm management device is present or if there was bacterial infection in the donor, antibiotics should be selected based on microbiological sensitivities. Antiviral prophylaxis for CMV should be initiated within 24 to 48 hours of transplantation. Antifungal prophylaxis to prevent mucocutaneous candidiasis should be commenced once the patient is weaned from mechanical ventilation, and antiprotozoal prophylaxis against *Pneumocystis jirovecii* (*P. carinii*) and toxoplasmosis should also be initiated in the early postoperative period.

Immunosuppression

Immunosuppressive therapy is required after heart transplantation to prevent rejection. Advances in immunosuppressive therapy have improved the long-term survival, functional status and quality of life of transplant recipients.

Induction immunosuppression is administered at the time of transplantation and in the early postoperative period, with the aim of reducing the risk of early acute rejection. Induction is generally achieved with high-dose intraoperative corticosteroids and the initiation of maintenance therapy with antibody preparations such as anti-thymocyte globulin and monoclonal interleukin-2 receptor antibodies.

Late Complications and Morbidity

The most significant complications contributing mortality in the first 3 years include: graft failure, multi-organ failure, infection and acute rejection. Thereafter, malignancy, renal dysfunction, cardiac allograft vasculopathy (CAV), graft failure, infection and acute rejection are the most significant direct contributors to mortality.

Immunosuppressive drug therapy predisposes patients to infection and malignancy, and the development of renal impairment, hypertension and DM. The prevalence of renal dysfunction is 50% at 5 years, with 4% of patients requiring chronic dialysis or renal transplantation (increasing to 9.5% at 10 years). Renal failure accounts for 5% of deaths at >5 years post-transplantation and 9% of deaths at >10 years.

CAV is the major limitation to long-term survival after heart transplantation. It is present in 30% of patients at 5 years post-transplantation, and in 50% by 10 years, although in studies using intravascular ultrasound it has been demonstrated in up to 75% of patients at 3 years post-transplantation. CAV is a significant direct contributor to mortality, accounting for 13% of all deaths occurring after more than 1-year post-transplantation.

Key Points

- A TPG above 15 mmHg is associated with higher postoperative mortality.
- RV failure is likely to occur if the recipient's PVR is above 5 Wood units.
- Early graft failure occurs in only 4% of recipients, but accounts for 40% of deaths within 30 days of transplantation.
- Renal failure accounts for 5% of deaths at >5 years post-transplantation and 9% of deaths at >10 years.

Further Reading

Banner NR, Bonser RS, Clark AL, *et al.* UK guidelines for referral and assessment of adults for heart transplantation. *Heart* 2011; 97: 1520–7.

Costanzo MR, Dipchand A, Starling R, *et al.* International Society for Heart Lung Transplantation Guidelines for the care of heart transplant recipients. *J Heart Lung Transplant* 2010; 29: 914–56.

Fischer S, Glas K. A review of cardiac transplantation. *Anesthesiology Clin* 2013; 31: 383–403.

International Society for Heart and Lung Transplantation. International Thoracic Organ Transplant (TTX) Registry data slides. https://ishltregistries.org/registries/slides.asp (accessed December 2018).

Kobashigawa J, Zuckermann A, Macdonald P, *et al.* ISHLT Consensus: report from a consensus conference on primary graft dysfunction after cardiac transplantation. *J Heart Lung Transplant* 2014; 33: 327–40.

Lund LH, Edwards LB, Kucheryavaya AY, *et al.* The Registry of the International Society for Heart and Lung Transplantation: Thirty-second Official Adult Heart Transplantation Report – 2015; focus theme: early graft failure. *J Heart Lung Transplant* 2015; 34: 1244–54.

Mehra MR, Canter CE, Hannan MM, *et al.* The 2016 International Society for Heart Lung Transplantation listing criteria for heart transplantation: a 10-year update. *J Heart Lung Transplant* 2016; 35: 1-23.

Messer S, Page A, Axell R, *et al.* Outcome after heart transplantation from donation after circulatory-determined death donors. *J Heart Lung Transplant* 2017; 36: 1311–18.

Petit SJ, Kydd A. Heart transplantation. In Valchanov K, Jones N, Hogue CW (eds), *Core Topics in Cardiothoracic Critical Care*, 2nd edn. Cambridge: Cambridge University Press; 2018. pp. 333–9.

Ramakrishna H, Jaroszewski DE, Arabia FA. Adult cardiac transplantation: a review of perioperative management Part I. *Ann Card Anaesth* 2009; 12: 71–8.

Ramakrishna H, Rehfeldt KH, Pajaro OE. Anesthetic pharmacology and perioperative considerations for heart transplantation. *Curr Clin Pharmacol* 2015; 10: 3–21.

Yancy CW, Jessup M, Bozkurt B, *et al.* 2013 ACCF/AHA Guideline for the Management of Heart Failure. *Circulation* 2013; 128: e20–e327.

Electrophysiological Procedures

Joseph E. Arrowsmith

Rhythm Management Devices

As the indications for these devices has widened, the prevalence of permanent pacemakers (PPMs) and ICDs has increased. The complexity of these devices makes them susceptible to perioperative interference and inadvertent reprogramming, placing patients at greater risk of perioperative morbidity. Management guidelines are largely based on case series and expert consensus rather than prospective, randomized studies.

Permanent Pacemakers

Over 1,000,000 PPMs are implanted every year world-wide. PPM systems comprise a generator (electrical circuits and a battery) and one or more leads, designed to sense cardiac electrical activity and deliver a stimulus. In unipolar lead systems the generator serves as an electrode for completing the electrical circuit. Unipolar pacing systems, which produce noticeable pacing spikes on the standard ECG, are more susceptible to interference (e.g. skeletal muscle contraction) than bipolar systems. The indications for PPMs are summarized in Box 18.1. Indications for pacing in children, adolescents and patients with congenital heart disease (CHD; not shown) are broadly similar.

Device classification provides a concise and consistent means of describing device function. The generic PPM code is shown in Table 18.1.

VVI systems, which have largely superseded VOO systems, are appropriate for chronic AF with slow ventricular rate. Dual-chamber devices (DDD), which are capable of sensing and pacing both the atrium and the ventricle, are more haemodynamically efficient than ventricle pacing alone. Rate-adaptive (DDDR) devices, which allow the HR to increase during exercise, are more physiological. Some PPMs have the ability to switch mode. Switching from DDD to VVIR or DDIR mode may be useful in patients with paroxysmal AF.

Cardiac Resynchronization Therapy

Cardiac resynchronization therapy (CRT) is used in advanced heart failure. An additional lead is placed in the coronary sinus to pace the LV independently from the RV. Resynchronizing ventricular contraction is thought to improve cardiac function.

Temporary Pacing

In patients with symptomatic bradycardia that is unresponsive to chronotropes (e.g. isoproterenol), emergency transvenous (internal jugular or femoral) VVI or VVO pacing can be used as a bridge to recovery or definitive treatment. A balloon-tipped floatation catheter is inserted through a haemostatic sheath and advanced into the RV, 'blind' or under fluoroscopic guidance.

In the setting of cardiac surgery, wires attached to the epicardial surfaces of the RA and RV are used for temporary pacing. Fixed-rate pacing (VOO, AOO, DOO) should be converted to demand mode (VVI, AAI, DDD) at the end of surgery. The anaesthetist must be familiar with both single- and dual-chamber pacing systems. Dealing with common pacing problems requires bedside monitoring of the ECG together with the CVP and arterial waveforms.

Implantable Defibrillators

ICDs have the ability to detect abnormal cardiac rhythms and deliver either antitachycardia pacing or a DC shock. The devices are used for the primary and secondary prevention of 'sudden cardiac death'. The indications for ICD therapy are shown in Box 18.2.

Device Implantation

Most PPM and ICD implants are performed in the cardiac catheter laboratory, on a day-case basis under local anaesthesia with conscious sedation. The

131

Table 18.1 The NASPE/BPEG five-position generic pacemaker code

Position	I	II	III	IV	V
Category	Chamber(s) paced	Chamber(s) sensed	Response to sensing	Rate modulation	Antitachycardia functions
Code letters	O	O	O	O	O
	A	A	T	R	P
	V	V	I		S
	D	D	D		D

NASPE, North American Society of Pacing and Electrophysiology; BPEG, British Pacing and Electrophysiology Group. O = None, A = atrium, V = ventricle, D = dual (A+V), T = triggered, I = inhibited, R = rate modulation, P = antitachycardia, S = shock

---

Box 18.1   ACCF/AHA/AATS/HFSA/STS guidelines for device-based therapy of cardiac rhythm abnormalities

Acquired atrioventricular (A-V) block (in adults)	Third-degree A-V block with symptomatic bradycardia or documented asystole, neuromuscular disorders, following A-V node ablation
Chronic bifascicular and trifascicular block	Intermittent second-degree (Mobitz type II) A-V block, intermittent third-degree A-V block
A-V block following acute MI	Persistent second-degree A-V block; transient third-degree A-V block; need not be symptomatic
Sinus node dysfunction	Documented symptomatic bradycardia; frequent sinus pauses
Prevention of tachycardia	Sustained, pause-dependent VT in which efficacy of pacing has been documented
Carotid sinus hypersensitivity	Recurrent syncope due to carotid sinus stimulation
Heart failure	Cardiac resynchronization therapy – symptomatic heart failure (NYHA class >2) with impaired ventricular function with widened QRS complex.
Specific conditions	Hypertrophic cardiomyopathy; idiopathic dilated cardiomyopathy; cardiac transplantation – persistent bradycardia

---

subclavian, cephalic or axillary veins are commonly used for lead insertion. The device is usually sited in the pre-pectoral region or in the sub-pectoral space.

In 2016, the FDA approved the first 'leadless' PPM (Micra^{TM}, Medtronic – VVIR) for clinical use. This small cylindrical device (6.7 × 25.9 mm, 1.75 g) is delivered percutaneously under local anaesthesia and attached to the RV apex by Nitinol tines. Concerns about lost telemetry and poor battery life have prompted the manufacturer of a similar device (NanoStim^{TM}, St Jude) to halt implantation.

ICD implantation is typically more complex because of the nature of the devices (larger devices and thicker leads) and the types of patients encountered. Device testing requires the deliberate induction of VF and measurement of the minimally effective defibrillation threshold (DFT). Newer, entirely subcutaneous systems (e.g. EMBLEM S-ICD, Boston Scientific) require a large axillary incision to accommodate the generator. Patients undergoing S-ICD implantation tend to be young and typically opt for general anaesthesia (Figure 18.1). The complications of device implantation are shown in Box 18.3.

Prophylactic, broad-spectrum antibiotics should be administered before device implantation. Antibiotics are mandatory in cases of PPM infection, lead-related endocarditis and prior to device extraction.

Device Explantation

The indications for explantation include: generator replacement (low battery charge), lead failure,

Box 18.2   Indications for ICD therapy

Primary prevention of sudden cardiac death

Coronary artery disease

Non-ischaemic dilated cardiomyopathy

Long-QT syndrome

Hypertrophic cardiomyopathy

Arrhythmogenic RV dysplasia/cardiomyopathy

Non-compaction of the LV

Primary electrical disease (idiopathic VF, short-QT and Brugada syndromes and catecholaminergic polymorphic VT)

Idiopathic VT

Advanced heart failure and cardiac transplantation

Secondary prevention of sudden cardiac death

Sustained VT

Coronary artery disease

Non-ischaemic dilated cardiomyopathy

Hypertrophic cardiomyopathy

Arrhythmogenic RV cardiomyopathy

Genetic arrhythmia syndromes

Syncope with inducible sustained VT

Source: American College of Cardiology/American Heart Association/Heart Rhythm Society 2008 Guidelines for Device-Based Therapy of Cardiac Rhythm Abnormalities (*Circulation* 2008; 117: e350–e408)

Box 18.3   Complications of PPM and ICD implantation

Early complications

Venous access	Pneumothorax, haemothorax, air embolus
Lead-related	Perforation, malposition, dislodgement
Pocket	Haematoma, infection

Delayed complications

Lead	Thrombosis, venous occlusion, infection, insulation failure
Generator	Erosion, migration, external damage

Device function issues

Pacing/sensing	Oversensing, undersensing, crosstalk, battery failure
ICD-specific	Failure to deliver shock, ineffective, inappropriate

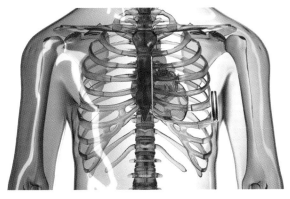

Figure 18.1 The subcutaneous ICD system (Boston Scientific).

infection, thrombotic complications and heart transplantation. Lead extraction using mechanical or laser-based cutting instruments has the potential to cause catastrophic damage to central veins, and the RA, TV and RV. The risk of injury, which is a function of the duration of implantation, must be discussed with the operating cardiologist in advance. Low-risk cases can be undertaken under local anaesthesia and sedation with minimal monitoring. High-risk cases tend to be undertaken under general anaesthesia with substantial venous access, arterial and CVP monitoring, endotracheal intubation and CPB standby. Where available, TOE is used for the early detection of a pericardial collection.

Perioperative Management

Perioperative assessment of patients with rhythm management devices is summarized in Box 18.4. It is essential to determine the device manufacturer and model as telemetric programming devices are manufacturer-specific and non-interchangeable. An ECG should be obtained in all patients and a pre-operative device check should be undertaken where possible. By definition, patients undergoing CRT have advanced heart failure and require additional investigation and perioperative precautions.

Reprogramming

The need to alter the device function is determined by the type of surgery being undertaken, the likelihood

---

Box 18.4 Perioperative considerations for patients with PPMs and ICDs

- Original indications for implantation – medical history and pre-pacemaker symptoms
- Recurrence of pre-pacemaker symptoms, particularly during exercise
- Device type and manufacturer – current mode of function:
  PPM/ICD identification card carried by patient; device may be identified on plain CXR
- Magnet effect? Conversion to fixed-rate pacing?
- Is device functioning properly? Recent PPM/ICD checks?
- CXR – location, type and continuity of leads
- Is patient pacemaker dependent? ECG: evidence of pacing spikes and capture?
- Is reprogramming necessary before surgery? – PPM usually reprogrammed to fixed-rate pacing prior to induction of anaesthesia for cardiac surgery; ICD therapies usually deactivated
- What are likely effects of anaesthesia and surgery on device? – Electromagnetic interference (EMI): diathermy may cause reprogramming to VVI or VOO; drugs, electrolytes, defibrillation
- What are likely effects of the device on anaesthesia and surgery? – Bipolar diathermy where possible, smallest possible currents, avoid unnecessary cautery less than 5 cm from device

---

of EMI and the underlying cardiac rhythm. Rate-responsive or adaptive PPMs should have these features disabled. ICDs should have therapies disabled and external defibrillation equipment made available.

Central Venous Access

Blind insertion of a central venous cannula may cause lead dislodgement or damage. Recently implanted leads (<1 year) and RV leads are particularly vulnerable to dislodgement. Preoperative venography or contrast CT, or procedural ultrasound, can be used to determine vein patency.

Magnet Application

Placing a permanent magnet over a PPM or ICD generator typically activates a predetermined behaviour (e.g. VOO or therapies off). Magnet responses are device-specific and can be altered or deactivated by reprogramming. A prolonged magnet application may have a time-limited effect or permanently disable some devices. The application of a magnet without knowledge of its effects is not recommended.

Electromagnetic Interference

All electronic devices are potentially susceptible to electromagnetic or radiofrequency interference. The principal sources of EMI are: diathermy, radiofrequency ablation devices and MRI. In the setting of cardiac surgery, temporary pacing systems and evoked potential monitors may generate EMI.

Diathermy: Most PPMs interpret diathermy EMI as cardiac electrical activity, which may induce asynchronous pacing or inhibition. Bipolar

diathermy should be used where possible. If unipolar diathermy is used, the grounding plate should be positioned as far away from the generator as possible. ICDs may interpret EMI as VF and could inappropriately deliver shocks if not deactivated.

Radiofrequency ablation: Delivery catheters can interfere with device function and induce currents in leads.

MRI: Magnetic interference can have unpredictable effects on PPMs and ICDs. Magnetic resonance-induced heating may damage generators and leads, and produce myocardial damage. New generation, MRI-compatible devices are increasingly available.

Electrophysiological Procedures

The availability of real-time anatomical and mapping equipment, and recent developments in catheter-based ablation technology have driven an enormous rise in the non-surgical treatment of arrhythmias.

Types of Disorders

These can be classified according to the underlying electrical problem, the underlying mechanism and whether the disorder is congenital or acquired (Box 18.5).

Preoperative Assessment

The following questions must be answered:

- What is the rhythm disturbance and what compromise results from it?
- Is the cardiac anatomy normal?

Table 18.2 Pitfalls of elective DCCV

Situation	Pitfall	Solution
Ever-present risk of LA thrombus in longstanding AF	Embolization and stroke	Therapeutic anticoagulation for 3 weeks prior to DCCV or TOE to exclude LA thrombus
Paroxysmal AF	Patient may be in NSR on arrival	Scrutinize monitored ECG Abandon procedure
Atrial flutter	Easy to convert to NSR	Start with 30 J biphasic shock
Presence of PPM or ICD	Interpretation of ECG may be difficult Potential device damage with DCCV	DCCV and expect ventricular depolarization change DCCV in an axis perpendicular to that of the lead system Post DCCV PPM/ICD check
Obesity	Anterolateral electrode position may result in reduced transmyocardial current	Position electrodes between scapulae and over left praecordium
After cardioversion	Hypotension in the setting of NSR	IV fluids
Slow ventricular response rate	Profound bradycardia after cardioversion	Temporary external pacing facility incorporated into the defibrillator

---

Box 18.5   Classification of electrophysiological disorders

Congenital	Anatomical	Disordered impulse generation
Acquired	Physiological	Disordered impulse conduction
		Disordered action potential

- If the anatomy is not normal, is there any history of progression of heart failure, cyanosis or chronic pulmonary disease?
- What is the ventricular performance?
- Are there any implanted devices?
- What is the anticoagulation status?
- Are serum electrolyte concentrations (especially potassium and magnesium) within acceptable ranges?
- What procedure is intended?

The patient population ranges between two extremes. At one end of the spectrum is the asymptomatic or minimally compromised patient with a structurally and functionally normal heart, who does not require specialized perioperative care. At the other end of the spectrum is the grossly compromised patient with palliated complex CHD who requires full invasive cardiovascular monitoring and postoperative admission to the ICU. Some procedures may last several hours, making general anaesthesia more desirable than prolonged sedation. Paediatric and many adult CHD patients require general anaesthesia.

DC Cardioversion

DC cardioversion (DCCV) is the most commonly performed electrophysiological intervention and is often performed on a day-case basis. The anaesthetist is often the most senior doctor present. In the vast majority of cases the underlying rhythm disturbance is either AF (90%) or atrial flutter. Common pitfalls are described in Table 18.2.

Elective DCCV requires at least 3 weeks of anticoagulation and a normal K^+ concentration. Nowadays, hands-free electrodes are used – these should be used to confirm the dysrhythmia *before* induction of anaesthesia. Following preoxygenation, propofol $(1–2 \text{ mg kg}^{-1})$ usually provides adequate sedation and ensures a rapid recovery. Where the referring physician requests pre-DCCV TOE to exclude LA thrombus, deeper anaesthesia and consideration of airway management are required. In suitable patients, the careful use of a supraglottic airway device may obviate the need for neuromuscular blockade and tracheal intubation.

Mapping and Ablation Procedures

Mapping is performed to characterize tachyarrhythmias, to locate arrhythmogenic substrates and pathways, and to guide subsequent ablation. Mapping typically entails deliberate electrical or pharmacological induction of the dysrhythmia under investigation. This may have profound haemodynamic consequences in patients with post-MI VT.

Cardiac ablation – freezing (cryoablation) or heating (radiofrequency ablation) – creates myocardial scarring that either obliterates an arrhythmogenic focus (e.g. ischaemic VT) or electrically isolates an arrhythmogenic focus from the rest of the heart (e.g. pulmonary vein isolation). The procedures are typically undertaken via the femoral vessels and may last several hours. While it is technically possible to use conscious sedation, many patients experience unpleasant cardiac pain and are unable to lie supine for prolonged periods – many patients (and operators) opt for general anaesthesia. In patients with persistent AF, it has been shown that ablation is more successful when conducted under general anaesthesia.

All patients have external defibrillator electrodes applied. Invasive arterial and CVP monitoring is reserved for higher-risk patients, and airway management is dictated by patient size and regurgitation risk. The choice of anaesthetic regimen is a matter of personal preference, although infusions of propofol (3–5 mg kg^{-1} h^{-1}) and remifentanil (0.04–0.1 µg kg^{-1} min^{-1}) provide stable anaesthesia and facilitate rapid recovery. IV fluid administration should be minimized during radiofrequency ablation as a significant volume of crystalloid (500–2,000 ml) may be given to cool the catheter. Where access to the LA is required (AF ablation), fluid loading may be required to permit safe intra-atrial septal puncture. Persistent hypotension is best treated with a low-dose vasopressor infusion. Despite the length of ablation procedures, the anaesthetist must maintain vigilance as drug-induced hypotension may be indistinguishable from pericardial tamponade secondary to cardiac puncture.

Inadvertent right phrenic nerve injury is a recognized complication of ablation (cryoablation 5%, radiofrequency ablation 1%). For this reason, neuromuscular blockade is usually confined to induction of anaesthesia or avoided altogether. If DCCV is undertaken at the end of the procedure, care should be taken to prevent arm injury.

Key Points

- Patients with implantable devices should be identified and referred to a cardiac technician at an early stage.
- ICD therapies should be deactivated before surgery and facilities for external defibrillation made available for the period that the device is disabled.
- Application of a magnet without knowledge of its effects is not recommended.
- Both IV and volatile anaesthetic agents have effects on the cardiac conduction system. These effects are of little clinical significance and play no role in determining anaesthetic technique.
- Persistent AF ablation is more successful when performed under general anaesthesia.

Further Reading

Dooley N, Lowe M, Ashley EMC. Advances in management of electrophysiology and atrial fibrillation in the cardiac catheter laboratory: implications for anaesthesia. *BJA Education* 2018; 18: 349–56.

Epstein AE, DiMarco JP, Ellenbogen KA, *et al.* ACC/AHA/HRS 2008 guidelines for device-based therapy of cardiac rhythm abnormalities: a report of the American College of Cardiology/ American Heart Association task force on practice guidelines. *J Am Coll Cardiol* 2008; 51: e1–62.

Martin CA, Curtain JP, Gajendragadkar PR, *et al.* Improved outcome and cost effectiveness in ablation of persistent atrial fibrillation under general anaesthetic. *Europace* 2018; 20: 935–42.

Tracy CM, Epstein AE, Darbar D, *et al.* 2012 ACCF/AHA/HRS focused update of the 2008 guidelines for device-based therapy of cardiac rhythm abnormalities: a report of the American College of Cardiology Foundation/American Heart Association task force on practice guidelines. *J Thorac Cardiovasc Surg* 2012; 144: e127–45.

Procedures for Structural Heart Disease

Cameron G. Densem and Andrew A. Klein

Historically, the cardiac catheterization laboratory has been used for blood sampling, contrast-enhanced imaging and intravascular pressure measurement to provide diagnostic and prognostic information and to guide surgical intervention. In recent years, technological advancements have made less invasive therapies feasible and driven tremendous growth in percutaneous procedures. While this now encompasses a wide range of cardiovascular interventions, this chapter will focus on percutaneous therapies for structural heart disease, where the anaesthetist is most likely to be involved.

Valvular Interventions

Transcatheter Aortic Valve Implantation

Percutaneous interventions have transformed the treatment of AS over the past decade. Following the 2002 report of the first successful percutaneous implantation of a prosthetic AV as a salvage procedure by Alain Cribier in France, and subsequent elective implantations via the femoral artery and the LV apex in 2005 by John Webb in Canada, the use of transcatheter aortic valve implantation (TAVI) has grown enormously. Although it was initially embraced as a therapeutic option for patients with an unacceptably high operative risk for surgical AV replacement (SAVR), advances in product design and improved operator skill and experience are driving its adoption as a viable alternative to SAVR for a much larger group of patients.

Current Devices and Techniques

Access routes for TAVI include: peripheral arteries (femoral, axillary), peripheral veins (trans-septal), the LV apex via a small thoracotomy, or the ascending aorta via a mini-sternotomy. According to international registries, the most commonly used approaches currently are transfemoral and transapical (Table 19.1).

A number of prosthetic valves are available. These are generally categorized as balloon-inflated or self-expanding (Figure 19.1). Current areas of focus for new valve design are the ability to retrieve and reposition after deployment, the expansion of the indications by facilitating safe deployment in non-calcified native valves or within bioprosthetic valves and to address some common complications observed with early devices.

Procedural Risks

The majority of patients undergoing TAVI are elderly, frail and have numerous co-morbidities. It is therefore crucial to consider not only procedural mortality but also the frequency of non-fatal complications, which are likely to significantly impact the quality of life.

Table 19.1 TAVI – most commonly used approaches

	Transfemoral	Transapical
Access	Usually percutaneous	Mini thoracotomy
Anaesthesia	Sedation or general anaesthesia	General anaesthesia
Regional anaesthesia	Ilioinguinal or fascia iliaca block	Serratus anterior, intercostal or paravertebral block
Echocardiography	TTE or TOE	TOE
Surgeon presence	Optional (standby)	Scrubbed

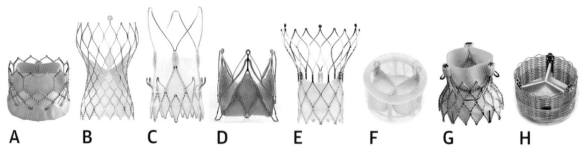

A   B   C   D   E   F   G   H

Figure 19.1 Valves available for TAVI in Europe. (A) Sapien 3 Valve (Edwards Lifesciences), (B) CoreValve Evolut R (Medtronic), (C) Acurate *neo* valve (Symetis), (D) JenaValve (JVT), (E) Portico valve (St. Jude Medical), (F) Direct Flow valve (Direct Flow Medical), (G) Engager valve (Medtronic), (H) Lotus valve (Boston Scientific).

Not surprisingly, TAVI is associated with considerable morbidity, ranging from mild acute kidney injury to catastrophic aortic root rupture. However, there are several complications in particular which are significantly more common with TAVI than with SAVR, and these continue to be a focus of study (Box 19.1). One of the most common complications with early devices was vascular injury, particularly femoral or aortoiliac injury when using large first-generation 22–24 Fr access devices. Design improvements have decreased current access systems to 14–16 Fr, increasing the number of eligible patients and reducing vascular complications. Technological advancements have also reduced the frequency of a paravalvular leak (PVL), a complication much more common with TAVI and, if significant, it is associated with increased mortality. Other important complications more common with TAVI include stroke and conduction block, requiring a permanent pacemaker.

It is important to note that the incidence of specific complications varies with the choice of valve and route of approach. As TAVI teams gain experience with multiple manufacturer systems, this allows a customized approach based on individual risk tolerance and anatomical considerations.

Patient Selection

Symptomatic severe AS has a poor prognosis that can be dramatically improved with valvular intervention. Traditionally, the option of SAVR has been offered on the basis that the risks of the underlying disease outweigh the risks of surgery. For patients with exceedingly high predicted surgical mortality, TAVI represents an alternative intervention that offers a lower risk than the natural history of the disease. As the populations of patients eligible for TAVI or SAVR

> **Box 19.1 Immediate complications of TAVI**
> - Poor recovery of cardiac function after rapid ventricular pacing
> - Haemodynamic instability
> - Incorrect stent placement:
>
>   Too high, may impair coronary flow, leading to myocardial ischaemia and infarction
>
>   Too low, may lead to device embolization
>
> - Embolization of aortic material or air, leading to neurological dysfunction
> - AR, especially paravalvular:
>
>   May need further device dilatation to improve moulding of device to aorta
>
> - Complete heart block
> - Transfemoral approach:
>
>   Vascular access damage (femoral/iliac artery or aorta), including dissection, rupture and haemorrhage
>
> - Transapical approach:
>
>   Difficulty closing ventricular apex, leading to haemorrhage
>
>   Post-thoracotomy pain

now overlap significantly, there is a clear role for a multidisciplinary team decision-making (Figure 19.2). Current guidelines recommend that the multidisciplinary team includes an anaesthetist. While the relative risk of the two approaches to valve intervention are generally based on age and risk score (e.g. EuroSCORE-II), TAVI can have a particularly useful role in patients with specific surgical risks such as previous sternotomy with patent coronary grafts or patients with a 'porcelain' aorta.

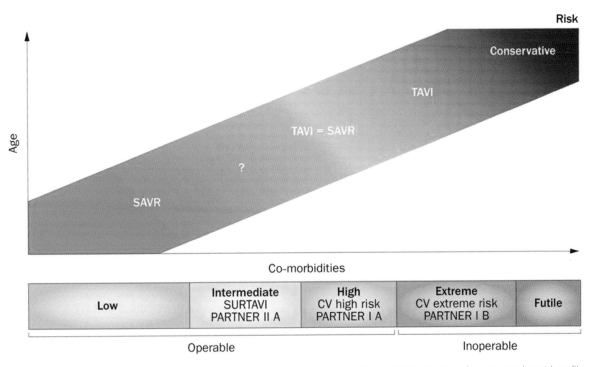

Figure 19.2 Cumulative patient-related risk in AS influences the decision between TAVI and SAVR. Patients with an intermediate risk profile are being studied currently to determine the optimal treatment strategy. Names of large trials providing the evidence underpinning this framework are listed within the risk categories at the bottom of the figure. From Grube *et al. Eur Heart J* 2014, 35(8): 490.

A common exclusion criterion for TAVI is the presence of severe co-morbid illness or frailty, indicating that the patient is unlikely to receive any meaningful benefit from a procedure targeted at the AV. This includes an anticipated life expectancy of less than a year after AV replacement. Anatomical constraints also exist – although the number of valve sizes has increased, the options remain much more limited than for SAVR. Furthermore, careful evaluation and sizing of the aortic root must be performed, often with multiple imaging modalities, and an appropriate access point through the peripheral vasculature, the left chest or the mediastinum must be available.

Finally, TAVI does not currently have an established role in patients with cardiac disease other than calcific AS. The presence of concurrent coronary or other structural heart disease reduces the anticipated benefit from TAVI relative to open surgery and could also significantly increase the risks of rapid ventricular pacing during valve deployment. The potential utility of TAVI for AR or bicuspid AV disease is questionable and these are currently considered

contraindications. This is largely because the most widely used valves depend on significant radial forces, applied against a calcified annulus, for proper anchoring and prevention of a PVL. Furthermore, the presence of concomitant aortic pathology in such patients may mandate surgery in itself. Nevertheless, the potential for TAVI using newer devices in these patients is being investigated.

Anaesthetic Technique

A standard preoperative cardiac anaesthetic assessment should be performed in all TAVI patients. As previously stated, they are often elderly and have numerous co-morbidities - these should be evaluated thoroughly and optimized as necessary. The procedure may take place in the cardiac catheterization lab or in a hybrid operating theatre. In either case, appropriate preparations for the emergency institution of CPB should be made. This includes an agreed plan for surgical rescue, the immediate availability of appropriate equipment and personnel, and clarification of the planned cannulation approach in patients chosen for TAVI because of difficult surgical access.

Furthermore, this includes the clear identification of patients for whom surgical intervention and CPB are not considered appropriate.

Knowledge of the planned approach is essential, as this can greatly influence the anaesthetic technique chosen. In many instances general anaesthesia, regional anaesthesia or sedation may be used. The advantages of general anaesthesia include a secured airway in case of respiratory or haemodynamic compromise, guaranteed immobility and access to TOE. In an effort to improve recovery and reduce the length of hospital stay, a regional nerve block supplemented with sedation is becoming increasingly common. Avoiding general anaesthesia minimizes the haemodynamic consequences of anaesthetic agents and positive pressure ventilation and reduces the incidence of arrhythmias and the requirement for vasoactive support. This can be one component of an enhanced recovery strategy, which minimizes benzodiazepines, avoids unnecessary invasive lines and urinary catheterization and promotes early mobilization once haemostasis is assured. When sedation is used, arterial monitoring can be achieved by 'sharing' the cardiologist's arterial access, eliminating the need for a separate arterial line. Central venous access – routinely obtained for rapid ventricular pacing – can be used by the anaesthetic team for drug and fluid administration.

Echocardiography

The use of echocardiography during the procedure is essential for confirming adequate valve seating, excluding a significant PVL and diagnosing aortic injury or new pericardial effusion. When TOE is not available, a preoperative assessment of the aortic annulus and root can be undertaken with CT or MRI, and an intraoperative assessment of the prosthesis can be made using fluoroscopy and TTE.

Balloon AV Dilation

Although not commonly performed, simple balloon dilatation of a stenotic AV may be considered as a bridge to a more definitive therapy (TAVI or SAVR) if it is not immediately available. This may be particularly helpful in a patient who requires urgent non-cardiac surgery, such as cancer resection. In addition, it can be used as a preliminary intervention where the contribution of AS to a patient's symptoms, and therefore the benefit of TAVI, is unclear.

Percutaneous Mitral Valve Intervention

Minimally invasive, catheter-based therapies exist for both MS and MR. For several reasons, progress has been much slower than AV interventions.

- MV repair is preferable to replacement
- The asymmetrical, saddle-shaped MV annulus poses great technical challenges – the use of radial force puts nearby structures at risk (e.g. coronary sinus, circumflex artery)
- MV replacement exposes patients to the risks of thrombosis and endocarditis
- Surgical repair typically combines several techniques – replicating this multifaceted repair with a minimally invasive approach requires multiple devices and routes of access

While several systems are currently under development, only clipping for MR and balloon commissurotomy for MS will be discussed in detail.

Mitral Valve Clipping

The MitraClip® system is a percutaneous technique which permanently joins the A2 and P2 segments of the MV in an edge-to-edge repair, analogous to the open repair technique described by Alfieri. Like the open technique, the MitraClip® creates a double-orifice MV.

The MitraClip® system employs a 24 Fr delivery catheter, approaching the valve from the LA via an interatrial septal puncture. Access is most often gained via a femoral vein. Because precise deployment is crucial to the procedural success, the clip delivery system not only allows manoeuvring, opening, grasping and eventual detachment of the clip, but the opening and grasping steps can be repeated as necessary with TOE guidance before final deployment onto the valve leaflets.

It follows that the use of echocardiography during MitraClip® application is essential to procedural success, and this includes several key steps through the procedure.

1. A detailed evaluation of the MV pathology and appropriate patient selection must be confirmed (Table 19.2).
2. TOE assists in guiding trans-septal puncture – a posterior/superior puncture site through the fossa ovalis, at least 3.0 cm from the mitral annulus, is ideal, providing adequate room for manoeuvre within the LA to optimize the approach trajectory.

Table 19.2 Patient eligibility criteria for MitraClip® repair

Echocardiography inclusion criteria	Anatomic inclusion criteria
Coaptation length ≥ 2 mm Coaptation depth ≤ 11 mm Flail gap < 10 mm Flail width < 15 mm	MR jet must be associated with A2 and P2 Absence of severe mitral annular calcification No leaflet calcification in the grasping area No significant leaflet cleft or perforation Leaflet thickness < 5 mm LVEF > 20% LVEDD < 6 cm MVA > 4 cm^2 No restricted posterior leaflet

LVEF, LV ejection fraction; LVEDD, LV end-diastolic dimension; MVA, MV area.

3. TOE is used to guide the system towards the valve in line with the axis of diastolic inflow, and position the clip arms at the central portion of the valve, perpendicular to the line of coaptation. Once the leaflet tips are grasped, the sonographer quantifies any residual MR and evaluates for iatrogenic valvular stenosis, bearing in mind the impact of significant residual MR on the assessment of MS parameters. Based on this assessment, the clip can be deployed, or the arms reopened and repositioned, increasing the likelihood of optimal repair.

4. A comprehensive TOE examination is undertaken to assess for any complications, including residual valve disease and haemodynamic consequences, partial clip detachment, atrial wall perforation and a residual ASD.

As in percutaneous AV therapies, patient selection is of utmost importance. Early evidence suggests that percutaneous mitral clipping has a lower procedural risk than surgical repair, but a significantly higher rate of moderate to severe residual MR (21% versus 3%). Currently, the device is FDA-approved for primary degenerative MR in patients deemed to be inoperable.

Balloon Mitral Valve Valvotomy

Chronic rheumatic heart disease remains the most common cause of MS worldwide. It is characterized by thickening of the leaflet tips with eventual fusion of anterior and posterior leaflet edges at the valve commissures. Rheumatic MS is frequently amenable to minimally invasive therapy using a catheter-directed balloon to mechanically separate fused commissures. The likelihood of success or of complications with percutaneous balloon mitral valvotomy (PBMV) can be made echocardiographically using one of several scoring systems, such as the Wilkins score.

Contraindications to PBMV include LA thrombus, moderate or severe MR and a Wilkins score predictive of a low success rate. An open surgical technique is an important alternative for these patients; however, for those with a very high predicted operative risk, PBMV is sometimes considered even if the valve anatomy is thought to be unfavourable. PMBV has no role in the management of senile calcific MS, where there is progressive calcification from leaflet bases to tips without commissural fusion.

Nonvalvular Interventions

Percutaneous Septal Closure

Percutaneous devices for septal closure, similar to that depicted in Figure 19.3, can be used for PFO, ASD and VSD closure. The same devices may also be used to close prosthetic PVLs. Patient-specific factors must be considered based on the characteristics of defect. For example, there may be a history of stroke associated with a PFO or the presence of an RV volume overload or PHT with an ASD. Patients with a congenital VSD may have associated cardiac or extracardiac anomalies. Patients with a post-infarction VSD may have significant cardiovascular compromise.

Depending on patient factors, the procedure can be undertaken under sedation or general anaesthesia with TOE. TOE is used so that the defect is suitable for percutaneous closure – an adequate rim of tissue on all sides for anchoring of the device (typically 4 to 5 mm) and a sufficiently large LA to accommodate the device in the case of PFO or ASD closure. Procedural complications include a residual or worsened shunt, embolism (air, thrombus or device), arrhythmia or conduction block, valvular dysfunction and pericardial effusion/tamponade.

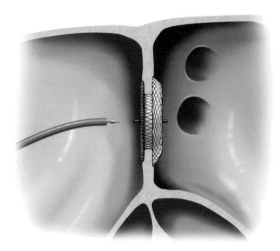

Figure 19.3 Percutaneous closure of the interatrial septum using the Amplatzer device (St Jude Medical)

Left Atrial Appendage Occlusion

Systemic thromboembolism, in particular embolic stroke, is a significant lifelong risk of AF. Patients unable to take anticoagulants and those who have repeated embolic events despite adequate anticoagulation may be suitable for LA appendage (LAA) occlusion. Exclusion of the LAA as a site of thrombus formation can help reduce the future risk of stroke. Several percutaneous devices are available.

TOE is generally considered mandatory for procedural guidance, so most patients require general anaesthesia. After ensuring the absence of LAA thrombus, the LAA anatomy is evaluated in detail. 3D TOE is particularly useful for assessing the LAA and guiding device selection – usually 2–4 mm greater than the maximum LAA diameter. The primary risk of device undersizing is device embolization, while oversizing may cause compression of the

circumflex coronary artery or the left superior pulmonary vein, and LAA perforation. Evaluation of the LAA using 3D TOE can also help to categorize its morphology as (1) chicken wing, (2) cauliflower, (3) windsock or (4) cactus. The morphological type may influence the thromboembolism risk as well as the choice of device type and sizing.

Conclusions

The cardiac catheter laboratory is increasingly being used to deliver advanced therapies for structural heart disease. The cardiac anaesthetist is likely to be involved in many of these procedures; to aid with sedation and anaesthesia, echocardiography, haemodynamic management and, where required, to perform resuscitation and facilitate conversion to surgery. As the indications for surgical and percutaneous treatments continue to overlap, the lines between open and minimally invasive therapies will likely blur with the increasing use of hybrid operating theatres and combined surgical and percutaneous techniques. The anaesthetist can take on a central role in this setting, bridging any divide that exists between potentially disparate or unfamiliar teams and overseeing a coordinated effort to maximize the patient benefit and optimize the outcomes.

Key Points

- Complex, catheter laboratory-based procedures require a multidisciplinary approach.
- TAVI is an established treatment for patients deemed to be unsuitable for surgical AV replacement.
- TOE guidance is required for the majority of structural heart procedures that are conducted under general anaesthesia.

Further Reading

Alfieri O, Maisano F, De Bonis M, *et al.* The double-orifice technique in mitral valve repair: a simple solution for complex problems. *J Thorac Cardiovasc Surg* 2001; 122: 674–81.

Feldman T, Kar S, Rinaldi M, *et al.* Percutaneous mitral repair with the MitraClip system: safety and midterm durability in the initial EVEREST (Endovascular Valve Edge-to-Edge REpair Study) cohort. *J Am Coll Cardiol* 2009; 54: 686–94.

Grube E, Sinning JM, Vahanian A. The year in cardiology 2013: valvular heart disease (focus on catheter-based interventions). *Eur Heart J* 2014; 35: 490–5.

Guarracino F, Baldassarri R, Ferro B, *et al.* Transesophageal echocardiography during MitraClip® procedure. *Anesth Analg* 2014; 118: 1188–96.

Klein AA, Skubas NJ, Ender J. Controversies and complications in the perioperative management of transcatheter aortic valve replacement. *Anesth Analg* 2014; 119: 784–98.

Klein AA, Webb ST, Tsui S, *et al.* Transcatheter aortic valve insertion: anaesthetic implications of emerging new technology. *Br J Anaesth* 2009; 103: 792–9.

Mack M, Smith RL. Transcatheter treatment of mitral valve disease: déjà vu all over again? *Circulation* 2016; 134: 198–200.

Shook DC, Savage RM. Anesthesia in the cardiac catheterization laboratory and electrophysiology laboratory. *Anesthesiol Clin* 2009; 27: 47–56.

Vahl TP, Kodali SK, Leon MB. Transcatheter aortic valve replacement 2016: a modern-day 'through the looking-glass' adventure. *J Am Coll Cardiol* 2016; 67: 1472–87.

Chapter

20

General Principles and Conduct of Paediatric Cardiac Anaesthesia

Isabeau A. Walker and Jon H. Smith

General Principles

Congenital heart disease (CHD) occurs in approximately 8:1,000 live births and may be associated with recognizable syndromes or chromosomal abnormalities in 25% of cases. Abnormalities are often complex, affecting structure and function. Surgery may be corrective or palliative and can be staged. Over half of these operations occur in the first year of life. The timing of surgery is dictated by the severity of the lesion, the need to avoid the development of pulmonary vascular disease or the complications of cyanotic heart disease.

There are significant differences in infant and adult physiology that have a bearing on the conduct of anaesthesia for children with CHD. This chapter will address these differences in physiology and some general principles of anaesthesia for paediatric cardiac surgery.

Normal Neonatal Physiology

Newborn infants have a high metabolic rate and oxygen consumption. This is reflected in a high resting RR and CI (neonate: 300 ml kg^{-1} min^{-1}, adult 70–80 ml kg^{-1} min^{-1}). They have a limited capacity to increase the SV in response to increased filling and the resting HR is near maximal (Table 20.1). Neonates are exquisitely sensitive to negative inotropic or chronotropic agents.

The sarcoplasmic reticulum in neonatal myocytes is poorly developed. Calcium for cardiac contraction is derived from the extracellular fluid and infants do not tolerate ionized hypocalcaemia. There is a relative imbalance of sympathetic and parasympathetic nervous systems at birth and neonates are prone to vagal reflexes.

The infant lung is very compliant, the ribs are also relatively compliant. The lower airways are small and easily obstructed by secretions. Infants are consequently prone to respiratory failure.

Table 20.1 Normal ranges for RR, HR and systolic BP according to patient age

Age	RR (bpm)	HR (bpm)	Systolic BP (mmHg)
Newborn	40–50	120–160	50–90
Infant (<1 year)	30–40	110–160	70–90
Preschool (2–5 years)	20–30	95–140	80–100
Primary school (5–12 years)	15–20	80–120	90–110
Adolescent (>12 years)	12–16	60–100	100–120

Other important factors to consider include immature renal function, temperature regulation, hepatic function and drug, particularly opiate, metabolism.

Transitional Circulation

In utero blood bypasses the foetal lung via two shunts, the foramen ovale and the ductus arteriosus (DA). With the first few breaths, there is a dramatic reduction in the PVR and closure of foetal shunts. Pulmonary vasodilatation continues during the first few weeks of life, due to thinning of smooth muscle in the media of the pulmonary arterioles. The PVR reaches adult levels by a few weeks of age (Figure 20.1). During this time the pulmonary vasculature remains reactive and stimuli such as hypoxia, hypercarbia and acidosis will cause pulmonary vasoconstriction and possibly reopen the DA (see below). Persistent PHT of the newborn may result; hypoxia may become critical and require treatment with inhaled NO or, in extreme cases, ECMO.

Closure of the DA occurs in two phases. Functional closure occurs within 2–4 days in nearly all healthy infants under the influence of increasing PaO$_2$, falling PaCO$_2$ and prostaglandins. Anatomical

145

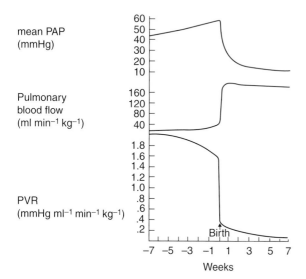

mean PAP (mmHg)

Pulmonary blood flow (ml min⁻¹ kg⁻¹)

PVR (mmHg ml⁻¹ min⁻¹ kg⁻¹)

Birth

Weeks

Figure 20.1 Perinatal changes in pulmonary haemodynamics. Reprinted with permission from Rudolph AM, 1996.

Table 20.2 Conditions dependent on continuing patency of the DA

Duct-dependent	Conditions
Systemic circulation	Critical coarctation, critical AS, HLHS
Pulmonary circulation	Pulmonary atresia, critical PS, tricuspid atresia
'Mixing'	Transposition of the great arteries

closure of the DA due to fibrosis occurs within the first 3 weeks of life.

Continued ductal patency may occur due to prematurity (inadequate ductal smooth muscle) or in sick infants under the influence of excessive endogenous prostaglandin, released in response to stimuli such as hypoxia (causing relaxation of the ductal smooth muscle). A large duct may result in cardiac failure due to excessive pulmonary blood flow (PBF); the diastolic BP will be low and may be associated with impaired renal or intestinal blood flow (possible renal impairment or necrotizing enterocolitis). Prostaglandin synthetase inhibitors such as indomethacin promote closure of the duct.

Duct-Dependent Circulation

In certain situations, continued ductal patency may be required for survival of the neonate (Table 20.2). In this situation prostaglandin E_2 (PGE_2) infusion will be required and should be continued until definitive surgery. High doses of PGE_2 can result in apnoea, fever and systemic vasodilatation. Where PGE_2 infusion has been continued long term (for instance, a premature neonate awaiting surgery), it should be remembered that prostaglandins are effective pulmonary vasodilators and may have to be weaned gradually after surgery.

Infants with a duct-dependent systemic circulation typically present with cardiac failure or collapse during the first week of life as the duct closes and shunting from the pulmonary to systemic circulation is lost. Treatment comprises resuscitation with inotropes and fluids, and institution of PGE_2 infusion prior to definitive surgery.

Infants with duct-dependent pulmonary circulation become cyanosed after duct closure and the loss of left-to-right shunting across the duct. Cyanosis will be unresponsive to an increased FiO_2 and the PBF must be restored with prostaglandin infusion before a definitive surgical procedure; for example, valvotomy or a systemic to pulmonary shunt is performed.

Infants with duct-dependent 'mixing' have two parallel closed-loop circulations and are dependent on mixing between the right and left side. PGE_2 infusion and balloon atrial septostomy will be required where there is inadequate intracardiac mixing.

Balancing Systemic and Pulmonary Circulations in Neonates

An appropriate balance between systemic blood flow and PBF can be crucial, particularly in the neonate when alteration in the direction of shunt blood flow may cause dramatic changes in saturation or CO.

Oxygen is a potent pulmonary vasodilator in neonates, while hypercarbia and acidosis cause pulmonary vasoconstriction. A high FiO_2 and hyperventilation may be beneficial in infants with reduced PBF. Conversely, they may have a detrimental effect in infants with high PBF, or with balanced systemic and pulmonary shunts.

Exposure of neonates with large left-to-right shunts (e.g. a large VSD) to a high FiO_2 will cause pulmonary hyperaemia and worsening cardiac failure. Infants in cardiac failure preoperatively should be given sufficient inspired oxygen to maintain the SaO_2 in the low 90s only. Similarly, neonates with a duct-dependent systemic circulation (see above) or with high-volume, high-pressure shunts (e.g. atrio-ventricular (A-V) septal defect, truncus arteriosus, a large Blalock–Taussig (B–T) shunt), may have balanced shunts between systemic and pulmonary circulation. Ventilation with 100% oxygen may cause a marked fall in the PVR, excessive left-to-right shunting and a fall in systemic perfusion, leading to hypotension and metabolic acidosis. Strategies should be adopted to improve the CO (e.g. fluids, inotropes) and reduce the PBF. Mechanical ventilation in the operating room should be with air (or for cyanotic lesions, sufficient oxygen to maintain the SaO_2 in the mid 80s), and with moderate hypercarbia. Conversely, a marked fall in the SVR should be avoided as this may result in increased right-to-left shunting and critical cyanosis. Inotropic support may be required to increase the SVR and CO, thus improving the PBF. Similar principles should be followed postoperatively in the ICU, particularly after the first-stage Norwood procedure for hypoplastic left heart syndrome (HLHS).

The SVR should be maintained in infants with large right-to-left shunts, such as tetralogy of Fallot. Excessive vasodilatation on induction of anaesthesia may result in worsening cyanosis; vasoconstrictors may be required. Extreme right-to-left shunting is seen in the 'spelling Fallot' due to spasm of the RVOT infundibulum in the presence of excess catecholamines. Measures to overcome infundibular spasm and increase the PBF are required. These include adequate sedation, hyperventilation with 100% oxygen, a fluid bolus, bicarbonate or phenylephrine – the latter to reverse the direction of the shunt across the VSD and improve forward flow to the lungs. Propranolol or esmolol may also be considered to reduce infundibular spasm.

The SVR must be maintained in infants with left (or right) ventricular outflow obstruction. A fall in the SVR may lead to critical hypoperfusion of the hypertrophied ventricle. A reduction in the PVR may be beneficial in infants with RVH.

Cardiopulmonary Interactions

Positive pressure ventilation is generally beneficial to infants in cardiac failure due to poor myocardial function or left-to-right shunts (reduced work of breathing and afterload, improved oxygenation and CO_2 clearance), with attention to the FiO_2, as described above. However, hyperventilation at high airway pressures or lung volumes may increase the PVR by distension of the lungs, disproportionately reducing the cross-sectional area of the pulmonary vasculature.

Spontaneous ventilation – where intra-pleural pressure is negative during inspiration – will augment systemic venous return to the right heart and improve the PBF. This fact is utilized in the postoperative management of patients with cavopulmonary connections.

Surgical Strategy

The timing of surgical repair is dictated by the functional impact of the cardiac lesion. Urgent balloon septostomy may be indicated in neonates with transposition of the great arteries. Duct-dependent lesions require corrective or palliative surgery within days of birth. Similarly, infants with obstructed total anomalous pulmonary venous drainage (TAPVD) may present with extreme cyanosis and cardiac failure, requiring urgent corrective surgery.

Systemic arterial to pulmonary shunts such as the B–T (subclavian artery-to-main PA) shunt are performed in infancy for conditions associated with a low PBF such as severe tetralogy of Fallot or pulmonary atresia. Definitive corrective surgery is performed, usually in the first year, after further growth of the pulmonary arteries.

Conditions involving left-to-right shunts increase the PBF and cause cardiac failure and PHT. Typically, high-volume shunts cause heart failure as the PVR falls to adult levels at a few weeks of age (e.g. a large VSD). A continued high PBF will result in irreversible changes in the pulmonary vasculature and will severely limit treatment options. Early surgery is therefore indicated. PA banding may be performed in infants with a high PBF not suitable for early definitive surgery (e.g. multiple VSDs). Low-volume shunts (e.g. ASDs) may be closed when the child is older to avoid irreversible PHT in adult life.

Palliative surgery to create a univentricular circulation is performed in conditions where there is only a single functional ventricle or great vessel (univentricular A-V connection – double-inlet ventricle, HLHS, tricuspid atresia or severe pulmonary atresia with intact ventricular septum). The PBF may initially be provided with a B–T shunt in the neonatal period while the PVR remains high. Systemic venous shunts are performed after the PVR

147

falls – initially a Glenn (SVC-to-PA) shunt, followed by an IVC-to-PA anastomosis to complete the Fontan circulation (or total cavopulmonary venous connection – see Chapter 21).

Closed Cardiac Surgery

Cardiac operations may be 'closed' or 'open'. Open operations are performed on CPB and are discussed in the next chapter. Closed operations are usually performed on the great vessels and do not require CPB. The four commonest indications for closed operation in neonates and infants are:

- Ligation of a patent ductus arteriosus (PDA) via left thoracotomy
- Repair of coarctation via left thoracotomy
- PA banding via sternotomy or thoracotomy; PA banding is a temporary measure to prevent PHT and is reversed at the time of definitive surgery
- Systemic to pulmonary shunts, for example, a B–T shunt via sternotomy or thoracotomy

Cyanosis

Children with cyanotic heart disease maximize the tissue oxygen delivery by becoming polycythemic and having a mild metabolic acidosis (causing a right shift of the Hb–O_2 dissociation curve). The progression of cyanosis is reflected in an increase in the haematocrit; venesection and haemodilution may be indicated. There is a risk of thromboembolism, including cerebral infarction, which is exacerbated by dehydration. Prolonged preoperative starvation must therefore be avoided. The prothrombotic tendency is partially compensated for by a mild coagulopathy – clotting factors should be available post CPB.

Conduct of Anaesthesia

The anaesthetist requires a thorough understanding of congenital cardiac lesions, the planned surgery, the management of CPB and familiarity with anaesthetizing small infants for major surgery – this is not for the occasional practitioner.

The anaesthesia plan should be formulated in the light of all preoperative investigations and discussions. The predominant cardiac lesion should be considered on the basis of the pathophysiology (Table 20.3), myocardial reserve and an assessment of the nature of the shunt or obstructive lesions and the impact of an alteration of the SVR or PVR.

Children with uncomplicated procedures, such as closure of the ASD, VSD or PDA, may be suitable candidates for a 'fast-track' approach and this should be taken into account in planning anaesthesia. A child having a cavopulmonary connection may benefit from early tracheal extubation as the PBF is improved with spontaneous ventilation. Children who are in cardiorespiratory failure preoperatively, are haemodynamically unstable or who have large left-to-right shunts and are at risk for postoperative PHT will require postoperative ventilation.

Preoperative Assessment

The child must be evaluated carefully in the light of cardiological investigations. Symptoms of cardiac failure should be sought – poor feeding, sweating and grunting in young infants, recurrent chest infections, failure to thrive and poor exercise tolerance in older children. Signs of cardiac failure in young infants include tachycardia, tachypnoea and hepatomegaly (but rarely oedema). In children with cyanotic heart disease, the baseline SaO_2 should be recorded and a history suggestive of hypercyanotic episodes in children with tetralogy of Fallot should be sought. It is obviously important to exclude intercurrent infection as a cause of worsening symptoms.

A note should be made of associated congenital disorders, particularly those affecting the airway. Di George syndrome (22q11 deletion) causes 5% of cardiac anomalies, is associated particularly with truncus arteriosus and interrupted aortic arch and often results in thymic aplasia and neonatal hypocalcaemia. The immunological defect necessitates the use of irradiated blood products to prevent graft versus host disease.

There should be a detailed and sympathetic discussion with the parents (and child if appropriate) concerning invasive monitoring, the need for postoperative intensive care, blood transfusion, analgesia and sedation. This is obviously a time of enormous stress for the family. It is our normal practice for the parents to accompany the child to the anaesthetic room with a member of the nursing staff, if they wish – discussions should focus on their role and what to expect.

Premedication

Premedication of the young infant is not necessary, although midazolam may be considered if the child

Table 20.3 Pathophysiology of congenital heart lesions

		Example	Comment
Acyanotic lesions	Left-to-right shunt Restrictive Non-restrictive	Small ASD, VSD, PDA Large ASD, VSD, PDA, A-VSD	May lead to congestive cardiac failure and PHT, depending on the magnitude of the shunting
	Obstructive	AS, coarctation of the aorta interrupted aortic arch, HLHS, PS, MS, TS	Severity of lesion determines age at presentation – neonates may be critically ill
	Regurgitant	AR, MR, MV prolapse, TR, pulmonary incompetence	
Cyanotic lesions	Transposition of the great arteries	With ASD, PDA or VSD, ±LVOT obstruction	May require balloon atrial septostomy for survival if inadequate mixing Presence of LVOT obstruction determines surgical options
	Right-to-left shunt	Tetralogy of Fallot, critical PS, pulmonary atresia (±VSD), tricuspid atresia	Severity of cyanosis depends on degree of obstruction through the right heart
	Common mixing	TAPVD (+ASD, ±VSD, PDA, coarctation of the aorta), truncus arteriosus, double-inlet ventricle ('single ventricle'), double-outlet ventricle	Cyanosis may not be severe if lung blood flow unobstructed, but congestive heart failure will be present

Modified from Archer and Burch, *Paediatric Cardiology: An Introduction*. 1998 Hodder Arnold)

has frequent hypercyanotic 'spells'. Older children may be premedicated with oral midazolam or temazepam, provided there are no contraindications, such as upper airway obstruction or limited cardiac reserve. Oral morphine (Oramorph 0.1-0.2 mg kg^{-1}) can be used if 'heavier' premedication is required. Topical local anaesthesia is routine; amethocaine gel (Ametop^{TM}) is suitable for infants from 6 weeks of age. No food or milk should be taken in the 6 hours prior to induction of anaesthesia. Clear fluids, however, are permitted up to 2 hours prior to induction to reduce preoperative discomfort and intraoperative hypoglycaemia.

Induction of Anaesthesia

Non-invasive monitoring is applied before induction; at minimum a SaO$_2$ monitor. Full monitoring should be applied as soon as the child will tolerate it. Infants who are unstable should be anaesthetized in the operating room.

The choice of induction agent depends on the cardiac lesion. Children with less severe lesions (e.g. ASDs, small VSDs) will tolerate induction with

judicious doses of propofol. Inhalational induction with sevoflurane is routine for infants, although extreme care should be taken in sick infants with severe cyanosis or cardiac failure as they will not tolerate the myocardial depressant effects of volatile agents. Anaesthesia may be maintained with isoflurane and continued during CPB. Inhalational induction of anaesthesia may be delayed in children with cyanotic heart lesions and be more rapid in children with left-to-right shunts, although this is of little clinical importance. N$_2$O is no longer used – it is a myocardial depressant and may increase the PVR. Air must be available on the anaesthetic machine as it is required for infants with balanced shunts.

Ketamine, a safe alternative to inhalational agents, is commonly used in sick patients. It causes an increase in the CI, SVR and PVR, although a rise in the PVR may be avoided with effective airway control. It has a direct myocardial depressant effect that is usually offset by inhibition of norepinephrine uptake. The myocardial depressant effect may be evident in children on long-term inotrope therapy with depleted catecholamine stores.

149

High-dose fentanyl anaesthesia is also suitable for infants with limited myocardial reserve. It will limit the stress response to surgery, but total doses of >50 $\mu g\ kg^{-1}$ probably confer no additional benefit and may result in hypotension. Doses higher than 1–2 $\mu g\ kg^{-1}$ should only be given incrementally with invasive monitoring.

Cuffed endotracheal tubes are used routinely in many centres. They are usually used a half size smaller than the uncuffed tubes. They diminish leakage and optimize ventilation. Our impression is that there has been no increase in airway problems because of this change.

Some practitioners advocate regional anaesthesia for paediatric cardiac surgery to reduce the stress response, improve postoperative recovery and reduce hospital costs. Others believe the risk of an epidural haematoma in a child who will be heparinized far outweigh the benefits. It is suggested that the risk of epidural haematoma is minimized by ensuring normal preoperative coagulation, abandoning difficult insertions or those where blood returns through the needle or epidural catheter. Heparin should be given no less than 60 minutes after needle placement and the catheter removed only in the presence of normal coagulation.

Vascular Access and Monitoring

The long saphenous vein is useful for peripheral vascular access. Sites for arterial access may be the radial, femoral, axillary or brachial arteries. Procedural ultrasound should be routine. The arterial line and SaO_2 monitor should be sited in the right arm for coarctation repair. Monitoring from the ipsilateral arm during a B–T shunt should be avoided. NIBP monitoring on the leg is useful after coarctation repair.

Central venous access is usually via the internal jugular vein (IJV); with ultrasound guidance. Double- or triple-lumen (4 Fr or 5 Fr) catheters are available in various lengths. The IJV should not be used in infants with univentricular physiology as thrombosis of the neck veins will make a subsequent Fontan procedure impossible. The femoral vein should be used as an alternative, with a small monitoring line in the IJV to reflect the PAP. The left IJV should be avoided in children with a persistent left SVC as it commonly drains into the coronary sinus. Transthoracic lines are commonly used in the USA;

they may be placed to measure the LA or PAP post CPB; their routine use might spare the central veins and is said to be associated with a low incidence of bleeding, once removed.

Core and peripheral temperatures are measured in all cases. The nasopharyngeal temperature gives a measure of brain temperature – a peripheral probe should be placed on the foot. Overhead radiant heaters may be useful in the anaesthetic or induction room, if used, although overheating should be avoided and moderate hypothermia may be protective in infants undergoing coarctation repair.

Cardiopulmonary Bypass

Differences in CPB management in children reflects a physiology that differs from adults and the complexity of intracardiac surgery. Cannulation will usually be bicaval for intracardiac surgery. Flow rates are relatively high, reflecting the increased metabolic rate of small infants. Perfusion pressures are maintained at 30–60 mmHg at normothermia and vasoconstrictors are rarely required. In the past, the volume of the pump prime was large relative to the circulating volume of infants; 800–1,000 ml of prime relative to a blood volume of 250–300 ml. Citrated blood is added to the pump prime to avoid excessive haemodilution. Calcium is added to avoid hypocalcaemia. In the current era there is much more emphasis on reducing the prime volume to minimize perioperative fluid overload. Paediatric oxygenators and cardiotomy reservoirs are smaller, the length and diameter of the bypass lines are reduced and, unlike in most adult surgery, venous drainage is enhanced by applying a negative pressure to the venous line.

CPB may be conducted at normothermia, moderate hypothermia (25–32 °C), deep hypothermia (15–20 °C), or deep hypothermia with circulatory arrest (DHCA). Moderate hypothermia is mainly used in adolescents – SVC and IVC cannulae do not obstruct the surgeon's view of the intracardiac anatomy and full flows are maintained. Modern practice is to cool to 32 °C for most operations, lower temperatures are reserved for complex lesions or excessive collateral flow.

Uniform cooling is important and an inadequate cooling time (<18 minutes) is associated with worse outcomes. Vasodilatation during cooling may be useful. Cerebral protection may be improved using pH-stat acid–base management prior to circulatory arrest (associated with cerebral vasodilatation). Alpha-stat acid–base management, which preserves cerebral autoregulation, is used at other times. Ice-packs are placed over the head during DHCA to prevent rewarming. Hyperglycaemia should be avoided.

Weaning from CPB

Rewarming after AXC removal allows for the spontaneous return of myocardial electrical activity. VF is uncommon in children and, if persistent, may reflect poor myocardial preservation. Intracardiac de-airing should be meticulous to avoid coronary and cerebral air embolism – the lungs are mechanically ventilated and the venous line partially occluded to increase the LA filling. As the heart starts to eject, endotracheal suction is performed and ventilation recommenced. Temporary pacing wires are routinely used as intra-cardiac surgery may affect the cardiac conducting system.

Inotropic support is usual in infants and should be started when the nasopharyngeal temperature reaches 30 °C after removal of the AXC. Epinephrine is the drug of choice, although dobutamine or a phospho-diesterase (PDE) inhibitor may be used if the PVR is increased. PDE inhibitors (e.g. milrinone) are commonly used when there is PHT or RV dysfunction. The combination of a PDE inhibitor with epinephrine or dopamine is useful in the presence of poor ventricular function or after ventriculotomy (Table 20.4). A volume overload in the small non-compliant ventricle must be avoided.

The use of vasoconstrictors in children after cardiac surgery is controversial. In the setting of systemic arterial hypotension and poor end-organ perfusion in the setting of good cardiac function and oxygen delivery, the authors' preference is to use vasopressin at a dose of 0.0003–0.002 IU kg^{-1} min^{-1}. Vasoconstrictors should not be used in the context of a low CO where peripheral limb ischaemia may result.

Measurement of the SvO_2, either by intermittent sampling of blood in the central veins or continuously using an oximeter that is integral to the central line, may be helpful in deducing the adequacy of the CO.

Increasingly, near-infrared oximetry has been used to monitor the adequacy of cerebral and, occasionally, visceral oxygenation throughout the course of cardiac surgery requiring CPB. There are several devices available with some technical differences beyond the scope of this chapter. It is a proxy measure of the CO but is susceptible to changes in the $PaCO_2$ and the perfusion pressure. A regional cerebral saturation of less than 50% usually

Table 20.4 Common cardiac drug dosages in paediatric cardiac practice

Drug	Dilution	1 ml hr^{-1} =	Dose range
Dopamine	3 mg kg^{-1} in 50 ml 5% dextrose	1 µg kg^{-1} min^{-1}	5–10 µg kg^{-1} min^{-1}
Dobutamine	3 mg kg^{-1} in 50 ml 5% dextrose	1 µg kg^{-1} min^{-1}	5–10 µg kg^{-1} min^{-1}
Epinephrine	0.03 mg kg^{-1} in 50 ml 5% dextrose	0.01 µg kg^{-1} min^{-1}	0.01–0.5 µg kg^{-1} min^{-1}
Norepinephrine	0.03 mg kg^{-1} in 50 ml 5% dextrose	0.01 µg kg^{-1} min^{-1}	0.01–0.5 µg kg^{-1} min^{-1}
Milrinone	0.3 mg kg^{-1} in 50 ml 5% dextrose	0.1 µg kg^{-1} min^{-1}	0.375-0.75 µg kg^{-1} min^{-1} Loading dose 50–100 µg kg^{-1} over 20 minutes
Isoproterenol	0.03 mg kg^{-1} in 50 ml 5% dextrose	0.01 µg kg^{-1} min^{-1}	0.01–0.5 µg kg^{-1} min^{-1}
Sodium nitroprusside	3 mg kg^{-1} in 50 ml 5% dextrose	1 µg kg^{-1} min^{-1}	0.5–5 µg kg^{-1} min^{-1}
GTN	3 mg kg^{-1} in 50 ml 5% dextrose Maximum 1 mg ml^{-1}	1 µg kg^{-1} min^{-1}	0.5–5 µg kg^{-1} min^{-1}
Calcium gluconate	10%		Bolus dose 0.1 ml kg^{-1}
Phenylephrine			Bolus dose 1 µg kg^{-1}
Vasopressin	3 IU kg^{-1} in 50 ml 5% dextrose	0.001 IU kg min^{-1}	

indicates that there is a major problem that requires intervention.

Management Post Bypass

Modified Ultrafiltration

Modified ultrafiltration is useful in children weighing less than 20 kg. It is started prior to protamine administration. Blood is taken from the aorta, passed through an ultrafilter and returned to the RA. The process usually takes 15–20 minutes and is continued until the haematocrit is ~40%. Between 150 and 500 ml of fluid may be removed, depending on the prime volume and starting haematocrit. In addition to increasing the haematocrit, modified ultrafiltration increases colloid osmotic pressure, removes extracellular water (including myocardial water), reduces transfusion requirements and improves the haemodynamic function. It also reduces the PVR, improves the cerebral function and may reduce the levels of circulating vasoactive cytokines. Some centres use continuous ultrafiltration during CPB to remove excess fluid; this may obviate the need for modified ultrafiltration.

Haemostasis

Diffuse coagulopathy is common in neonates after CPB. This is due to a combination of immature hepatic function, haemodilution by the CPB prime and activation of clotting by the large non-endothelialized surface of the bypass circuit. Operations tend to be long, they may require DHCA, pump flow rates are high and relatively large volumes of blood are salvaged and returned to the bypass circuit. Thrombocytopenia and hypofibrinogenaemia are common, and platelets and cryoprecipitate (or FFP) are ordered routinely. Mild coagulation defects are also common in children with cyanotic heart disease. CPB prime volumes have been reduced to limit the coagulation problems of neonatal CPB. It is now common to order a thromboelastogram in patients who continue to bleed after heparin reversal.

Aprotinin is not used routinely, being reserved for complex surgery, transplants and reoperations (see Chapter 36). It may reduce bleeding after reoperation but its use in patients undergoing DHCA or venous shunts (e.g. a bidirectional Glenn shunt) is controversial. It may have a useful anti-inflammatory effect, but a test dose should be given because of the risk of anaphylaxis. Tranexamic acid (TXA) and ε-aminocaproic acid may also be useful although the optimal dose of TXA is unknown.

Transoesophageal Echocardiography

TOE is useful before the onset of CPB to exclude additional defects and in the post-CPB period to assess myocardial contractility and the integrity of the surgical repair. Considerable expertise is required to interpret TOE images in the setting of complex lesions. Smaller infants should have epicardial echocardiography. Images should be obtained and stored routinely prior to leaving the operating room.

Delayed Sternal Closure

The chest may be left open after neonatal surgery or if there is evidence of cardiac tamponade after primary chest closure. Delayed primary closure is usually possible on the ICU after 24–72 hours.

Pulmonary Hypertensive Crisis

All newborns and those with high PBF (e.g. truncus, A-V septal defect and TAPVD) are at risk of postoperative PHT. For this reason, a monitoring line may be inserted into the PA during surgery. During a pulmonary hypertensive crisis there may be a sustained rise in the PAP (>2/3 systemic) or the PAP may be suprasystemic. It will usually respond to inhaled NO (20 ppm), although doses up to 80 ppm may be required. Standard management also includes moderate hypocapnia, avoidance of acidosis, ventilation with 100% oxygen and additional sedation and paralysis. The usual duration of therapy is 24-48 hours.

Right Heart Failure

Right heart failure may be a consequence of surgical ventriculotomy, poor myocardial preservation (particularly with pre-existing RVH), transient PHT, raised TPG or anatomical problems subsequent to the surgery, such as an obstructed outflow tract. It is important to rule out the latter with on-table echocardiography or early postoperative right heart catheterization.

Treatment strategies include those for PHT, if indicated, careful volume loading (RA pressures of 15–16 mmHg) and norepinephrine combined with a PDE inhibitor. Failure to respond to high-dose inotropes may be an indication for the use of ECMO or a mechanical ventricular assist device.

Transfer to Intensive Care

The transfer of the child back to intensive care may be a hazardous process – lines may be displaced and haemodynamic instability may occur due to bleeding (Chapter 22). The child should be fully monitored at all times. Finally, it is important that the anaesthetist transfers the wealth of information they have gleaned about the patient during the perioperative period to the intensive care team in an effective manner.

Key Points

- Neonates have a limited cardiopulmonary reserve and reactive pulmonary vasculature during the first weeks of life.
- Prostaglandin infusion is required for duct-dependent circulation prior to surgery.
- Manipulations of the PVR and SVR have an important effect on balanced circulation; ventilation strategies should be carefully considered.
- Children with cyanotic heart disease require careful perioperative care.
- The conduct of anaesthesia and CPB strategy are determined by patient age, the pathophysiology of the cardiac lesion and the planned surgical procedure.
- Recent advances include reducing the pump prime volume and monitoring of tissue oxygenation.
- Modified or continuous ultrafiltration improves the fluid balance and cardiac function after bypass in infants.
- Neonates with a high PBF are at risk of pulmonary hypertensive crisis post bypass.

Further Reading

Davis PJ, Cladis FP (eds.). *Smith's Anesthesia for Children and Infants*, 9th edn. Philadelphia, PA: Elsevier; 2016.

Durandy Y. Warm pediatric cardiac surgery: European experience. *Asian Cardiovasc Thorac Ann* 2010; 18: 386–95.

Goldman AP, Delius RE, Deanfield JE, Macrae DJ. Nitric oxide is superior to prostacyclin for pulmonary hypertension after cardiac operations. *Ann Thorac Surg* 1995; 60: 300–6.

Hirsch JC, Charpie JR, Ohye RG, Gurney JG. Near-infrared spectroscopy: what we know and what we need to know – a systematic review of the congenital heart disease literature. *J Thorac Cardiovasc Surg* 2009; 137: 154–9.

Laussen P. Optimal blood gas management during deep hypothermic paediatric cardiac surgery: alpha stat is easy, but pH stat may be preferable. *Paediatr Anaesth* 2002; 12: 199–204.

May LE. *Paediatric Heart Surgery: A Ready Reference for Professionals*, 5th edn. Children's Hospital of Wisconsin: MaxiShare; 2012.

Romlin BS, Wåhlander H, Synnergren M, Baghaei F, Jeppsson A. Earlier detection of coagulopathy with thromboelastometry during pediatric cardiac surgery: a prospective observational study. *Paediatr Anaesth* 2013; 23: 222–7.

Shah A, Carlisle JB. Cuffed tracheal tubes: guilty now proven innocent. *Anaesthesia* 2019; 74: 11186–90.

Wypij D, Jonas RA, Bellinger DC, *et al.* The effect of hematocrit during hypothermic cardiopulmonary bypass in infant heart surgery: results from the combined Boston hematocrit trials. *J Thorac Cardiovasc Surg* 2008; 135: 355–60.

Chapter

21

Common Congenital Heart Lesions and Procedures

David J. Barron and Kevin P. Morris

It is not unusual for the cardiac anaesthetist to encounter adults with palliated, corrected or newly diagnosed congenital heart disease (CHD). It is essential, therefore, that the anaesthetist has an appreciation of the types of CHD, surgical procedures and perioperative management.

Arterial Shunts

Variants to arterial shunts include the modified Blalock–Taussig (B–T) shunt (Figure 21.1), the systemic-to-pulmonary shunt and the central shunt.

Physiology

Arterial shunts are used to augment pulmonary blood flow (PBF) in a variety of conditions with inadequate PBF. Some conditions have biventricular anatomy (e.g. Fallot's, pulmonary atresia/VSD, transposition of the great arteries (TGA)/VSD/PS). Others have functionally single ventricle anatomy (e.g. tricuspid atresia/TGA/PS, pulmonary atresia/intact ventricular septum). Behaviour following the shunt is influenced by the underlying anatomy; patients with biventricular anatomy are usually more stable and tolerate the volume load of the shunt better.

Many neonates are duct-dependent preoperatively and receiving a prostaglandin E_2 (PGE_2) infusion (Chapter 20). The duct is usually tied at the time of shunt placement. Blood flow through the shunt will be influenced by the shunt radius and length:

$$\text{Flow } \alpha \; \frac{\text{Radius}^4}{\text{Length}}$$

Typical shunt sizes are 3.5–4.0 mm in diameter, although these may need to be modified in light of the PA size and the PVR.

Surgery

The most widely used procedure is the modified B–T shunt, which can be performed via either by thoracotomy or midline sternotomy. This involves placement of a small-calibre Gore-Tex® tube graft between the innominate artery and the PA (the original description anastomosed the subclavian artery directly to the PA). This is generally performed on the right side without CPB unless the child is very unstable or a more complex repair is required. The term 'central shunt' involves a similar procedure but implies a shunt between the aorta and the PAs, usually with a short Gore-Tex® graft. It is usually performed via sternotomy and delivers a higher blood flow.

Postoperative Management

It is important to establish the underlying anatomy:

- Single or biventricular anatomy?
- Any other source of pulmonary blood supply other than the shunt (is the ductus arteriosus still open)?

A shunt procedure requiring CPB implies unstable haemodynamics and the need for careful monitoring. Shunts with underlying biventricular anatomy tend to be more stable but all neonates with arterial shunts can be unstable with a low diastolic pressure and the risk of sudden coronary 'steal', leading to unheralded

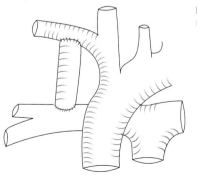

Figure 21.1 The modified B–T shunt

cardiac arrest. There is a need to balance the pulmonary:systemic blood flow (Q_P:Q_S) in a functionally single ventricle. If the shunt is the only source of PBF, aim for an SaO_2 of ~75–80% and Q_P:Q_S = 1:1 (see Figure 21.13). Too small a shunt or an obstructed shunt results in hypoxaemia; a trial of inhaled NO may be helpful in differentiating a structural shunt problem from an elevated PVR. Only the latter is reactive and responds to inhaled NO. Too high a shunt flow leads to a low diastolic pressure, pulmonary congestion and a ventricular volume overload. Attempts to reduce the PBF by increasing the PVR are seldom effective. Lowering the SVR with vasodilators is more effective at balancing the Q_P:Q_S ratio. Surgical revision of the shunt may be necessary.

Start heparin infusion on return to the ICU when the patient is stabilized and not bleeding (10 IU kg^{-1} h^{-1}).

Atrial Septal Defects

Incidence and Associations

ASDs account for 8% of all CHD. Most occur in isolation, but recognized associations include Holt-Oram, Turners and maternal rubella syndromes, as well as Down syndrome in the specific case of primum ASDs.

Anatomy

Defects occur at different sites (Figure 21.2):

Secundum ASDs are the most common – the majority can be closed with a device in the catheter laboratory. Features making device closure unlikely are: a very large defect, the lack of an inferior or lateral rim of tissue and relatively large defects in smaller children. All other types of defect require surgical closure.

Primum ASDs are part of the spectrum of atrioventricular (A-V) septal defects (AVSDs, see below) and are more correctly called 'partial AVSDs'. They are always associated with a cleft in the left A-V ('mitral') valve, which is repaired as part of the procedure.

Sinus venosus ASDs are associated with anomalous drainage of the upper right pulmonary veins into the root of the SVC (Figure 21.3). These can be baffled back to the LA with a patch repair

Coronary sinus ASDs are very rare, and are associated with unroofing of the coronary sinus, thus, closing the defect leaves the CS draining into the LA creating a small, haemodynamically insignificant right-to-left shunt.

Physiology

Left-to-right shunts cause a volume load on pulmonary circulation. Most children are symptomless but plethoric

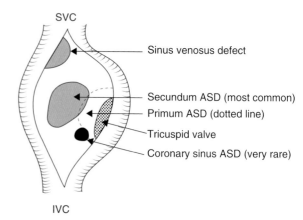

Figure 21.2 View inside the RA

lungs may predispose to chest infections and failure to thrive. Very large shunts may result in effort intolerance. PHT is *not* associated with isolated ASDs in children.

Surgery

Small detects can be repaired by simple suture closure. Larger defects require patch repair with either autologous pericardium or prosthetic patch material. Intraoperative echocardiography should focus on pulmonary venous drainage in a sinus venosus ASD and on the left A-V valve function in partial AVSD repair.

Postoperative Care

Surgery is generally of low risk and children can be weaned from ventilation and extubated shortly after surgery. Sinus venosus ASD repair involves the root of the SVC and there is a risk of causing SVC obstruction. If the face looks plethoric or the SVC pressure is high, arrange echocardiographic or contrast evaluation. Nodal rhythms may occur with high atrial incisions (e.g. sinus venosus ASD).

Some units 'fast-track' ASD repairs to a monitored 'step-down' facility on the day of surgery.

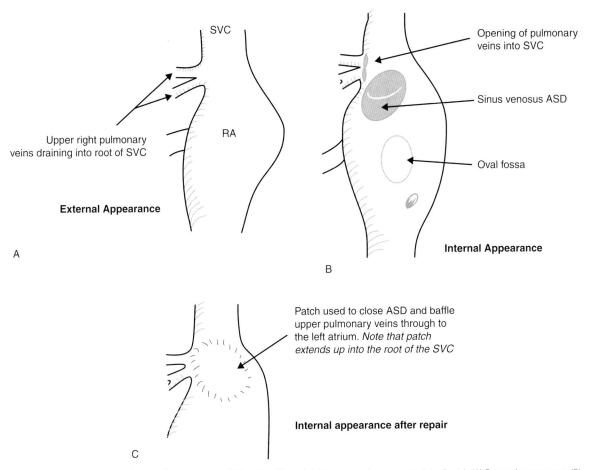

Figure 21.3 Surgical patch closure of sinus venosus ASD and baffling of right upper pulmonary vein into the LA. (A) External appearance, (B) internal appearance, (C) internal appearance after repair.

Atrioventricular Septal Defects

AVSDs are also called A-V canal defects or endocardial cushion defects. They may be complete or partial.

Incidence and Associations

AVSDs account for 4% of all CHD. Both complete and partial AVSD are strongly associated with Down syndrome.

Anatomy

There is a defect in the centre of the heart with a single valve (the common A-V valve), straddling both ventricles, and a hole above and below it. In partial AVSD, the VSD component has closed, leaving only an ASD (see Figure 21.4).

Physiology

A *complete AVSD* behaves like a large VSD (i.e. a left-to-right shunt, leading to a high PBF and heart failure in neonates). In addition, the common A-V valve can be regurgitant, adding to the heart failure. All require surgical closure before 6 months of age. Later repair is associated with significant risk of irreversible PHT.

In *partial AVSDs* (also called primum ASDs), the ventricular component has closed, there is less of a left-to-right shunt and a lower likelihood of heart failure. Repair is generally undertaken before 5 years of age.

Surgery

Operative mortality for repair of complete AVSD is ~ 4%, whereas that for partial AVSD repair is ~ 1%.

Usually, the VSD is closed with one patch, the ASD with another, sandwiching the valve between them (Figure 21.5) – alternatively the procedure can be performed with a single patch, fixing the valve to the crest of the ventricular septum, particularly if the VSD is relatively shallow. Surgery recreates two separate A-V valves. However, anatomically the valve between the LA and LV is not a true 'mitral' valve and is referred to as the 'left A-V valve'. The cleft in the left A-V valve is closed as part of the repair to create a competent valve. The repair of cAVSD in babies without Down syndrome is typically more complicated (poor A-V valve function) compared to babies with Down syndrome. Intra-operative echocardiography should focus on looking for any residual VSD, assessing left and right A-V valve function and ensuring that the LVOT is unobstructed.

Postoperative Management

An LA line is useful and a PA line is inserted where concern exists about PHT. Echocardiography is repeated to exclude a residual VSD, and to assess ventricular and A-V valve function. The cardiac rhythm should be confirmed as there is a risk of heart block. Babies are usually in marked heart failure preoperatively with pulmonary congestion and may take time to wean from the ventilator. The risks and management of PHT are described below. Partial AVSD repairs are generally uncomplicated. All have had left A-V valve repair and should have an echocardiogram to document the AV-valve function.

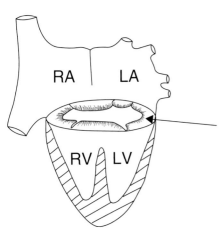

Figure 21.4 Anatomy of an AVSD

There is a defect in the centre of the heart with a single valve (the common AV valve) straddling both ventricles and a hole above and below it. In partial AVSD the VSD component has closed leaving only an ASD

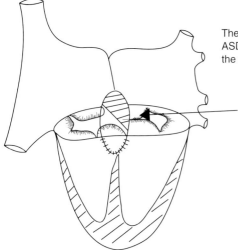

Figure 21.5 Surgery for an AVSD

The VSD is closed with one patch, the ASD with another, sandwiching the valve between them

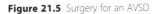

The cleft in the left AV valve is then closed to make the valve competent

Bidirectional Cavopulmonary Shunt

The bidirectional cavopulmonary shunt (BCPS) is also called a cavopulmonary (CP) shunt, a modified Glenn shunt and Hemi-Fontan shunt. It represents one of the staged palliative procedures for children with a functionally single ventricle circulation (see Staged Palliation of the Functionally Univentricular Heart). It accounts for 3–4% of all CHD (e.g. tricuspid atresia, double-inlet LV, hypoplastic left heart syndrome (HLHS)), unbalanced AVSD, PA/interventricular septum (IVS)). It is usually the second stage after an initial Norwood operation, B–T shunt or PA band but it may be the first operation if the Q_P: Q_S ratio is balanced and no surgery is required in the neonatal period.

A BCPS is carried out at around 4–6 months of age. The SVC is anastomosed to the PA, and the IVC remains connected to the RA (Figure 21.6). If the patient has previously had an arterial shunt, this is usually taken down. In other patient groups, a decision is taken as to whether to ligate the main PA or to leave some antegrade PBF. The original Glenn operation involved direct anastomosis of SVC to the surgically isolated right PA.

Physiology

These procedures involve connecting the systemic veins directly into the pulmonary circulation, thus bypassing the right side of the heart completely. They rely on venous pressure to drive the PBF and are only possible if the PVR is low. A failing ventricle or a high PVR may preclude these procedures. If a CP ('venous') shunt was created in the early neonatal period, the high PVR would result in an excessively high SVC pressure and a low PBF – hence an arterial shunt is initially needed, which provides a higher driving pressure and guarantees an adequate PBF.

Postoperative Management

Arterial saturation is typically 80–85%. An SVC line and IVC (or common atrial) line is typically required. The SVC pressure equates to the PAP (typically 14–18 mmHg). The difference between the PAP and atrial/IVC pressure gives the TPG. A TPG of 8–10 mmHg generally implies a low PVR and a favourable outcome. If the TPG is greater than 15 mmHg a mechanical holdup (e.g. anastomotic narrowing, anastomotic thrombosis or PA narrowing) must be excluded before considering inhaled NO to reduce the PVR. The SVC and PA pressures may be elevated (>20 mmHg) with a normal TPG as a consequence of a high atrial pressure, secondary to ventricular dysfunction. Management is aimed at lowering the atrial pressure (vasodilators, inotropes), which will lead to a lowering of the SVC and PA pressures. Haemodynamics are generally good since the volume loading of the ventricle is substantially reduced by this procedure. Hypertension is common and may require treatment.

Ideally, infants are weaned from positive-pressure ventilation as soon as possible to reduce intrathoracic pressure and improve the PBF. Any SVC line should be removed as soon as possible to reduce the risk of thrombosis. A high SVC pressure may result in pleural effusions (sometimes chylothorax), venous congestion of the head and neck, and headaches.

Certain congenital heart lesions are associated with an interruption of the IVC and azygous vein continuation such that IVC blood enters the SVC. A BCPS in this setting (called a Kawashima operation) results in all venous blood other than hepatic venous return contributing to the PBF – the SaO_2 is higher at around 85–90%.

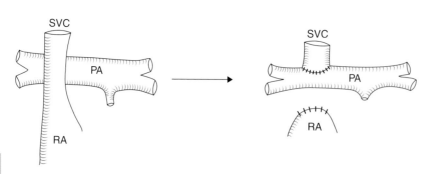

Figure 21.6 The BCPS

Coarctation of the Aorta

Incidence and Associations

Coarctation of the aorta (CoA) accounts for 6% of all CHD. It is associated with Turner syndrome, bicuspid AV (up to 40% of cases) and VSDs.

Anatomy

CoA is narrowing of the aorta in the region of the ductal insertion, i.e. distal to the left subclavian artery. It can occasionally occur proximal to the left subclavian artery.

Aortic interruption is an extreme form of coarctation where there is complete separation of the aortic components, the distal component being supplied by the ductus. Interruption is (almost) always associated with some sort of intracardiac shunt, usually a VSD or aorto-pulmonary window. It is commonly associated with 22q11 deletion. Interruption is a much more complex lesion, requiring repair on CPB and carrying much higher risk.

Physiology

The presentation depends on the severity of narrowing:

- Severe CoA typically presents in the neonatal period as the duct closes – the aorta is virtually occluded, causing circulatory collapse, acute LV failure and loss of lower limb pulses
- Moderate CoA presents more subtly with a degree of LV failure in childhood (rare)
- Less severe CoA presents with chance finding of a murmur, an abnormal CXR or upper-limb hypertension/radio-femoral delay

Management of the Neonate

Administration of prostaglandin E_2 (PGE_2) by infusion reopens the duct and re-establishes flow to the lower body. Ductal tissue is often involved in CoA, and the severity of CoA may also be reduced with PGE_2. Neonates with severe CoA usually have considerable heart failure. They may require full resuscitation with ventilation/inotropic support. The condition can usually be stabilized with these measures. Rarely, the duct will not reopen and emergency surgery is required.

Surgery

Surgery is carried out via a left thoracotomy, and is associated with ~1% perioperative mortality. It is repaired either with resection and end-to-end anastomosis or with subclavian flap angioplasty (Figure 21.7). Both have excellent results although the former is regarded by most as being the 'gold standard'. Sacrificing the subclavian artery in the neonate does not cause limb ischaemia and at worse may result in reduced limb growth. Repair of the associated hypoplastic aortic arch may require CPB via sternotomy. An arterial line should be placed in the right brachial/radial artery to ensure monitoring can be continued with a clamp on the aortic arch. Ideally, two arterial lines, one in the right arm and one femoral, can be placed.

Older children/adolescents are now mostly treated by interventional catheterization with covered stenting rather than a surgical approach.

Complications: The risk of recurrence is 2-4%; the majority can be successfully dilated with balloon angioplasty. Injury to recurrent laryngeal nerve or thoracic duct is rare. There is also a risk of paraplegia (due to spinal ischaemia <0.5% – virtually unknown in neonates). Protective measures include core cooling to 35 °C and keeping the clamp time to less than 30 minutes. Full or partial CPB can be used, allowing for more profound cooling.

Postoperative Management

The femoral pulses should be monitored. Echocardiography is used to assess LV function and confirm adequate arch repair. Patients may have hypertension, requiring treatment (β-blocker). Limb function should be documented once the effects of muscle relaxants have worn off.

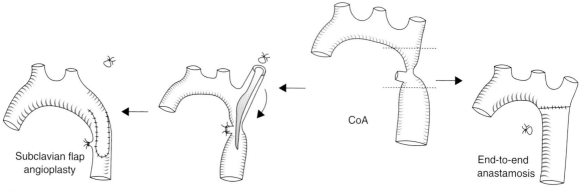

Subclavian flap
angioplasty

CoA

End-to-end
anastamosis

Figure 21.7 Surgery of CoA

Fallot's Tetralogy

Fallot's tetralogy is also called tetralogy of Fallot, ToF and Fallot.

Incidence and Associations

Fallot's tetralogy accounts for 6% of all CHD. It is associated with many syndromic conditions, affecting 20% of patients with Di George syndrome/22q11 deletion, CHARGE (coloboma, heart defects, choanal atresia, retardation of growth or development, genital or urinary abnormalities, and ear abnormalities and deafness) association, VACTERL (vertebral anomalies, anal atresia, cardiovascular abnormalities, tracheo-oesophageal fistula, oesophageal atresia, renal, limb defects) and Down syndrome.

Anatomy

The key anatomical features are a perimembranous VSD with aortic override and multilevel RV outflow obstruction (Figure 21.8). The degree of right outflow tract obstruction is variable and tends to worsen with time as the RVH progresses. Important variants are tetralogy of Fallot with multiple VSDs and the presence of an anomalous left coronary artery (2–5%) – in the latter, repair usually requires a conduit to jump over the coronary artery as it crosses the outflow tract.

Absent PV syndrome is a rare type of Fallot with similar intracardiac anatomy but no true PV. The PAs beyond the valve have marked post-stenotic dilatation and may cause compression of the airways and bronchomalacia. Treatment is similar but involves plication of the aneurysmal central PAs and respiratory assessment.

Physiology

Management depends on the degree of cyanosis at presentation and associated lesions. Cyanotic neonates are usually palliated with a systemic-to-pulmonary shunt procedure (usually a B–T shunt), or with an RVOT stent placed in the cardiac catheter laboratory. Although some centres favour complete neonatal repair, the majority favour delaying surgery in stable infants until they are 3-9 months of age.

Cyanotic 'spelling' typically develops in the first 6 months of life and is treated with β-blockers, which relieve infundibular muscle spasm and reduce the degree of cyanosis. Patients can 'spell' severely on induction of anaesthesia and if this fails to respond to oxygen therapy and volume infusion then a systemic vasoconstrictor (epinephrine/norepinephrine/phenylephrine) may be required to increase the systemic afterload and so improve the PBF.

Surgery

Surgery results in 2–3% early mortality. Muscle bundles in the RVOT are resected and the VSD is closed, usually via the RA. The PV and main PA usually need to be opened out and patched to enlarge the outflow tract sufficiently, requiring a 'transannular' incision and patch. This relieves obstruction but leaves significant PR (Figure 21.9).

The presence of an anomalous LAD coronary artery usually requires the placement of an RV–PA conduit to avoid the vessel. Intraoperative echocardiography should be used to exclude any residual VSD (or additional VSD) and to carefully assess the RVOT, looking for residual obstruction and to quantify the degree of PR.

Postoperative Management

Rhythm disturbances and a low CO can occur. Junctional tachycardias are common and may be nodal or His bundle in origin. An atrial wire study may identify dissociated P-waves, suggesting His bundle tachycardia. The management of junctional ectopic tachycardia is discussed in Chapter 22.

Restrictive physiology may lead to a low CO state due to a non-compliant, stiff RV chamber, leading to predominantly diastolic dysfunction:

- A pathognomonic echocardiography finding is forward flow in the PA during ventricular diastole; atrial systole results in opening of the PV

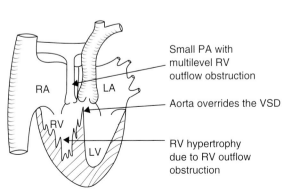

Figure 21.8 Anatomy of tetralogy of Fallot

Small PA with multilevel RV outflow obstruction

Aorta overrides the VSD

RV hypertrophy due to RV outflow obstruction

RA

LA

RV

LV

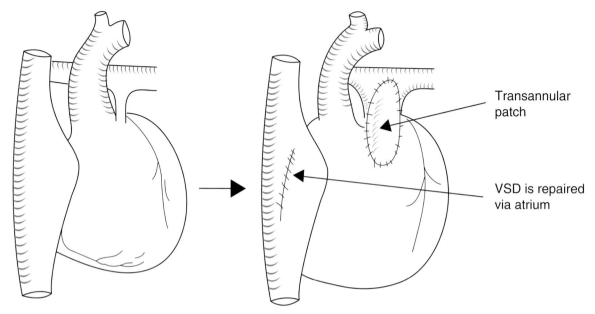

Figure 21.9 Surgery for tetralogy of Fallot

as a consequence of pressure transmission through the stiff, non-compliant RV

- Residual structural RVOT obstruction must be excluded by echocardiography
- Treatment is by increasing preload – RA pressure 10–15 mmHg
- Inodilators such as milrinone are preferred to epinephrine, which may worsen RV diastolic function
- PA forward flow and PR are adversely affected by positive-pressure ventilation; shorten inspiratory time relative to expiratory time, possible role for negative-pressure ventilation

- There is a marked capillary leak often with high ascitic losses – a peritoneal drain is important and dialysis may be needed
- Consider return to operating room if the residual RVOT obstruction cannot be overcome, the placement of a competent valve into the RVOT or the creation of an ASD to allow a right-to-left shunt

Fontan Procedure

The Fontan procedure is also called total cavopulmonary connection (TCPC). It is the final staged palliative procedure for children with a functionally single ventricle circulation (see Staged Palliation of the Functionally Univentricular Heart). TCPC accounts for 3–4% of all CHD (e.g. tricuspid atresia, double-inlet LV, HLHS, unbalanced AVSD, PA/IVS). Children have almost always had a previous BCPS. It is very rarely performed in one step, i.e. without a previous CP shunt. There is 3–5% early mortality.

The completion of the Fontan circulation, usually before school age, directs IVC blood flow to the PA (SVC return is already connected to the PA through the BCPS). Surgery has evolved over time from the original Fontan (direct RA-to-PA connection) to the TCPC, which is now achieved in one of two ways:

1. *Lateral tunnel TCPC*: a baffle is placed inside the atrium to redirect IVC blood into the PAs
2. *External conduit TCPC*: a Gore-Tex® tube is placed outside the atrium to divert IVC blood into the PAs

The TCPC is usually fenestrated which in the setting of a high PVR preserves an adequate ventricular output at the expense of a degree of hypoxaemia (Figure 21.10).

Postoperative Management

This involves similar principles to the management of BCPS (see above). The SVC and IVC pressures are now equal and are equivalent to the PAP (typically 12–16 mmHg). A low PVR is essential and the TPG should ideally be less than 10 mmHg. The SVC/IVC pressure is no longer a marker of ventricular preload and so a direct atrial line is needed to monitor the filling pressure. These patients often require a lot of volume, which should be titrated to atrial pressure. The interpretation of haemodynamics following the Fontan procedures is shown in Table 21.1.

Fenestration causes some obligate right-to-left shunt, the degree of shunting being proportional to the TPG and the size of the fenestration. A low PVR and favourable haemodynamics are generally associated with an SaO_2 greater than 90%.

Ideally, haemodynamically stable children should undergo early weaning from mechanical ventilation to decrease the intrathoracic pressure and increase the flow through the Fontan circuit, thus increasing the CO. Haemodynamic instability, by contrast, is an indication for continued mechanical ventilation.

A high PAP with a low CO requires careful review – optimization of ventricular function and cardiac rhythm. A therapeutic trial of inhaled NO may be used but is rarely effective. In this setting, an

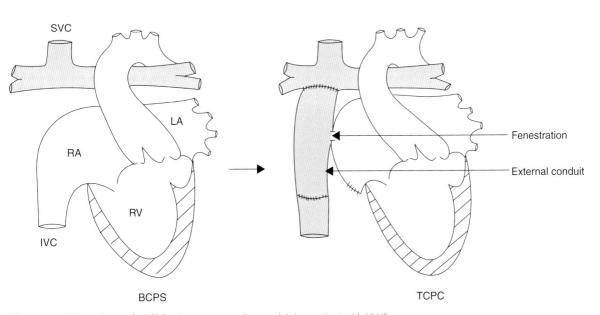

Figure 21.10 Completion of a TCPC using an extracardiac conduit in a patient with HLHS

Table 21.1 Interpretation of haemodynamics after the Fontan operation

	SVC/IVC ('PA') pressure	LA pressure	TPG
Hypovolaemia	↓	↓	Normal/low
High PVR	↑	↓	High
Systemic venous pathway obstruction	↑	↓	High
Pump failure	↑	↑	Normal/high

urgent cardiac catheter may be required to assess flow pathways and determine the need for enlargement of any fenestration or surgical revision.

Early postoperative anticoagulation is mandatory due to the sluggish nature of the venous circulation.

Echocardiography should be used to assess the ventricular function, ensure non-obstructed pulmonary venous return and exclude any ventricular outflow tract obstruction (a reduced ventricular volume load may unmask an outflow tract obstruction).

Hypoplastic Left Heart Syndrome and Norwood Procedure

Incidence and Associations

HLHS accounts for 1.5% of all CHD, but causes 40% of all neonatal cardiac deaths. There are no proven associations, although potential gene loci have recently been identified.

Anatomy

There are a variety of subtypes with varying degrees of hypoplasia of the LV and LVOT. It classically occurs with mitral and aortic atresia together with a hypoplastic ascending aorta.

Physiology

HLHS is characterized by an inability of the LV to support the systemic circulation. Thus the RV supports the systemic circulation via the PDA. The condition is fatal without surgery. Problems balancing parallel circulations are discussed in Chapters 22 and 23.

Preoperative Management

HLHS is often present with profound circulatory collapse, requiring preoperative mechanical ventilation together with inotropes and vasodilators to improve systemic circulation and limit the PBF. A PGE_2 infusion is used to keep the PDA open. The goal is a balanced circulation (i.e. $Q_P:Q_S = 1:1$, aiming for $SaO_2 \approx 75–80\%$ if there is no forward flow through the LVOT).

Surgery

Surgery involves the Norwood procedure (Figure 21.11). There is significant risk, with 25–30% perioperative mortality. The RV supports both the systemic and pulmonary circulations. Surgery secures a controlled source of pulmonary blood supply via Gore-Tex® shunt and repairs any systemic outflow tract stenosis.

There is an increasing use of an RV–PA conduit to supply the PBF instead of modified B–T shunt (Sano modification, Figure 21.12). The RV directly supports both systemic and pulmonary circulations. This maintains the diastolic BP better than the modified B–T shunt. The 'hybrid' technique is a further recent option, placing bilateral PA bands and a stent in the PDA to mimic the Norwood circulation without the need for CPB. There has been some early success, but longer-term outcome studies are awaited.

Postoperative Management

The patient is fragile postoperatively and the chest is usually left open. CVP line monitoring gives the common atrial pressure. Hyperventilation and high FiO_2 should be avoided as these lead to pulmonary vasodilatation, an increased $Q_P:Q_S$ ratio and a

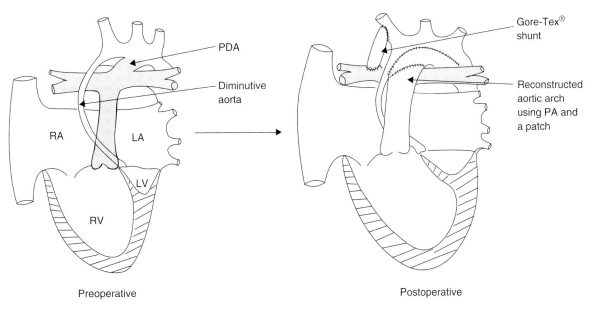

Preoperative   Postoperative

Figure 21.11 The Norwood procedure

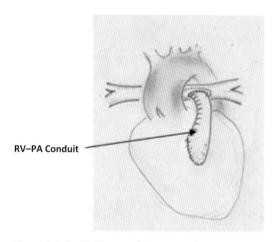

Figure 21.12 Modification of the Norwood procedure using a RV–PA conduit

compromised systemic circulation. Aim for an SaO_2 of 75–80%. It is important to monitor blood lactate and SvO_2 to assess systemic perfusion, aiming for an SvO_2 of 45–60%, which requires $Q_P:Q_S \approx 1:1$ (see Figure 21.13 and Table 21.2). Vasodilators and inotropes are used to improve systemic perfusion. Echocardiography is required to assess the RV function, the degree of TR and the arch repair. Manual ventilation with 100% oxygen should be avoided. An air/oxygen mix should be used to match the FiO_2 used during mechanical ventilation. Chest closure can decrease the RV compliance and cause deterioration over subsequent hours. Repeat echocardiography and maintain high vigilance following chest closure.

$$Q_P : Q_S \approx \frac{SaO_2 - SvO_2}{SpvO2 - SpaO2}$$

Note that the pulmonary arterial oxygen saturation ($SpaO_2$) is the same as the SaO_2 after the Norwood procedure.

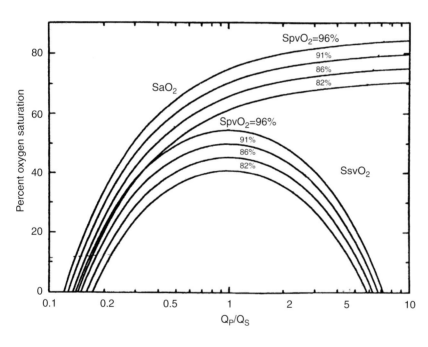

Figure 21.13 Balancing systemic and pulmonary flow in a Norwood circulation. The hyperbolic relationship between SaO_2 and $Q_P:Q_S$ and the parabolic relationship between systemic venous saturation ($SsvO_2$) and $Q_P:Q_S$ are not often appreciated. SaO_2 and $SsvO_2$ as a function of $Q_P:Q_S$ is shown for different values of pulmonary venous oxygen saturation ($SpvO_2$). It is often assumed that SaO_2 ~75% equates to the ideal $Q_P:Q_S$ of ~1:1. This will be the case if there is good systemic perfusion (oxygen extraction resulting in SvO_2 ~50%) and normal lung function ($SpvO_2$ ~100%). It is dangerous to infer $Q_P:Q_S$ from SaO_2 alone as an SaO_2 of 75% may represent a $Q_P:Q_S$ of >>1:1 in certain situations.

Table 21.2 Interpretation of SaO_2 in the presence of different physiological states

SaO_2	Physiological status	Consequences	$Q_P:Q_S$	Treatment
75%	Balanced Q_P and Q_S	None	~1:1	None
	↓CO	↑O_2 extraction, ↓SvO_2	>1:1	↑CO ↑PVR ↓SVR
	Lung disease	↓$SpvO_2$	>1:1	Optimize ventilation ↑PVR ↓SVR
>85%	Shunt too big	↑PBF	>1:1	↑PVR, ↓SVR, revise shunt
<65%	Shunt too small or blocked	↓PBF	<1:1	Revise shunt
	↑PVR	↓PBF	<1:1	↓PVR ↑MAP
	↓CO	↑O_2 extraction, ↓SvO_2	~1:1	↑CO
	Lung disease	↓$SpvO_2$	~1:1	Optimize ventilation

SvO_2, mixed venous saturation; $SpvO_2$, pulmonary venous oxygen saturation

Patent Ductus Arteriosus

Incidence and Associations

A patent ductus arteriosus (PDA) is common: its persistence is inversely proportional to gestational age. The incidence is greater than 80% in infants of less than 1 kg birth weight. It is associated with prematurity, diaphragmatic hernia, TGA, Fallot's tetralogy and pulmonary atresia.

Anatomy

A PDA is a remnant of the distal portion of the sixth left aortic arch. It connects the main PA to the descending thoracic aorta (Figure 21.14).

Physiology

A PDA carries ~90% of the RV output *in utero*. The left-to-right shunt increases as the PVR falls following birth. Functional (reversible) closure occurs within 15 hours of birth, and permanent closure occurs by 3 weeks in term infants. The haemodynamic impact of PDA is dependent on size. A small PDA may go undetected although there is a very small risk of endarteritis (often termed duct-related infective vasculitis). A large PDA may cause severe heart failure. An excessive PBF may exacerbate respiratory distress syndrome, precipitate pulmonary haemorrhage and compromise weaning from mechanical ventilation. 'Run-off' from the aorta results in a low diastolic pressure and 'steal' from the systemic circulation. Reduced mesenteric blood flow may result in necrotizing enterocolitis.

Diagnosis

A continuous machinery murmur is characteristic of a PDA. Echocardiography confirms the diagnosis and

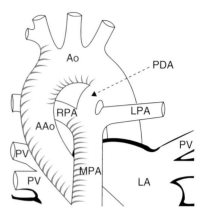

Figure 21.14 The PDA. AAo, ascending aorta; MPA, main pulmonary artery; RPA, right pulmonary artery; LPA, left pulmonary artery.

the direction of shunting; the LA to aortic diameter ratio reflects the degree of left-to-right shunting.

Management

Medical: Treatment with indomethacin or another NSAID may result in duct closure. This is often combined with fluid restriction and diuretics.

Trans-catheter closure: This may be undertaken in the catheter laboratory in larger infants (usually >3 kg) or children.

Surgical: Necessary if medical treatment fails or is contraindicated (renal impairment, GI or other haemorrhage). Almost exclusively in low birth weight, premature babies (<1.5 kg). The duct is ligated or closed with a clip via left thoracotomy without CPB. Pre- and post-ductal oximetery is required.

Complications: Inadvertent ligation of the left PA or descending aorta, damage to the recurrent laryngeal nerve or thoracic duct. Anaesthetic expertise is required in the management of small and premature babies. Lung compliance is typically poor and worsened by thoracotomy positioning.

Pulmonary Artery Banding

PA banding is performed in a variety of different conditions. The major indication is to limit the PBF. The band protects the lungs from high pressure and flow in the following situations:

(1) Biventricular heart with multiple VSDs that are not suitable for surgical closure or for a large VSD/AVSD in a neonate if felt to be a high risk to repair.

(2) CoA + VSD where the CoA is the critical lesion and is repaired via a thoracotomy; the band can also be placed via the thoracotomy (increasingly uncommon, usually both lesions are repaired as a neonate via median sternotomy).

(3) Functionally single ventricle anatomy with an excessive (unobstructed) PBF (e.g. tricuspid atresia with TGA/VSD) (commonest indication) – see Staged Palliation of the Functionally Univentricular Heart.

Rarely, PA banding is performed to 'train' the subpulmonary ventricle in infants with TGA in preparation for an arterial switch procedure. This may be required in late presentations in which the LV muscle mass has regressed. The band places an afterload on the ventricle and stimulates hypertrophy.

Physiology

The physiology depends on the underlying anatomy. In groups 1 and 2 (above), the band reduces the degree of heart failure by reducing the left-to-right shunt across the VSD. Any shunting remains predominantly left-to-right and so the SaO_2 will remain 95–100%. In group 3 (above), there is obligate mixing of the circulation and aim for a $Q_P:Q_S$ ratio of 1:1 with an SaO_2 of 75–80% (Figure 21.15).

Surgery

PA banding does not require CPB. It can be placed either via midline sternotomy or via left thoracotomy.

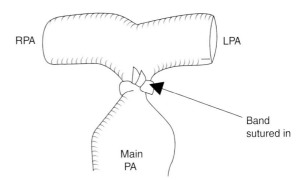

Figure 21.15 PA banding

Postoperative Management

This depends on the underlying anatomy. In groups 1 and 2 (above) a target SaO_2 of 95–100% is generally well tolerated. Group 3 (above) will be cyanotic and may be haemodynamically unstable, so aim for an SaO_2 of 75–80%. Echocardiography is used to quantify the gradient across the band, to assess the ventricular function (you can cause rapid ventricular failure if the band is too tight) and to assess the A-V valve function (the band can increase A-V valve regurgitation in an AVSD). Bands placed for VSDs are tighter (Doppler flow velocity 3–4 m s^{-1}) than bands in the single ventricle setting (velocity 3–3.5 m s^{-1}). Babies with a high PVR may show a deceptively small gradient because the distal PAP is high rather than the PA band being loose.

PA banding that is performed to 'train' the LV in a baby with TGA may be complicated by hypoxaemia due to a failure of mixing of the systemic and pulmonary circulations. They may need the addition of a modified B–T shunt. The stressed subpulmonary (left) ventricle may fail postoperatively as a result of an excessive afterload. Echocardiography is used to assess the degree of ventricular dilatation and to monitor for a rise in the LA pressure or signs of a falling CO.

PA banding patients can be very unstable. Since the procedure is relatively minor, there is a tendency to regard the patients as low risk when the converse can be true.

Pulmonary Atresia

Pulmonary atresia encompasses a complex group of conditions. Patients may have areas of lung supplied by major aorto-pulmonary collateral arteries (MAPCAs). Pulmonary atresia can be divided into three groups:

(1) those with an intact ventricular septum

(2) those with a VSD, without MAPCAs

(3) those with a VSD and MAPCAs

Incidence and Associations

Pulmonary atresia accounts for 1.5% of all CHD. It is associated with a 22q11 deletion.

Pulmonary Atresia With an Intact Ventricular Septum

This is characterized by a so-called 'dead-end' ventricle, which can vary in size from normal to hypoplastic. Management depends on the size of the RV.

- *Normal size*: Perforation and balloon dilatation of the PV (in cardiac catheter laboratory) with or without surgical opening of the RVOT
- *Small*: Modified B–T shunt (or ductal stent) with opening of the RVOT to encourage forward flow through the RV
- *Very small (hypoplastic)*: Modified B–T shunt or ductal stent

Adequate mixing at the atrial level is important – ensure a good-sized ASD, consider septostomy if not.

A 'dead-end' ventricle generates enormous intracavity pressures that may squeeze blood backwards into the coronary arteries and create coronary fistulae or sinusoids. This is fortunately rare, but if present relieving the RVOT obstruction (with resultant lowering of the RV pressure) will cause coronary ischaemia (RV-dependent coronary circulation).

Pulmonary Atresia With VSD, Without MAPCAs

This is effectively an extreme form of tetralogy of Fallot. Patients are duct-dependent at birth and require PGE_2 infusion and a modified B–T shunt or ductal stent. Complete repair is managed as per tetralogy of Fallot but using an RV-to-PA valved conduit to restore continuity.

Postoperative management: This is similar to that of tetralogy of Fallot, but the valved conduit reduces the risk of restrictive physiology.

Pulmonary Atresia With VSD and MAPCAs

In this group, pulmonary blood supply is derived from large collateral vessels arising from the aorta. There are variable patterns of blood supply from the native PAs and from MAPCAs, with some areas supplied by both, one vessel only, or neither.

Surgery aims to join the MAPCAs together ('unifocalization'), reconnect them to the native PAs (if present), insert an RV–PA conduit and close the VSD (Figure 21.16). This may require a combined thoracotomy and sternotomy.

Several staged procedures may be required. The VSD may be left open until you are confident that the PVR will be low enough for the RV to cope.

Postoperative management: These patients will remain cyanotic after surgery if the VSD is left open, with the degree of cyanosis being dependent on the quality of the vessels. There may be considerable collapse or contusion of the lung, especially if additional thoracotomy is performed. Previously poorly perfused areas may suffer reperfusion injury with localized oedema, congestion and haemorrhage. Management includes PEEP and diuretics. Any increase in the PAP or PVR is usually a consequence of small PAs and is seldom reactive; i.e. the patient is unlikely to respond to inhaled NO. The RV may be non-compliant and may show restrictive physiology.

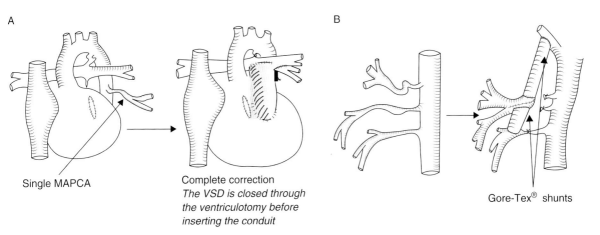

A

Single MAPCA

Complete correction
*The VSD is closed through
the ventriculotomy before
inserting the conduit*

B

Gore-Tex® shunts

Figure 21.16 (A) Repair of a PA/VSD with a single MAPCA. (B) Example of unifocalization of three major MAPCAs to the right lung.

Ross Procedure

The Ross procedure (Figure 21.17) is an alternative approach to conventional AV replacement using the patient's own PV in the aortic position and replacement of the PV with a homograft. It has the advantage of providing a living valve replacement that will grow with the child – thus, it is suitable for neonates, infants and children.

Anatomy

Indications are similar to adult AVR: AR, AS or commonly a combination of both. It is often related to a congenitally bicuspid AV. Significant aortic root dilatation is a contraindication to the Ross procedure as there is a risk that the new valve will also dilate. Complex sub-AS can also be addressed by extension of the procedure to widen the outflow septum – the so-called Ross–Konno procedure.

Surgery

The risk of surgery is 2–3%. It is a complex procedure, requiring excision of the PV as a complete root and implanting this into the aortic position with reimplantation of the coronary arteries. The PV is replaced with a homograft (allograft).

Intraoperative echocardiography should focus on the regional ventricular wall function and on the new AV to look for any regurgitation or stenosis.

Postoperative Care

An LA line is useful to monitor the LV preload. The ECG should be checked for evidence of coronary ischaemia. Echocardiography should be used early to assess the ventricular function and the 'new' AV function. The procedure entails extensive suture lines so hypertension should be avoided and the patient kept sedated and mechanically ventilated until all bleeding has settled.

Long-term concerns over dilatation of the neo-aortic root have led to a decreasing enthusiasm for the procedure – but it remains a valuable technique in smaller children and infants where prosthetic valve replacement is not feasible.

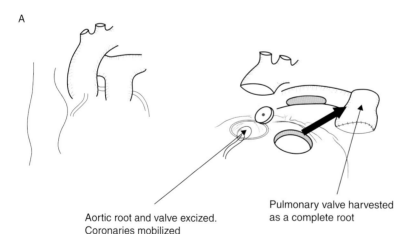

A

Aortic root and valve excised. Coronaries mobilized

Pulmonary valve harvested as a complete root

B

Pulmonary autograft reimplanted as aortic root

Homograft used to reconstruct RV–PA continuity

Figure 21.17 The Ross procedure (pulmonary autograft). (A) Preoperative and intraoperative appearances. (B) Completed appearance.

Staged Palliation of the Functionally Univentricular Heart

A number of lesions are not suitable for a two-ventricle repair and are managed with a series of two or three palliative procedures. Examples include tricuspid atresia, some forms of pulmonary atresia, a double-inlet LV, an unbalanced AVSD, isomerism and HLHS.

In the neonatal period, surgery may be required to optimize the PBF:

- If there is an inadequate PBF, an arterial shunt (such as a modified B–T shunt) may be necessary (or occasionally a PDA stent)
- If the PBF is high, a band is placed around the PA and tightened to limit the PBF and balance the circulation

There must be no obstruction to systemic and pulmonary venous mixing (atrial septostomy or surgical septectomy may be necessary). There must be unobstructed outflow to the systemic circulation (any associated CoA or arch hypoplasia must be repaired). Pathways of palliative operations for a univentricular heart are summarized below.

Once the neonatal circulation has become balanced, all of these patients join a common pathway to a 'Fontan circulation', where the systemic venous

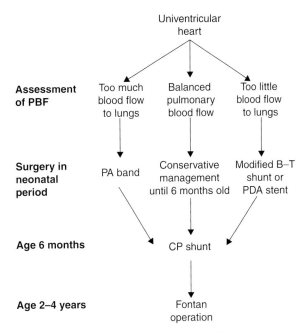

Figure 21.18 Pathways of palliative operations for a univentricular heart

return is redirected directly into the pulmonary circulation (Figure 21.18). This is usually done in two further stages – the CP shunt and then the Fontan completion (TCPC). These are covered in the relevant sections of this chapter.

Total Anomalous Pulmonary Venous Drainage

Total anomalous pulmonary venous drainage (TAPVD) is also sometimes known as total anomalous pulmonary venous connection (TAPVC).

Incidence

TAPVD accounts for 1.5% of all CHD.

Anatomy

In TAPVD, the pulmonary veins do not drain back to the LA, but to a separate collecting chamber that drains into the systemic venous circulation (Figure 21.19). Supracardiac TAPVD is commonest, draining into the innominate vein. Infracardiac TAPVD drains into the IVC and is the most likely variant to be obstructed. Cardiac TAPVD drains into the coronary sinus and is usually unobstructed.

Physiology

The infant is cyanotic due to mixing as pulmonary venous drainage re-enters the systemic venous system. The LV filling and systemic output is dependent on a PFO allowing right-to-left flow at atrial level. Key to the condition is whether or not the drainage is obstructive. When the pathway is unobstructed, the infant will be cyanosed but well. Obstructed pathways lead to PHT, pulmonary congestion (diffuse pulmonary oedema on CXR), tachypnoea and profound cyanosis.

Cor triatriatum is a condition in which there is a membrane within the LA between the pulmonary veins and the MV. If the opening in this membrane is small or absent, presentation will be similar to TAPVD. Treatment is surgical resection of the membrane.

Management

Unobstructed cases are stable but cyanosed and need elective surgical repair. Obstructed cases present in the neonatal period; mechanical ventilation and urgent surgical decompression are often required.

Surgery

All types can be surgically repaired by restoring the pulmonary vein-to- LA blood flow. There is 5–10% perioperative mortality, dependent on the degree of obstruction. There is a risk of recurrent pulmonary vein stenosis, which is associated with a poor outcome. Intraoperative echocardiography should focus on pulmonary venous blood flow, looking for stenosis and/or turbulence.

Postoperative Care

PHT is inevitable in obstructed cases and is an additional operative risk. Consequently, it is an indication for PAP monitoring. The surgeon may leave a small PFO if there is concern about PHT; the right-to-left shunt may reduce the PAP but will also lead to arterial desaturation. The LV tends to be non-compliant because it has not been exposed to a normal preload. For this reason, high LA pressures are generally expected. Small fluid challenges, however, may produce a large increase in the LA pressure. Obstruction at the level of the anastomosis will lead to pulmonary venous congestion. Reoperation should be considered if the pulmonary vein (Doppler) flow appears obstructive.

A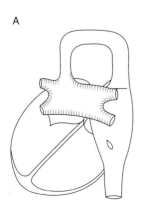

B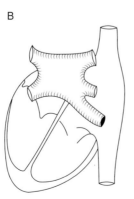

C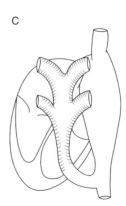

Figure 21.19 Three anatomical variants of TAPVD as seen from behind the heart. (A) Supracardiac: the most common, drain into an ascending vertical vein. (B) Cardiac: drain to coronary sinus; least likely to be obstructive. (C) Infracardiac (note not intracardiac): less common, drain into a descending vein, usually below the diaphragm, most likely to get obstructed.

Transposition of the Great Arteries

Transposition of the great arteries (TGA) is frequently referred to as just 'transposition'. D-TGA is the most common variety and the type requiring neonatal correction. L-TGA, commonly called congenitally corrected transposition (ccTGA), is rare, more complex and not covered in this chapter.

Incidence

TGA accounts for 5% of all CHD.

Anatomy

The aorta arises from the RV and the PA arises from the LV. The great vessels usually lie in an anterior–posterior relationship, with the aorta anterior and to the right. There are many associated features, but 'simple' transposition (the commonest) implies the ventricular septum is intact (as opposed to TGA/VSD, Figure 21.20).

Circulations are in parallel rather than in series. Coronary arteries arise from the aorta from the sinuses that face the main PA and come off in a variety of patterns. Risk factors for a more complicated surgical course include:

- Unusual coronary artery patterns, especially intramural coronaries (running in the wall of the aorta in an oblique course) and those with a single coronary origin
- Side-by-side great vessels (rather than anterior–posterior)
- Presence of additional lesions, e.g. CoA or VSDs
- Age >10 days, slight risk; age >42 days, major risk

Physiology

Infants are cyanotic and reliant on the PFO and the PDA to allow mixing. The presence of a VSD may improve mixing. In TGA with an intact IVS, the LV muscle mass will begin to regress once the PVR falls. The presence of a VSD prevents this as ventricular pressures are both at a systemic level. Rare combinations such as TGA/VSD/PS may be well-balanced cyanotic circulations and may not require any early intervention.

Initial Management

A PGE$_2$ infusion maintains patency of the PDA and mechanical ventilation may be required. Cardiologists may perform balloon atrial septostomy (which can be done under echocardiographic guidance on the ICU), to enlarge the PFO and improve mixing. In cases with an intact IVS, the aim is to perform surgery within the first 10 days of life, before the LV muscle mass regresses. In late presentations (>4 weeks) PA banding may be considered to 'train the LV' (i.e. increase the muscle mass) prior to a switch procedure.

Surgery

The arterial switch procedure is used, and there is 2-4 % perioperative mortality. The great arteries are divided and switched. The coronaries are transferred separately onto the neo-aorta. Note from Figure 21.21 that the PA ends up in front of the aorta (the 'Lecompte manoeuvre'). Additional lesions such as VSDs or CoA are usually repaired at the same time, although this increases operative complexity and risk.

Intraoperative echocardiography should focus on the LV and RV function. The LVOT and RVOT

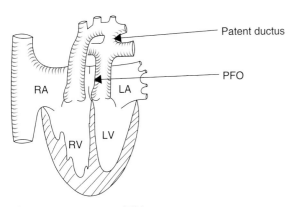

Figure 21.20 Anatomy of TGA

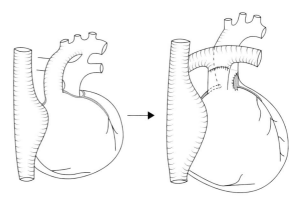

Figure 21.21 The arterial switch procedure

should be examined to assess the severity of any AR or PR. An LA line is placed routinely.

Postoperative Care

The LV tends to be non-compliant and small changes in the preload cause marked changes in the LA pressure. Kinking or malposition of the coronary arteries can result in coronary ischaemia. If the ECG suggests ST changes or rhythm problems, a formal 12-lead ECG should be obtained. Echocardiography should be performed on return to ICU to:

- Assess the LV function and regional contractility
- Examine the LVOT and RVOT, and exclude any residual VSD
- Exclude neo-AR

Vasodilators may help a non-compliant LV to relax. Infants with a large PDA may have had a high pre-operative PBF and require regular diuretics. Older switch patients (>4 weeks) may require prolonged inotropic support to 'retrain' the LV. Branch PA stenosis may develop as a late complication.

Truncus Arteriosus

Truncus arteriosus is also called common arterial trunk and 'truncus'.

Incidence and Associations

Truncus arteriosus accounts for 1.5% of all CHD. It is associated with a 22q11 deletion (Di George syndrome).

Anatomy

In truncus arteriosus there is a single ventricular outflow tract (arterial trunk) with a multi-leaflet truncal valve and VSD. PAs arise from the arterial trunk via a main PA (type 1) or via separate origins for the right and left PAs (types 2 and 3) – see Figure 21.22.

Complex variants include:

- Truncus with interrupted arch
- Disconnection of the left PA (supplied by a ductus)

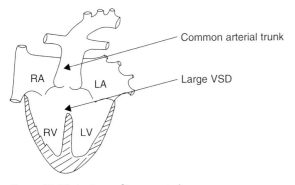

Figure 21.22 Anatomy of truncus arteriosus

Physiology

There is unrestricted PBF, which causes heart failure in the neonatal period. Infants have cyanosis due to mixing of bloodstreams – this is usually mild because of the high PBF.

Surgery

Surgery has a high risk, with 10–15% early mortality. The procedures comprises VSD closure, disconnection of PAs from trunk, and formation of an RV–PA conduit (Figure 21.23).

Surgical risk factors include:

- A regurgitant truncal valve
- Severe heart failure at presentation
- Complex variants

Postoperative Management

This is a high-risk procedure and the chest may be left open. LA and PAP monitoring lines are useful. There is a risk of PHT (especially if the infant is older than 6 weeks) – aim for a mean PAP of less than 50% of the mean systemic pressure. Management of PHT includes control of the $PaCO_2$, inhaled NO and phenoxybenzamine, which may have been given perioperatively. Echocardiography should focus on: truncal valve regurgitation, any residual VSD and blood flow into the RV–PA conduit. Irradiated blood products should be used unless a 22q11 deletion has been excluded. In the absence of a PAP monitoring line, the PAP can be estimated from the velocity of a regurgitant TR jet and CVP ($PAP \approx CVP + (4 \times Velocity_{TR}^2)$).

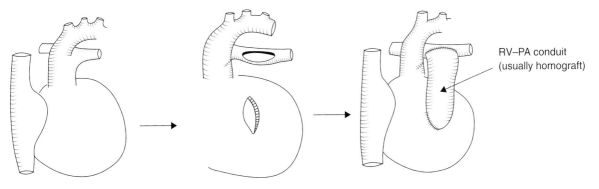

Figure 21.23 Surgery of truncus arteriosus.

RV–PA conduit (usually homograft)

179

Ventricular Septal Defects

Incidence and Associations

VSDs account for 30% of all CHD. Associations include coarctation and the VACTERL syndrome (see above). It should be borne in mind that many other complex forms of CHD include a VSD (e.g. truncus, pulmonary atresia, Fallot's tetralogy).

Anatomy

A schematic view of the ventricular septum viewed from the right side is shown in Figure 21.24.

Physiology

The majority of VSDs do not require intervention and either close spontaneously or are so small as to not warrant closure. Perimembranous VSDs are unlikely to close spontaneously and are the most likely to need surgical closure. Large VSDs, causing heart failure and failure to thrive, are the commonest indication for repair.

An 'unrestrictive' VSD means that there is no Doppler gradient across the VSD on echocardiography. This means that the VSD must be large and that the pressure in the RV is at a systemic level, leading to PHT. The PHT should completely reverse as long as the defect is closed before 6 months of age.

Less common indications for closure are:

- Moderate VSDs in older children, which have failed to close and continue to produce a significant shunt ($Q_P:Q_S > 1.5:1$)

- Small VSDs that have been associated with an episode of endocarditis (usually a jet lesion on the TV)
- Small perimembranous VSDs that have resulted in AV prolapse into the defect, with AR

Surgery

Surgery is associated with 1–2% mortality. Most VSDs are closed via the RA using a prosthetic patch. Intraoperative echocardiography should focus on looking for any residual VSD, ensuring the LVOT is unobstructed and assessing the TV function.

Postoperative Management

Patients are usually neonates/young infants with considerable preoperative heart failure. Regular diuretics and vasodilators help offload the LV.

It is important to monitor the cardiac rhythm as the A-V node is adjacent to perimembranous VSDs and variable degrees of heart block can be seen. All patients should have atrial and ventricular pacing wires available. An A-V block is usually transient (a few hours) but can be permanent (1–2%). Postoperative echocardiography should be used to reassess the LV function, exclude any residual VSD and estimate the RV pressure. Pulmonary hypertensive crises are a potential risk but are uncommon after simple VSD repair, although older children (>6 months) with large VSDs are at a greater risk.

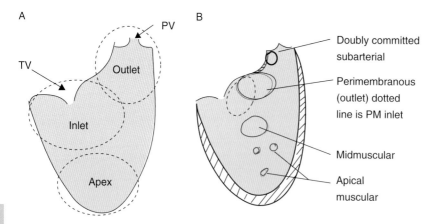

Figure 21.24 Schematic of ventricular septum, viewed from the right side. (A) The ventricular septum can be divided into inlet, apical and outlet portions. (B) Sites at which VSDs are found.

Chapter 22

Postoperative Paediatric Care

Jane V. Cassidy and Kevin P. Morris

This chapter highlights key aspects of management and potential complications in children following cardiac surgery. Critical to this is an understanding of diagnosis, physiology, appropriate physiological targets and multidisciplinary collaboration.

Routine Postoperative Care

Structured Handover

Transfer from the operating theatre to the ICU is one of the most vulnerable times in the patient's postoperative course. Information transfer must include the child's preoperative status, intraoperative management (anaesthetic, perfusion and surgical management), concerns regarding residual anatomic or physiological states, potential complications and anticipation of the postoperative course. During the time of handover, the anaesthetist is primarily responsible for the care of the patient. After the transfer of information and assessment, the intensivist assumes responsibility.

Generally, the child falls into one of three groups:

1. Uncomplicated and relatively straightforward surgery. A rapid recovery is anticipated and the child can be rapidly weaned from mechanical ventilation and the trachea extubated.
2. Children where surgery has been more complex. Whilst they may currently appear stable with satisfactory clinical and echocardiographic findings, they may be vulnerable to a low CO state (LCOS) or a worsening systemic inflammatory response. Until the clinician is satisfied that the period of vulnerability is over, these children are kept ventilated and sedated with progression following a period of stability.
3. Unstable children with an established LCOS. Multidisciplinary discussion and planning is essential. Important considerations include: has a residual lesion been excluded, are there other physiological problems, for example PHT and is extracorporeal life support (ECLS) indicated?

Mechanical Ventilation

Most children will be extubated relatively quickly. It is important to have an understanding of the source of the pulmonary blood flow (PBF) and the cardiopulmonary interactions of different circulations. Whilst oxygenation targets are tailored to an individual child, an SaO_2 of 75–80% in a single ventricle circulation will usually equate to a $Q_P:Q_S$ ratio of approximately 1.

In children with a limited PBF, particularly when dependent on passive systemic venous return, early extubation is helpful. In contrast, the volume-loaded single ventricle or the impaired LV may struggle with the associated increase in systemic afterload, particularly in the setting of coexisting atrioventricular (A-V) valve regurgitation. Management of $PaCO_2$ is particularly important in the setting of PHT.

Metabolic State

Infants are at a particular risk of hypothermia. Hyperthermia may occur with LCOS, increasing oxygen demand and myocardial work, putting the child at greater risk of neurological injury.

Fluid and Electrolyte Management

Derangements are common. The clinical spectrum ranges from mild fluid overload to severe oedema, capillary leak, vasodilatation and hypotension, merging into the systemic inflammatory response state. The stress response, triggered as a normal response to surgical stimulation and bypass, leads to antidiuretic hormone (ADH) production.

With prolonged surgery and significant capillary leak, or where there is felt to be a significant chance of the child requiring postoperative renal replacement therapy (RRT), a peritoneal dialysis (PD) catheter may be placed in theatre. Even if PD is not required the continuous drainage of peritoneal (ascitic) fluid may benefit renal perfusion and mechanical ventilation.

Maintenance fluids are restricted to 25% in the initial 24 hours after surgery. Oliguria is common but diuretics are unlikely to be effective during this time until the CO increases and ADH levels fall.

The fluid management plan is reviewed and adjusted according to the clinical status. Avoidance of hypokalaemia and hypocalcaemia is important. Hyperglycaemia is common but there is no evidence that tight glycaemic control improves outcomes.

Blood transfusion may be required for adequate oxygen delivery, particularly with single ventricle circulations where the target Hb is generally 120–140 g l^{-1}.

Nutrition

Adequate nutrition is critical as these children may be malnourished preoperatively. The basal metabolic rate is raised proportionally to the illness severity with high caloric requirements – up to 150 kcal kg^{-1} per day in infants.

Ideally, nutrition is enteral. Where there has been gut ischaemia or concern regarding splanchnic perfusion, then caution is indicated and, occasionally, a period of parenteral nutrition is needed.

Postoperative Problems

Systemic Inflammatory Response

An exaggerated inflammatory response is commoner in infants, especially following protracted complex surgery. This leads to endothelial failure, capillary leak and multi-organ dysfunction. Clinical manifestations include generalized tissue oedema, third-space fluid losses (peritoneal and pleural), a persistent volume requirement, vasoplegia and increasing vasoactive infusion requirements.

Low Cardiac Output Syndrome

LCOS affects up to 25% of infants post CPB. The nadir typically occurs 6–18 hours post surgery. In high-risk cases, the sternum is left open to minimize any mechanical tamponade effect on the heart. Equally, where the chest is closed and there is a significant LCOS, consideration should be given to reopening.

Postoperative bleeding may be significant with a dilutional coagulopathy. This should be corrected and a low threshold maintained for surgical review and/or

re-exploration if bleeding continues despite appropriate product replacement. In managing LCOS consider:

Preload: Children with passive systemic venous return as their source of PBF or who have restrictive physiology or diastolic dysfunction require higher preload.

Heart rate: Neonates have a fixed SV and thus are critically dependent on adequate chronotropy. Loss of A-V synchrony reduces the CO by 30%. Excessive tachycardia compromises coronary perfusion. Loss of rate variability is an important early sign of impending arrhythmia, reduced ventricular function or circulatory collapse.

Contractility: Consider potential residual lesions, particularly if the reduction in function persists beyond the first 24 hours.

Afterload: Consider in the context of both biventricular and univentricular circulations, and the potential benefit of positive pressure ventilation on afterload reduction, versus the preload impact.

In the univentricular circulation, the adequacy of systemic oxygen delivery is dependent on the balance between Q_P and Q_S, which in turn is dependent on the PVR and SVR. In the setting of a high SVR relative to PVR, the $Q_P:Q_S$ ratio will often be greater than 1 and the infant will have a high SaO_2 (often >90%) at the expense of inadequate systemic perfusion. Manipulation of the SVR is important in this situation and is in general easier to control than manipulating the PVR.

Extracorporeal Life Support

In severe LCOS with end-organ dysfunction, ECLS allows time for the heart to recover without further injury and provides a predictable 'CO' to vulnerable organs.

Modalities of ECLS include ECMO, or a ventricular assist device (VAD), with multiple different types available. Overall survival to discharge after postoperative ECMO is 35–50%. ECMO is also used as rescue therapy for refractory cardiac arrest – E-CPR.

The expectation must be recovery to a reasonable level of function with or without further intervention. Where the reason for instability is uncertain, ECLS may buy time for further investigation. Indications for ECLS include serum lactate of >10 mmol l^{-1}, lactate rising >3 mmol l^{-1} h^{-1} or increasing vasoactive support (e.g. epinephrine >0.2 μg kg^{-1} min^{-1}). The overall trajectory of the child is the most important determinant of the need for ECLS.

ECMO provides biventricular and pulmonary support (gas exchange). It is rapidly deployed with low priming volumes. Disadvantages include significant risks of both bleeding and thromboembolism, the requirement to decompress the left heart and a high incidence of infective complications. It is also time-limited, with complications increasing exponentially after 7 days of support.

A VAD may be used to support one or both ventricles. It does not offer pulmonary support so lung function must be adequate. Equally, where only a left-sided VAD is used, the right heart must function. All VADs require systemic anticoagulation with attendant bleeding and thromboembolic risks. VADs have a role where the heart is expected to recover but where this may take longer than the time period that ECMO can offer, for example following repair of an anomalous coronary artery with significant LV dysfunction. They may also be used as a bridge to cardiac transplant if appropriate, with success rates of more than 70%. Children with single ventricle circulations, however, are much more difficult to support using a VAD, with very few long-term support successes.

Rhythm Disorders

Rhythm disorders are common. Complete heart block is the commonest problem postoperatively, often following A-V or VSD repairs, subaortic resection and tetralogy of Fallot.

Tachyarrhythmias are commonly due to perioperative A-V node injury. Many congenital cardiac lesions are also associated with accessory pathways or ectopic foci. Postoperative arrhythmias may be due to this rather than operative injury.

Accurate diagnosis is the key to determining appropriate therapy. A 12-lead ECG, supplemented with an atrial ECG (from temporary pacing wires) may yield the diagnosis. An atrial ECG amplifies atrial activity, allowing easier differentiation between atrial and ventricular excitation (Figure 22.1).

Junctional ectopic tachycardia (JET) is common and potentially life-threatening, occurring 24–48 hours postoperatively, resulting from abnormal automaticity of the A-V node or His bundle. ECG shows A-V dissociation with a rapid QRS rate (160–260 min^{-1}) and narrow QRS morphology. The overall goal of treatment is to slow the ectopic rate allowing restitution of A-V synchrony at a physiological rate, using pacing set at a rate above the JET rate. Active

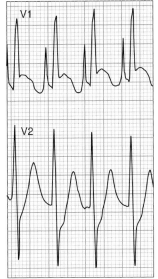

Atrial ECG taken by connecting atrial pacing wires to V1

P-wave precedes every QRS

P-waves on corresponding surface ECG are too small to be identified

Figure 22.1 Atrial (V1) and surface (V2) ECGs in NSR – P-waves are amplified by atrial ECG.

cooling to 34–35 °C with the use of muscle relaxation may be required. Catecholamines should be weaned to minimize sympathetic nervous system activation. Antiarrhythmic drug therapies are second line. Amiodarone is commonly used, but with a significant risk associated with its negative inotropy and potential refractory A-V block.

Ventricular dysrhythmias are rare and generally reflect myocardial ischaemia. DC cardioversion should be considered for haemodynamic instability. ECLS may occasionally be required to buy time for pharmacological rhythm control.

Pulmonary Hypertension

PHT may be due to:

- Intra- or extracardiac shunts to the pulmonary circulation, resulting in a high PBF
- Elevated pulmonary venous pressure: e.g. anomalous pulmonary venous drainage, LA hypertension or elevated LV end-diastolic pressure from outflow obstruction
- Distal branch PA narrowing/obstruction

PHT may be exacerbated following CPB. The expectation is that it will improve with time as the effect of the high PBF and CPB wear off. The critical feature in management is the exclusion of residual lesions such as a left-to-right shunt or pulmonary

183

venous obstruction, as pulmonary vasodilator therapy here may only worsen the situation.

The ventilation strategy depends on the cause of PHT – a single ventricle circulation will be managed entirely differently from a postoperative complete A-V septal defect repair, for example. In general, high airway pressures should be avoided, the effect of PEEP on the RV preload and septal deviation considered and, whilst hypercarbia should be avoided, remember that the evidence for hypocarbia in reducing the PVR is limited and a low $PaCO_2$ significantly reduces cerebral perfusion and increases the SVR.

Inhaled NO has an important role to play in reducing PVR in the acute postoperative stage as long as residual shunts and pulmonary venous hypertension are excluded. Withdrawal of inhaled NO as the child improves may result in rebound PHT, which can be ameliorated by oral sildenafil.

Acute Kidney Injury

This is common after cardiac surgery (~40%) and is independently associated with increased mortality and morbidity. Infants appear particularly vulnerable. Risk factors include application of an AXC, CPB duration, nephrotoxic drugs and postoperative LCOS. Continuous infusion of a diuretic is often used to manage associated fluid overload but RRT may be needed. In infants, this is typically peritoneal dialysis, while continuous veno-venous haemofiltration and diafiltration are reserved for older children.

Necrotizing Enterocolitis

Rates of necrotizing enterocolitis (NEC) in infants with congenital heart disease (CHD) are significantly higher than in the general neonatal population, particularly in single ventricle circulations. The pathophysiology differs from that of NEC in the preterm population, with gut ischaemia predominating. Contributory factors include CPB-related hypothermic stress and inflammatory response, LCOS and diastolic steal – e.g. with a systemic to PA (Blalock–Taussig) shunt.

Any child with poor systemic perfusion should be assumed to be vulnerable and should not be fed enterally until resolution of LCOS. Medical management is supportive: gut rest, antibiotics, parenteral nutrition and ventilator/vasoactive support. Surgical intervention may be required.

Neurological Injury

Infants with CHD are vulnerable to neurological injury. The aetiology is multifactorial and includes existing genetic defects, co-morbidities, impaired foetal neurodevelopment and acute perioperative hypoxic-ischaemic injury. Up to 40% of those with complex cardiac disease have neurological injury.

The highest operative risk is with aortic arch obstruction, requiring a period of deep hypothermic circulatory arrest. Although strategies such as antegrade cerebral perfusion are used to reduce the risk, neurodevelopmental follow-up studies are not supportive. Particulate and gaseous emboli may also contribute.

Secondary neurological injury may occur with the combination of a postoperative LCOS and the increased cerebral metabolic demands of hyperthermia. Catastrophic neurological insult after cardiac surgery with CPB is now uncommon. The spectrum of neurological injury ranges from focal or generalized seizures, to peripheral nerve injury and frank stroke. Infants are particularly vulnerable to subependymal or intraventricular haemorrhage.

Phrenic Nerve Injury

This may result from direct trauma, thermal (cold) injury or stretch injury – it may be temporary or permanent. Infants are dependent on diaphragmatic function so may not wean off respiratory support and may require diaphragmatic plication ('tucking' and shortening of diaphragm) to increase the lung volume on the affected side). Bilateral phrenic injury is rare, but results in the need for prolonged ventilatory support.

Laryngeal Nerve Injury

Injury to the recurrent laryngeal nerve, either thermal or traumatic, is commonest during aortic arch surgery. Clinically, the signs will be of a vocal cord palsy, which may lead to extubation failure. If the child tolerates extubation there may be ongoing hoarseness, weak cry and issues with secretions and airway protection. With bilateral vocal cord palsy, tracheostomy is almost inevitable.

Chylothorax

Postoperative chylothorax may result from:

- Damage to the thoracic duct
- Increased production of lymph secondary to increased filling (systemic venous) pressures

- Impaired lymph drainage due to obstruction to head and neck systemic venous drainage

It is commonest following cavopulmonary connection, aortic arch or RV outflow tract surgery.

Chylothorax is associated with significant morbidity and increased mortality. Clinical features include malnutrition, immune compromise and coagulation anomalies if the chest drain losses are large and persistent.

Management includes exclusion of thrombus, a trial of a medium chain triglyceride diet, moving to parenteral nutrition if this is unsuccessful, together with supportive therapy for associated immune and coagulation issues. With refractory cases, the use of a somatostatin analogue (octreotide) has been suggested but evidence is limited and potential adverse effects are significant. Surgical therapies include thoracic duct ligation, direct closure of leaking lymphatics or pleurodesis, and are a last resort.

Thrombosis

Inherent coagulation abnormalities and the polycythaemia and hyperviscosity associated with cyanotic CHD increase the risk of spontaneous thrombosis (3–11%). This is particularly important in single ventricle circulations, not least because venous thrombus can embolize to both systemic and venous circulations.

Outcome

Overall operative mortality for the correction of CHD is now less than 3% in developed countries. The perioperative mortality for surgical ASD closure is less than 1%, whereas mortality for first-stage palliation of hypoplastic left-heart syndrome is around 10%. Coexisting congenital and acquired conditions are important co-determinants of outcome.

Key Points

- Paediatric and adult cardiac surgical critical care have many facets in common. The variety of conditions encountered is much greater in paediatric practice.
- A detailed knowledge of anatomy and pathophysiology is needed, as management of individual complex lesions is very different.
- Good outcomes depend on multidisciplinary collaboration.
- A low CO or deviation from the expected clinical course should prompt exclusion of a residual lesion.

Further Reading

Barach PR, Jacobs JP (eds.). *Pediatric and Congenital Cardiac Care. Volume 1: Outcomes Analysis.* London: Springer-Verlag; 2014.

Barach PR, Jacobs JP (eds.). *Pediatric and Congenital Cardiac Care. Volume 2: Quality Improvement and Patient Safety.* London: Springer-Verlag; 2014.

Bronicki RA, Chang AC. Management of the postoperative pediatric cardiac surgical patient. *Crit Care Med* 2011; 39: 1974–84.

Joint Statement on Mechanical Circulatory Support in Children: A consensus review from the Pediatric Cardiac Intensive Care Society and Extracorporeal Life Support Organization. *Ped Crit Care Med* 2013; 14: S1–S118.

Pediatric Cardiac Intensive Care Society 10th International Conference 2014 Consensus Statement: Pharmacotherapies in cardiac critical care. *Ped Crit Care Med* 2016; 17: S1–S108.

Chapter

23

Adult Congenital Heart Disease

Craig R. Bailey and Davina D. L. Wong

Introduction

Heart disease is a common congenital abnormality, affecting 5–9 per 1,000 newborns. Successful evolution of treatment strategies has led to a significant reduction in the number of deaths from congenital heart disease (CHD) in children and this dramatic success has led to increased adult survivors with adult congenital heart disease (ACHD). Survival into adulthood is now more than 90% and estimates suggest that there are more than 2 million adults in the USA with ACHD; three times the number of children with CHD.

Approximately 40% of adults with CHD have simple lesions or have undergone curative procedures and thus require little specialist care. Between 35% and 40% require access to specialist consultation and 20–25% have complex lesions requiring lifelong specialist input. It is important to note that these patients have a significantly increased risk of premature death if managed inappropriately.

Although a small proportion (~10%) of first presentations may occur as an adult, most patients with ACHD have begun their medical care as a neonate or child. Transition from paediatric to adult congenital services can be difficult as adolescent patients start to take charge of their own medical condition.

Anaesthesia for ACHD patients relies on a multidisciplinary team approach with a thorough understanding of the original cardiac anatomy and knowledge of any procedures already performed. The functional capacity of individuals varies, and management should be tailored accordingly. ACHD can be divided into low-, moderate- and high-risk lesions (Box 23.1).

Patients may be broadly divided into those who have had corrective or palliative surgery and those with unoperated CHD. The focus of this chapter is anaesthesia for moderate- and high-risk patients with ACHD.

Special Considerations

Fontan Circulation

A fully complete Fontan circulation necessitates surgery to create a direct connection between the venous return and the PA, excluding the subpulmonary ventricle. Blood flow through the lungs is passive and depends on a relatively high CVP, low PVR and low systemic atrial and ventricular diastolic pressures. Patients are delicately balanced between an inadequate blood supply to the lungs, causing cyanosis, and an excessive pulmonary blood flow (PBF) causing pulmonary oedema. Over time, these patients develop chronically increased venous pressure, leading to hepatic congestion, pulmonary venous congestion, an increased PAP and, eventually, cardiac failure.

Box 23.1   Classification of ACHD according to risk

Low risk

Repaired lesions: PDA, ASD, VSD

Unrepaired lesions: Isolated mild AV or MV disease, isolated PFO, small ASD or VSD, mild PS

Moderate risk

Prosthetic valve or conduit

Intracardiac shunt

Moderate left-sided obstructive lesions

Moderate systemic ventricular dysfunction

Previous transposition of the great arteries

High risk

PHT

Cyanotic CHD

NYHA class 3 or 4

Eisenmenger syndrome

Severe systemic ventricular dysfunction (ejection fraction < 35%)

Severe left-sided obstructive lesions

Pulmonary Hypertension

PHT, defined as a mean PAP above 25 mmHg at rest, is a major perioperative risk factor. Strategies to manage PHT include avoidance of triggering agents, minimizing increases in the PVR with good oxygenation, avoidance of acidosis and limiting peak ventilatory pressures. Some patients are already taking conventional medications such as β-blockers, diuretics, digoxin or ACE inhibitors and may also require specific pulmonary vasodilators such as inhaled NO, prostacyclin (e.g. iloprost), calcium channel antagonists (e.g. diltiazem), phosphodiesterase-5 inhibitors (e.g. oral/IV sildenafil) or endothelin receptor antagonists (e.g. bosentan). Anaesthetic management must be tailored to the underlying cause of PHT in the ACHD patient.

1. *Systemic-to-pulmonary shunt* with an increased PVR or primary PHT – this may respond to pulmonary vasodilators.
2. *Eisenmenger syndrome* – Long-standing systemic-to-pulmonary shunts, leading to systemic pulmonary pressures, reversal of the right-to-left shunt and cyanosis. This is an anaesthetic challenge as both PHT and an exacerbation of the cyanosis must be addressed. This may respond to oral pulmonary vasodilators. The RV is accustomed to high afterload.
3. PHT due to left heart disease – this may require inotropic support and systemic afterload reduction.

Unrestricted Shunts

Patients with ASDs, VSDs, aortopulmonary collaterals or surgically created systemic-to-pulmonary shunts (e.g. Blalock–Taussig (B–T), Waterston and Potts) may have pulmonary to systemic blood flow ($Q_P:Q_S$) of 2:1 or 3:1 in room air, at rest. Breathing 100% oxygen reduces the PVR, leading to increased $Q_P:Q_S$, results in reduced systemic oxygen delivery and metabolic acidosis. Patients with single ventricles and pulmonary circulation supplied by aortopulmonary collaterals have a precarious balance between PBF and systemic oxygen delivery. Ideally, these patients should be maintained on an inspired oxygen concentration that recreates their normal room air oxygen saturations at rest, with the minimum ventilator settings, to maintain a normal $PaCO_2$.

Preoperative Assessment

History

Details of the original congenital lesion, previous percutaneous or open surgical interventions, anaesthetic records and subsequent cardiological investigations should be reviewed. It is important to understand the patient's current anatomy, any residual structural defects and the extent of any physiological adaptation. Many patients are accustomed to poor exercise tolerance, so it is important to determine what is *normal for them*. A history of prolonged periods of ventilation or prior tracheostomy should be elicited, as well as details of any associated pulmonary disease.

Episodes of syncope, chest pain, cyanosis or arrhythmias should be noted.

Cyanotic patients are at risk of thrombosis and details of anticoagulation therapy should be obtained. Patients may be taking other medications such as β-blockers and ACE inhibitors – details of these should be sought.

CHD is associated with a number of genetic syndromes, such as Trisomy 21 and 22q11 deletion – relevant associated features should also be elicited.

Physical Examination

The presence of clubbing, cyanosis and signs of congestive heart failure (jugular venous distension, pulmonary crackles, hepatomegaly and peripheral oedema) should be sought.

Problems associated with the airway should be highlighted as these can substantially increase the risk, especially in the setting of cyanotic heart disease or PHT. Previous cardiac surgery may have resulted in damage to the vocal cords, recurrent laryngeal nerve or phrenic nerve palsy, or Horner syndrome. Prolonged postoperative mechanical ventilation of the lungs may have led to subglottic stenosis.

Peripheral pulses may be diminished, unequal or absent following surgery or previous shunt placement. The presence of additional or abnormal heart sounds are evidence of residual disease.

Neurological assessment may reveal developmental delay and learning difficulties. This may be due to associated congenital disorders, chronic hypoxaemia or following complex cardiac surgery, with long bypass or deep hypothermic circulatory arrest times or prolonged intensive care. Cerebrovascular events occur in up to 14% of patients with cyanotic heart disease, especially in the presence of AF and hypertension.

Investigations

Blood tests: Polycythaemia occurs as a compensatory mechanism in patients with cyanosis. Normal levels of Hb in patients with cyanosis can mean the patient is relatively anaemic. Polycythaemia increases blood viscosity and the risk of thromboembolic events. An Hb concentration above 180 g l^{-1} may be an indication for preoperative venesection, and preoperative hydration is important, including IV fluids if necessary. Conversely, it also leads to a deficiency in vitamin K-dependent clotting factors, fibrinogen and platelets, increasing the risk of perioperative coagulopathy.

Renal function should be assessed because 41% of patients have mild renal dysfunction and 9% moderate or severe dysfunction. Patients with a Fontan circulation, Glenn shunt, Ebstein's anomaly or cardiac failure may have hepatic congestion and impaired synthetic function.

CXR: This may reveal a reason for oxygen desaturation such as a pleural effusion, an acute chest infection or pulmonary oedema. There may be kyphoscoliosis or calcification of a shunt.

ECG: Perioperative arrhythmias are common and may be symptomatic, especially in a failing heart. These are more common in patients with a Fontan circulation and may indicate end-stage cardiac failure or annular dilatation in the setting of atrioventricular valve regurgitation. VT is rare but is more common in patients following ventriculotomy, for example after a repair for tetralogy of Fallot. A preoperative QTc prolongation interval indicates susceptibility to VT.

Echocardiography: For cooperative patients with good acoustic windows, echocardiography alone can define the diagnosis and guide management and prognosis. It is used to identify the anatomy and assess ventricular and valvular function. In addition, an assessment of flow across shunts and conduits, and the degree of PHT, can be undertaken. TTE is of limited value when acoustic windows are poor, particularly for the assessment of extracardiac vascular structures. TOE is usually performed to exclude intra-atrial clots prior to cardioversion.

Angiography: This is used to gain direct information regarding pressures and patterns of blood flow within the heart. It gives information on the responsiveness of the pulmonary vasculature to oxygen and vasodilators and the coronary artery anatomy, and it is useful to assess the suitability of the patient for Fontan completion. In addition, interventional procedures can be undertaken in the cardiac catheter laboratory.

CT: This complements echocardiography in evaluating ACHD. Despite radiation exposure, it is useful in providing information on both the intra- and extracardiac anatomy, coronary arteries and vascular structures. It can also be used to diagnose airway and pulmonary co-morbidities.

MRI: This provides 3D anatomical and physiological information. Extracardiac anatomy, including the great arteries, systemic and pulmonary veins, can be delineated with high spatial resolution. Blood flow can be assessed, shunts can be quantified and myocardial function accurately quantified with high reproducibility, regardless of ventricular morphology. It is probably the best investigation for an assessment of the right side of the heart: RV volumes, degree of PR, RV outflow tract and proximal PAs. The aorta, including aneurysms of the root, and the site of any coarctation can also be visualized.

Cardiopulmonary exercise testing: This provides an integrated assessment of cardiac, pulmonary and metabolic function. It can identify the source of exercise limitation in many patients. The ACHD population often has restrictive lung disease, especially following neonate surgery via thoracotomy or sternotomy.

Anaesthetic Management

Most medications are continued up to the time of surgery. Diuretics and ACE inhibitors should be omitted on the day of surgery. Antiplatelet agents should be considered carefully as the risk of bleeding should be weighed against the risks of thromboembolism and shunt occlusion. Anticoagulants should be stopped according to their half-lives. Warfarin therapy should be bridged with heparin in consultation with a haematologist.

Sedative premedication should be considered, especially in patients who may be anxious from previous hospital experiences, although caution should be exercized in those with cyanosis.

External defibrillator pads are placed on patients undergoing reoperation as access with internal paddles is usually impossible during chest opening. All of our patients have depth-of-anaesthesia monitoring (bispectral index). Use of near-infrared spectroscopy monitoring is increasing.

Vascular access may be difficult. Previous vascular thromboses, catheterizations or vascular cut-downs may lead to scarring. Placement of shunts may have sacrificed peripheral arteries, for example, the right subclavian for a modified B–T shunt. SVC lines may be useful, but if used in patients with a Glenn shunt or a Fontan circulation they should be single lumen and removed as soon as possible due to the increased risk of thrombosis. The use of ultrasound guidance for the insertion of both peripheral and central vascular cannulae is standard practice.

All IV lines, infusions and intravascular transducer monitors should be checked thoroughly to ensure that no air bubbles are present. In-line filters and non-return valves should be used to reduce the risk of air embolism.

Opioid-based techniques are preferred for patients with poor ventricular function, although the choice of anaesthetic agents used is personal and less important than the achievement of appropriate haemodynamic goals. Meticulous attention should be paid to maintaining preload, contractility and sinus rhythm. IV induction may be slowed if the circulation time is prolonged. Right-to-left shunts theoretically prolong inhalational induction, but this is offset by a slower circulation time. The SVR and PVR must be balanced in order to avoid hypoxia or systemic hypoperfusion. Vasodilatation may increase the right-to-left shunt and reduce oxygen saturation, but this is partially offset by a reduced metabolic rate. If mechanical ventilation is required, then the PBF is less compromised if the inspiratory time is shortened, even at the expense of higher peak inspiratory pressures.

All of our non-diabetic patients receive a single IV dose of dexamethasone, and tranexamic acid is given to most patients. Vasoconstrictors, nitroglycerine and inotropes are drawn up and ready for administration as required.

Intraoperative TOE is almost always performed. It confirms preoperative findings, excludes previously undiagnosed lesions and aids optimization of cardiac function, guiding fluid and inotrope therapy. At the end of surgery, TOE is useful for confirming de-airing and assessing the quality of anatomical repairs.

Regional and neuraxial anaesthesia are rarely employed as a profound decrease in the SVR may reverse a left-to-right shunt and lead to hyperaemia, which can be difficult to reverse.

Blood Management

The risks associated with the administration of blood and blood products are well known and we aim to restrict their use whenever possible. Although blood is routinely cross-matched for use in our patients, the use of cell salvage, re-infusion of heparinized cardiotomy blood and individualized management guided by near-patient testing (thromboelastography (TEG)), means that fewer than 10% of our patients receive RBCs or component therapy.

Antibiotic Prophylaxis

NICE produced guidelines for prophylaxis against infective endocarditis in March 2008. (www.nice.org.uk/guidance/cg64) These state that healthcare professionals should regard people with the following cardiac conditions as being at increased risk of developing infective endocarditis:

- Acquired valvular heart disease with stenosis or regurgitation
- Hypertrophic cardiomyopathy
- Previous infective endocarditis
- Structural CHD, including surgically corrected or palliated structural conditions, but excluding an isolated ASD, a fully repaired VSD or a fully repaired patent ductus arteriosus (PDA), and closure devices that are judged to be endothelialized
- Valve replacement

Antibiotic prophylaxis should be given according to local, national or international guidelines. In our institution, the protocol is to administer single doses of teicoplanin and gentamicin.

Postoperative Care

We have a 'fast-track' policy for patients who require a relatively simple cardiac repair. Their procedure is

189

performed first on the operating list so that they can be extubated and transferred from the ICU to a high-dependency unit later the same day. Most patients, however, require a period of elective postoperative mechanical ventilation. In our unit we complete a comprehensive, bespoke handover sheet and communicate directly with the intensive care doctors and nurses (see Chapter 22). Those with a Fontan circulation fare better when breathing spontaneously but must not be allowed to become hypercarbic or develop post-extubation airway obstruction.

Postoperative inhaled NO is useful for patients with PHT. If mechanical ventilation is continued postoperatively then PBF is less compromised if the inspiratory time is shortened even if it is at the expense of a higher peak inspiratory pressure. The treatment of postoperative bleeding should be guided by point-of-care tests such as TEG. Good analgesia, review by the ACHD team, resumption of anticoagulants, continuation of oral pulmonary vasodilators and reintroduction of preoperative medication should take place as soon as possible.

Key Points

- ACHD presents as a spectrum ranging from well patients with corrected minor defects to those with extreme deviations from normal physiology.
- Anaesthesia should include careful attention to preservation of the CO by preserving sinus rhythm and adequate fluid balance.
- In complex patients, the balance between systemic and pulmonary blood flows should be maintained.
- Effective antibiotic prophylaxis and the prevention of either excessive bleeding or thromboembolism are essential.
- Those with high-risk lesions are at extremely high risk of death in the perioperative period, and should always be cared for by a fully informed multidisciplinary team.

Further Reading

Bennett JM, Ehrenfeld JM, Markham L, Eagle SS. Anesthetic management and outcomes for patients with pulmonary hypertension and intracardiac shunts and Eisenmenger syndrome: a review of institutional experience. *J Clin Anesth* 2014; 26: 286–93.

Maxwell BG, Posner KL, Wong JK, *et al.* Factors contributing to adverse perioperative events in adults with congenital heart disease: a structured analysis of cases from the closed claims project. *Congenit Heart Dis* 2015; 10: 21–9.

Nasr VG, Kussman BD. Advances in the care of adults with congenital heart disease. *Semin Cardiothorac Vasc Anesth* 2015; 19: 175–86.

Nasr VG, Faraoni D, Valente AM, DiNardo JA. Outcomes and costs of cardiac surgery in adults with congenital heart disease. *Pediatr Cardiol* 2017; 38: 1359–64.

Navaratnam D, Fitzsimmons S, Grocott M, *et al.* Exercise-induced systemic venous hypertension in the Fontan circulation. *Am J Cardiol* 2016; 117: 1667–71.

Chapter

24

Temperature Management and Deep Hypothermic Arrest

Charles W. Hogue and Joseph E. Arrowsmith

Temperature Control

In animals that maintain body temperature within a tight range (homeotherms), thermoregulation represents the balance between heat production (thermogenesis) and heat loss. Thermogenesis occurs as a result of metabolic activity, particularly in skeletal muscle, the kidneys, the brain, the liver and (in infants) adipose tissue. Body heat is lost by conduction, convection, radiation and evaporation (Table 24.1). Cold-induced hypothalamic stimulation activates autonomic, extra-pyramidal, endocrine and

Table 24.1 Mechanisms of heat loss during anaesthesia and surgery, and measures that may be used to reduce heat loss

Mechanism	Comments	Countermeasures
Conduction	Cold IV and irrigation fluids	Fluid warmer
Convection	Ventilation and laminar airflow ('wind-chill')	Surgical drapes and blankets
Radiation	Most significant factor – human skin is an efficient emitter of infrared energy Dependent on surface area: body mass ratio	Reflective (foil) blanket Window blinds/curtains
Evaporation	Vaporization requires considerable energy Skin preparation solutions, surgical site and airway	Heat and moisture exchanger

behavioural mechanisms to maintain the core temperature.

Anaesthesia and surgery interfere with many facets of thermoregulation – heat is lost by: vasodilatation and conduction to adjacent materials and through surgical drapes, convection of adjacent air and through open wounds, radiation of heat to enclosing surfaces, and evaporation of liquid from tissues. Radiant losses, which are the most important, are dependent on the fourth power of the temperature difference (in kelvins) between skin and the enclosing surface. Because of their high surface area-to-volume ratio, neonates are more vulnerable to hypothermia than adults. Minimizing passive heat loss and active warming are required to maintain normothermia (Box 24.1). Preoperative warming can prevent intraoperative cooling in patients undergoing anaesthesia <30 minutes in duration increasing the mass of tissues at core temperature. This strategy is ineffective for longer procedures as vasodilatation increases heat loss.

Hypothermia

Hypothermia is defined as a core temperature of less than 35 °C and occurs when heat losses overwhelm thermoregulatory mechanisms (e.g. during cold immersion) or when thermoregulation is impaired by pathological conditions (e.g. stroke, trauma, endocrinopathy, sepsis, autonomic neuropathy, uraemia) or drugs (e.g. anaesthetic agents, barbiturates, benzodiazepines, phenothiazines, ethanol). The pathophysiology of hypothermia is shown in Table 24.2.

Therapeutic Hypothermia

Multicentre studies have demonstrated that mild, deliberate hypothermia may improve neurological outcome in comatose patients who have a return of spontaneous circulation after cardiac arrest.

191

Box 24.1 Passive and active measures used during anaesthesia and surgery to maintain normothermia

Thermal insulation (e.g. blankets)	Static air, trapped within a blanket, is a poor conductor of heat Limited ability to insulate the legs and torso in cardiac surgery
Forced air warmer	Prevent radiant heat loss by covering the body with a warm outer shell The contact of warm air and skin reduces convective more than conductive losses Warming in proportion to the area of skin covered Considerably more effective than passive measures and heated mattresses
Heated mattress	Modern operating tables are well insulated, therefore most heat is lost through the front of the body Limited skin contact with mattress minimizes transfer of thermal energy Risk of pressure–heat necrosis (burns) at temperatures >38 °C
Radiant heaters	Generate infrared energy – most efficient when placed close to the body and when the direction of radiant energy is perpendicular to the body surface Allow heat transfer without the need for protective coverings Convective losses continue unimpeded Most commonly used in neonatal practice
Fluid warming	The effect of fluid warming is greatest for refrigerated fluids (e.g. blood) and the rapid administration of fluids at room temperature (i.e. 20 °C) Warming of maintenance fluids (administered slowly) is of little benefit Packed red cells at 4 °C represent a thermal stress of 120 kJ l^{-1} (30 kcal l^{-1}) One unit of red cells at 4 °C may reduce adult core temperature by ~0.25 °C
Humidification	Respiratory tract heat losses account for ~10% of total Passive (i.e. heat and moisture exchangers) measures are less effective but more convenient to use than active humidification systems

Hypothermia must be induced as soon as practicably possible. External (e.g. cooling pads, cooling blankets and ice packs) or internal techniques (e.g. endovascular cooling device) are used to reduce the core body temperature to 32–36 °C for 12–24 hours.

Cardiopulmonary Bypass

CPB offers the means to produce greater and more rapid changes in core temperature than can be achieved by other means. While rapid cooling can be achieved with few deleterious effects, rewarming must be undertaken gradually with a small gradient (e.g. <5 °C) between the warmed blood entering the circulation and the nasopharyngeal temperature. Gradual rewarming ensures more even rewarming and reduces the magnitude of the temperature gradient between the core and peripheral tissue, thought to be responsible for post-CPB 'after-drop'. Vasodilatation during rewarming reduces the core–periphery gradient and slows the rate at which the core temperature rises, albeit at the expense of hypotension.

Deep Hypothermic Circulatory Arrest

In certain situations, the nature of the surgical pathology or procedure necessitates a complete cessation of blood flow (Box 24.2). Preservation of organ function during circulatory arrest is achieved by reducing the core body temperature. Core cooling and cessation of blood flow is known as deep hypothermic circulatory arrest (DHCA).

DHCA provides excellent operating conditions – albeit for a limited duration – whilst ameliorating the major adverse consequences of organ ischaemia. The brain is the organ most at risk during circulatory arrest. Hypothermic neuroprotection is thought to be mediated, at least in part, via a reduction in oxygen-dependent neuronal activity and excitatory neurotransmitter release.

Table 24.2 The pathophysiology of hypothermia

	Mild (33–35 °C)	Severe (<28 °C)
Neurological	Confusion Amnesia Apathy – delayed anaesthetic recovery Impaired judgement	Depressed consciousness Pupillary dilatation Coma Loss of autoregulation
Neuromuscular	Shivering Ataxia Dysarthria	Muscle and joint stiffening Muscle rigor
Cardiovascular	Tachycardia Vasoconstriction Increased BP, CO	Severe bradycardia Increased SVR, reduced CO ECG changes: J (Osborn) waves, QRS broadening, ST changes, T-wave inversion, A-V block, QT prolongation VF → Asystole
Respiratory	Tachypnea Left-shift in the Hb oxygen dissociation (HbO$_2$) curve	Bradypnoea Bronchospasm Right-shift HbO$_2$ curve
Renal **Metabolic**	ADH resistance Cold-induced diuresis Reduced drug metabolism	Reduced GFR Reduced H$^+$ and glucose reabsorption Metabolic (lactic) acidosis
GI		Ileus Gastric ulcers Hepatic dysfunction
Haematology **Immunological**	Increased blood viscosity and haemoconcentration (2% increase in haematocrit/°C) Increased infection risk	Coagulopathy – inhibition of intrinsic/extrinsic pathway enzymes, platelet activation, thrombocytopenia (liver sequestration) Leucocyte depletion, impaired neutrophil function and bacterial phagocytosis

ADH, antidiuretic hormone; A-V, atrioventricular.

Box 24.2   Cardiac and non-cardiac indications for DHCA

Cardiac

Repair of complex congenital cardiac anomalies

Aortic aneurysm, rupture or dissection

Aortic arch reconstruction

Non-cardiac

Hepatic and renal cell carcinoma

Repair of giant cerebral aneurysms

Resection of cerebral arteriovenous malformations

Pulmonary (thrombo)endarterectomy

Anaesthetic Considerations

DHCA is commonly used for complex surgery on the thoracic aorta and PAs. In the emergency setting (e.g. aortic dissection) there may be little or no time to undertake exhaustive preoperative investigations. Significant co-morbidities (e.g. coronary and cerebrovascular disease, DM, renal dysfunction) should be anticipated on the basis of clinical history and physical examination.

Monitoring

Standard peripheral venous, arterial and central venous access is required in all cases. In addition, the following should be considered:

- Cannulation of the right radial artery and a femoral artery permits pressure monitoring proximal and distal to the aortic arch – a femoral arterial cannula serves as an anatomical marker should an IABP be required for separation from CPB

- Venous cannulae should be sited in the right arm if division of the innominate vein (to improve surgical access) is anticipated
- A central venous sheath provides a route for rapid fluid administration and the subsequent insertion of a PAFC
- TOE is invariably used to assess the great vessels and cardiac function, and to assist de-airing
- Temperature monitoring at two or more sites is essential – in most cases, nasopharyngeal or tympanic membrane monitoring provides an indication of brain temperature and bladder or rectal monitoring provides an indication of core temperature

Anaesthetic Drugs

The choice of anaesthetic drugs is largely a matter of personal and institutional preference. In theory, using propofol and opioid-based anaesthesia, in preference to volatile agents, reduces cerebral metabolism whilst preserving flow–metabolism coupling. The impact of hypothermia on drug pharmacokinetics should be considered and drug infusion rates adjusted accordingly.

Patient Care

The use of DHCA is invariably accompanied by prolonged CPB and anaesthesia. Careful attention must be paid to prevent pressure sores and inadvertent injury to the eyes, nerve plexuses, peripheral nerves and pressure points. Cannulae, lines, tubes, cables and other equipment should be padded to prevent pressure necrosis of the skin.

Devices to assist rewarming (e.g. heated mattress, forced-air warming blanket) should be placed before induction of anaesthesia.

Surgical Considerations

In some cases, such as an acute type A aortic dissection, femoral or right axillary arterial cannulation may initially be necessary, together with femoral venous cannulation. Femoro-femoral or axillo-femoral CPB permits systemic cooling *prior* to sternotomy and affords a degree of organ protection should chest-opening be accompanied by inadvertent damage to the aorta or heart and exsanguination. After completion of the aortic repair, placement of the arterial line directly into the prosthetic graft permits restoration of anterograde flow. Cannulation of the mid or distal aortic arch may be required in cases of a degenerative aortic aneurysm to reduce the risk of atheroembolism associated with retrograde flow via femoral arterial cannulation.

The choice of venous drainage site and cannula type is largely dictated by surgical preference and the degree of access required. For example, bicaval cannulation is required if retrograde cerebral perfusion (RCP) is to be used with reversal of blood flow in the SVC. If selective anterograde cerebral perfusion (SACP) is to be used, with selective arterial cannulation of the carotid arterial circulation, then adequate cerebral venous drainage must be ensured, again using bicaval cannulation, to optimize the cerebral perfusion pressure and prevent cerebral oedema. Removal of a renal tumour from the IVC requires the use of an RA basket – in preference to a caval or two-stage cannula – to permit full visualization of the cava and to prevent pulmonary tumour embolism.

DHCA during surgery of the distal aorta via left thoracotomy presents several problems. Access to the proximal aorta is limited and femoral arterial cannulation may be required initially. Access to the RA typically requires an extensive thoracotomy that traverses the sternum. Alternatively, venous drainage may be achieved using PA cannulation or a long femoral cannula advanced into the RA.

Extracorporeal Circulation

DHCA requires modifications to be made to the standard CPB set-up:

- Infusions bags for the storage of heparinized blood during haemodilution (see below)
- Use of a centrifugal pump – in preference to a roller pump – to reduce damage to the cellular components of the circulation and reduce haemolysis
- Incorporation of a haemofilter to permit haemoconcentration during rewarming
- Incorporation of a leucocyte-depleting arterial line filter (see below)
- Selection of a cardiotomy reservoir of sufficient capacity to accommodate the circulating volume during exsanguination, immediately before DHCA
- Arteriovenous bypass and accessory arterial lines – to permit RCP or SACP (see below)

- An efficient heat exchanger
- Consideration of the use of heparin-bonded circuits

Cooling

CPB is instituted with a constant flow rate of 2.4 l min^{-1} m^{-2} and cooling is immediately commenced with a water bath–blood temperature gradient of less than 10 °C. The application of external ice packs or a cooling cap to the head assists cerebral cooling. Vasoactive drugs are used to ensure a MAP of 50–60 mmHg. The onset of hypothermia-induced VF signals the need for either application of an AXC and administration of cardioplegia or, more commonly, insertion of a vent to prevent LV distention.

As much of the planned surgical procedure as possible (e.g. surgical dissection and preparation of any prosthetic grafts) is carried out during the cooling to minimize the duration of DHCA.

Cooling continues until the brain and core temperatures have equilibrated at the target temperature for 10–15 minutes. In some centres, continuous monitoring of the EEG, evoked potentials or jugular venous saturation is used as a guide to the adequacy of cerebral cooling.

Circulatory Arrest

The operating table is then placed in a slightly head-down position, the pump stopped and the patient partially exsanguinated into the venous reservoir. Once isolated from the patient, blood within the extracorporeal circuit is then recirculated via a connection between the arterial and venous lines in order to prevent stagnation and clotting. The surgical repair then proceeds with heed to the duration of circulatory arrest.

As the IV administration of drugs during DHCA is at best pointless and at worst potentially dangerous, all infusions should be discontinued when the CPB pump is switched off.

The removal of the AXC and opening the aorta to the atmosphere exposes both the coronary and cerebral arteries to the risk of air embolism. At the end of DHCA, therefore, adequate de-airing and measures such as head-down tilt and flooding of the surgical field with crystalloid at 4 °C should be undertaken. At the end of DHCA, infusions of anaesthetic agents should be restarted to avoid the risk of inadvertent awareness during rewarming.

Safe Period of Circulatory Arrest

Determining the duration of DHCA that any particular patient will tolerate without sustaining disabling neurological injury is, at best, an inexact science. Neonates and infants generally tolerate longer periods of DHCA than adults. Current practice makes it difficult to separate the neurological risks of the prolonged CPB, reperfusion and rewarming – all unavoidable consequences of DHCA – from those of DHCA alone.

Most patients tolerate 30 minutes DHCA at 18 °C. The incidence of neurological injury rises sharply when DHCA exceeds 40 minutes and only three-quarters of patients tolerate 45 minutes of DHCA at this temperature. On the basis of animal experimentation and clinical observation, unmodified DHCA is typically limited to no more than 60 minutes at 18 °C. Frustratingly, while some patients appear to tolerate DHCA more than 60 minutes without apparent injury, others sustain major brain injury after less than 20 minutes DHCA. In many centres, near-infrared spectroscopy (NIRS) is used to limit the duration of circulatory arrest when intermittent DHCA is feasible.

Rewarming

Animal evidence suggests that a period of 10–20 minutes of 'cold reperfusion' (i.e. rewarming is delayed) at the end of DHCA may improve the outcome. Rewarming after DHCA entails considerable transfer of energy (Figure 24.1). Excessively rapid rewarming is known to worsen neurological outcome. In patients undergoing CABG surgery, maintaining a temperature gradient of less than 2 °C between inflow temperature and nasopharyngeal temperature improves the cognitive outcome. The inflow temperature should not exceed 37 °C and CPB is terminated when the core body temperature reaches 35.5–36.5 °C. A significant 'after-drop' is inevitable and patients are sometimes admitted to the ICU with temperatures as low as 32 °C. Using a slow rate of rewarming with adequate time for even distribution of heat between core and peripheral tissues helps to reduce the extent of this after-drop.

During the period of rewarming, attention should be given to the correction of metabolic abnormalities, particularly the metabolic acidosis that inevitably accompanies reperfusion following circulatory arrest. Correction of the acid–base balance may require the

195

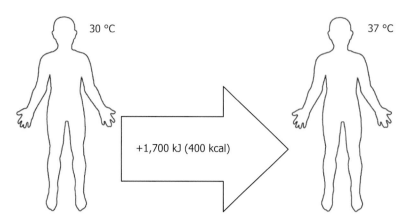

Figure 24.1 Energy transfer during rewarming. Assuming that human tissue has an average specific heat capacity of ~3.5 kJ kg^{-1} °C^{-1} (0.83 kcal kg^{-1} °C^{-1}), raising the temperature of a 70 kg adult from 30 °C to 37 °C requires a minimum energy transfer of ~1,700 kJ (400 kcal) – the same energy required to raise the temperature of 5 litres of water from 20 °C to 100 °C. In practice, ongoing heat losses dictate that greater overall energy transfer is required.

titrated administration of sodium bicarbonate or use of haemofiltration (ultrafiltration).

Haemostasis

Prolonged CPB and hypothermia produce a coagulopathy. Haemostasis is facilitated by meticulous surgery, the use of autologous blood (removed at the onset of CPB) and administration of allogenic blood components under the guidance of laboratory tests of coagulation and thromboelastography. Despite safety concerns, antifibrinolytic agents (e.g. tranexamic acid, ε-aminocaproic acid) and aprotinin have been shown to be efficacious in aortic arch surgery with DHCA.

Cerebral Protection

Hypothermia is the principal neuroprotectant during DHCA. Additional strategies that may reduce the likelihood of neurological injury include acid–base management strategy, haemodilution and glycaemic control. Surgical manoeuvres, such as intermittent cerebral perfusion, SACP and RCP, may also be used to both protect the brain and extend the operating time available to the surgeon.

Temperature

Cerebral metabolism decreases by 6–7% for every 1 °C fall in temperature below 37 °C, with consciousness and autoregulation being lost at 30 °C and 25 °C, respectively. At temperatures below 20 °C, ischaemic tolerance is around ten times that at normothermia. DHCA at 15–20 °C provides the longest safe period of circulatory arrest. The application of external ice packs or a cooling cap to the head delays brain rewarming during DHCA.

Haemodilution

Vasoconstriction, increased plasma viscosity and reduced RBC plasticity secondary to hypothermia leads to impairment of the microcirculation and ischaemia. Progressive haemodilution during hypothermic CPB (haematocrit = 18–20%) is thought to partially mitigate against this phenomenon. A degree of normovolaemic haemodilution is undertaken prior to the onset of CPB in some centres. The optimal haematocrit for a particular individual at a specific temperature remains unclear. Gross anaemia (haematocrit <10%) may result in inadequate tissue oxygen delivery, particularly during rewarming.

Acid–Base Management

Cerebral vasodilatation associated with pH-stat blood-gas management improves the brain cooling and ensures a more homogeneous cooling of deeper brain structures. The pH-stat strategy may, however, induce a cerebral metabolic acidosis and increase microembolization secondary to increased cerebral blood flow. In neonates undergoing DHCA for repair of congenital heart defects, pH-stat management prior to DHCA appears to be associated with fewer complications than α-stat management, and better developmental outcomes. In adults, however, the superiority of one strategy over another in the setting of DHCA is unproven. On theoretical grounds, using pH-stat during cooling and α-stat during rewarming (the so-called 'crossover' management) has some appeal.

Glucose Management

Insulin resistance and hyperglycaemia are common during DHCA. Whilst tight glycaemic control during cardiac surgery appears to reduce mortality and infective complications, any neuroprotective effect is unproven.

Selective Antegrade Cerebral Perfusion

This technique involves selective cannulation of the brachiocephalic, axillary or carotid arteries. Oxygenated blood is pumped via a separate arterial line at 10–20 ml kg^{-1} to maintain a perfusion pressure – measured in the right radial artery – of 50–70 mmHg. Although SACP permits surgery to be conducted at lesser degrees of systemic hypothermia (e.g. 22–25 °C) it often requires greater mobilization of the epiaortic vessels and division of the innominate vein. In addition to increasing complexity and crowding the surgical field with cannulae, SACP is accompanied by the risk of cerebral embolization. An intact circle of Willis is required when unilateral SACP is employed. A misplaced cannula may result in inadequate cerebral perfusion while giving a false sense of security.

Intermittent Cerebral Perfusion

Intermittent systemic perfusion punctuated by less than 20 minute periods of DHCA has been used as an alternative strategy to prolong the total duration of DHCA. It is suggested that intermittent reperfusion preserves neurological tissue by replenishing cerebral high-energy phosphates and removing accumulated waste products. In some centres, NIRS is used to guide the durations of DHCA and reperfusion.

Retrograde Cerebral Perfusion

RCP, which relies on the fact that cerebral veins have no valves, involves the continuous administration of cold (10–15 °C) oxygenated blood via an SVC cannula. Blood flow to the brain is most likely to occur via the azygos veins because the internal jugular veins possess valves. The azygos vein has connections to the vertebral venous system and the venous plexus of the foramen magnum and intracranial sinuses. Massive shunting via the superficial and deep venous systems, including the internal and external jugular veins, may result in only a small fraction of the blood entering the SVC actually reaching the cerebral arteries. For this reason, the exact levels of cerebral blood flow and metabolic substrate delivery provided by RCP have yet to be defined. Suggested blood flow rates for RCP are 200–300 ml min^{-1} with an SVC pressure of <25 mmHg.

Theoretical advantages of RCP include: more homogeneous brain cooling; wash-out of air bubbles, embolic debris and metabolic waste products; prevention of cerebral blood cell microaggregates; and delivery of O_2 and metabolic substrates to the brain. The prolongation of safe DHCA that can be achieved with RCP is less than that with SACP. RCP for more than 60 minutes is a significant predictor of permanent neurological dysfunction.

Neurological Monitoring

For a monitor to be useful it must prompt a corrective intervention before the onset of an irreversible neurological injury. The cost and lack of level 1A evidence of efficacy means neurological monitoring has yet to be universally adopted as 'standard of care'.

Spinal Cord Protection

Surgery involving the descending thoracic aorta may interrupt blood flow to the spinal cord via the anterior spinal artery (of Adamkiewicz) and cause paraplegia. Spinal cord protection is discussed further in Chapter 13.

Postoperative Care

Postoperative care is similar to that for any patient undergoing cardiac surgery. Every effort should be made to ameliorate the impact of secondary brain injury – hyperthermia, hypoxaemia, hypotension and hypoperfusion should be aggressively treated. Even mild degrees of hyperthermia, a common occurrence after cardiac surgery, have been shown to be detrimental after DHCA.

The incidence and severity of postoperative complications associated with DHCA are largely determined by the pathology being treated, the presence of significant co-morbidities and the urgency of surgery.

Key Points

- The most significant cause of intraoperative hypothermia is radiant heat loss.
- Clinical decision-making should be based on the core temperature rather than the gradient between the core and peripheral temperatures.

- Hypothermia is the single most important mechanism of cerebral protection during DHCA.
- The use of continuous or intermittent cerebral perfusion techniques during DHCA may prolong the safe duration of circulatory arrest.

- Infusions of anaesthetic drugs should be discontinued prior to the onset of DHCA and restarted soon after the commencement of rewarming.

Further Reading

Arrowsmith JE, Hogue CW. Deep hypothermic circulatory arrest. In Ghosh S, Falter F, Perrino AC (eds), *Cardiopulmonary Bypass*, 2nd edn. Cambridge: Cambridge University Press; 2015, pp. 152–67.

Dorotta I, Kimball-Jones P, Applegate R 2nd. Deep hypothermia and circulatory arrest in adults. *Semin Cardiothorac Vasc Anesth* 2007; 11: 66–76.

Ginsberg S, Solina A, Papp D, *et al.* A prospective comparison of three heat preservation methods for patients undergoing hypothermic cardiopulmonary bypass. *J Cardiothorac Vasc Anesth* 2000; 14: 501–5.

Grigore AM, Murray CF, Ramakrishna H, Djaiani G. A core review of temperature regimens and neuroprotection during cardiopulmonary bypass: does rewarming rate matter? *Anesth Analg* 2009; 109: 1741–51.

Hogue CW Jr, Palin CA, Arrowsmith JE. Cardiopulmonary bypass management and neurologic outcomes: an evidence-based appraisal of current practices. *Anesth Analg* 2006; 103: 21–37.

Khaladj N, Shrestha M, Meck S, *et al.* Hypothermic circulatory arrest with selective antegrade cerebral perfusion in ascending aortic and aortic arch surgery: a risk factor analysis for adverse outcome in 501 patients. *J Thorac Cardiovasc Surg* 2008; 135: 908–14.

National Institute for Health and Care Excellence. Clinical Guidance 65. Perioperative hypothermia (inadvertent). April 2008. www.nice.org.uk/guidance/CG65 (accessed December 2018).

National Institute for Health and Care Excellence. Intervention Practice Guideline 386. Therapeutic hypothermia following cardiac arrest. March 2011. www.nice.org.uk/guidance/ipg386 (accessed December 2018).

Nielsen N, Wetterslev J, Cronberg T, *et al.* Targeted temperature management at 33°C versus 36°C after cardiac arrest. *N Engl J Med* 2013; 369: 2197–206.

Polderman KH, Varon J. How low should we go? Hypothermia or strict normothermia after cardiac arrest? *Circulation* 2015; 131: 669–75.

25

The Effects of Cardiopulmonary Bypass on Drug Pharmacology

Jens Fassl and Berend Mets

The institution of CPB has profound effects on the plasma concentration, distribution and elimination of drugs. The major factors responsible for this are haemodilution, altered plasma protein binding, altered regional blood flow, hypothermia, isolation of the lungs from the circulation and sequestration of drugs into components of the extracorporeal circuit. These changes, which are influenced by physicochemical and pharmacokinetic characteristics, result in an alteration in free drug and effector-site concentration.

Factors during CPB Affecting Drug Pharmacokinetics

Haemodilution

The CPB circuit is primed with 1,500–2,000 ml of crystalloid solution, corresponding to a potential 30% increase in circulating blood volume, with associated haemodilution occurring when CPB is instituted. The immediate effect of this haemodilution is a decrease in circulating free drug concentration, a reduction in the concentration of plasma proteins and a reduction in the haematocrit.

The eventual plasma concentration of a drug is dependent on its plasma protein binding (PPB), its original volume of distribution and the extent of equilibration between tissue and plasma at the time of institution of CPB. An important consideration is the distinction between the total plasma concentration and the 'free' or unbound fraction. The free concentration of the drug is that which moves to the effector site and can be eliminated. The impact of haemodilution on the unbound fraction of drugs tends to be greater for drugs that have high PPB. This may result in a greater transfer of drug from the blood–prime mixture to the tissues, and thus a lower eventual circulating drug concentration. The volume of distribution (V_D) is another factor determining the circulating concentration of drugs during CPB. Drugs with a large inherent V_D tend to be less affected by haemodilution, as there is a large tissue reservoir from which the drug can diffuse back into the circulation to plasma.

Heparin administration can result in the displacement of plasma-protein-bound drugs (e.g. propofol). The mechanism appears to be heparin-induced lipase release, leading to the hydrolysis of plasma triglycerides to form non-esterified fatty acids, which bind competitively to plasma proteins. The administration of protamine reverses this effect.

The acute effects of haemodilution only (disregarding the effects of altered distributional changes from changed PPB and so increased free fractions) can be established from the formula:

$$\Delta Css = \frac{Css \times Vpp}{V1 + Vpp}$$

where ΔCss is change in drug concentration, Css is the drug concentration prior to haemodilution, Vpp the volume of pump prime and $V1$ is the V_D of the central compartment or the α phase.

The effects of haemodilution mean that the apparent V_D and effective (free) concentration of a drug are greater if administered during, rather than before, CPB.

Hypotension and Altered Blood Flow

CPB is associated with hypotension and altered regional blood flow, particularly at the onset of CPB, during aortic cross-clamping and declamping, and during cardioplegia administration. This is due to reduced blood viscosity and SVR. Associated alterations in hepatic and renal blood flow may affect the metabolism and elimination of drugs.

Hypothermia

The solubility of gases in blood is inversely proportional to temperature. Changes in inhaled or sweep

199

> **Box 25.1** The impact of hypothermia on drug pharmacokinetics
>
> - ↓ Absorption of drugs administered other than by the IV route
> - ↓ Drug distribution from central to peripheral compartments (↓V_D)
> - Altered CNS drug penetration
> - ↓ Rate of reuptake of drug from peripheral tissues to the central compartment and subsequent reductions in hepatic clearance, leading to prolonged elimination half-time
> - ↓ Biotransformation rate with decreased clearance and increased elimination half-time
> - Altered renal drug excretion as a result of ↓ renal perfusion, ↓ GFR and ↓ tubular secretion

gas volatile anaesthetic concentration will therefore take longer to alter the effect-site partial pressure.

Hypothermia may affect the hepatic metabolism and elimination of drugs by direct (enzymatic) inhibition and altered intrahepatic blood flow. Moreover, hypothermia may interfere with the binding affinity of some drug receptors and increase the relative potency of volatile anaesthetic agents (Box 25.1).

Acid–Base Status

CPB using pH-stat blood-gas management increases drug delivery by increasing the cerebral blood flow, and alters the degree of ionization and protein binding of some drugs, leading to altered free (active) drug concentrations.

Lung Isolation

Exclusion of the lungs during CPB interrupts the normal PA blood flow, although bronchial blood flow remains intact. The lungs act as a reservoir for basic drugs such as lidocaine, propranolol and fentanyl that are administered prior to CPB and so, with re-establishment of the pulmonary circulation, upon separation from CPB, the sequestered drug may return to the circulation. This may raise the systemic concentration above earlier levels or re-establish plasma concentrations sufficient to exert a pharmacological effect.

Sequestration in the CPB Circuit

In vitro experiments have demonstrated that a significant amount of fentanyl, alfentanil, volatile anaesthetic agents, propofol, barbiturates and GTN can be sequestered in bypass equipment. While theoretically there is a possibility for reducing the plasma concentration due to circuit uptake, there was no evidence that this has any clinical relevance.

Factors during CPB Affecting Drug Pharmacodynamics

Changes in drug effects secondary to CPB are poorly described.

Temperature: Hypothermia reduces anaesthetic requirements and decreases opioid and nicotinic receptor affinity.

Acid–base status: Acidosis is associated with alterations in plasma electrolyte concentrations, which may increase susceptibility to arrhythmias and enhance digoxin toxicity.

Specific Drugs

Propofol

Propofol exhibits a high degree of PPB (unbound fraction <4%) and has a high hepatic extraction ratio (>0.8). Changes in PPB can lead to clinically significant changes in the anaesthetic effects of propofol. The use of propofol infusions (3–6 mg kg^{-1} h^{-1}) during CPB has been extensively studied. There is a decrease in total concentration following the onset of CPB, associated with a small increase in the free fraction.

Sequestration may decrease the total circulating concentration initially, although the plasma concentration may rise during CPB as a result of decreased clearance. The impact of heparin on the concentration of free propofol (as mentioned above) is reversed by protamine. In a recent study, Takizawa *et al.* found a significantly increased anaesthetic effect of propofol during normothermic CPB. This was thought to be due to an increased unbound concentration, rather than a change in total drug concentration. Using two propofol administration regimens (4 mg kg^{-1} h^{-1} and 6 mg kg^{-1} h^{-1}) the total blood propofol concentration was unchanged during CPB relative to the pre-CPB value in both groups (2–5 μg ml^{-1}), although the unbound concentration increased two-fold (0.04 → 0.08 μg ml^{-1} – lower propofol infusion rate) during CPB. The enhanced efficacy of propofol may be caused by a reduction in the number of PPB sites during CPB.

Volatile Anaesthetics

The circulating concentration of volatile anaesthetic agents administered via the CPB circuit is governed by three factors:

- The blood:gas solubility coefficient of the agent – hypothermia increases solubility
- The tissue:gas solubility coefficient of the agent – hypothermia increases tissue uptake
- Uptake by the oxygenator – depends on the agent and the type of oxygenator

Taking a number of studies together it is evident that there may be a delay in achieving therapeutic partial pressures when volatile agents are first administered during CPB. Nussmeier *et al.* demonstrated that, after 32 minutes of isoflurane administration (1% at 32 °C), the blood partial pressure had only reached 51% of the inlet partial pressure. Using desflurane, which has lower blood-gas solubility, Mets *et al.* demonstrated that the initial wash-in was significantly faster. Although the arterial partial pressure reached 50% of the inlet partial pressure within 4 minutes, it took a further 28 minutes to reach 68%. Desflurane wash-out during CPB was also rapid; the arterial partial pressure fell by 82% within the first 4 minutes, and by 92%, 20 minutes after discontinuation of desflurane and rewarming the patient.

In contrast to these studies, where the volatile agent was first administered during CPB, Goucke *et al.* examined the effect of enflurane (1%) administration both before and during hypothermic CPB. Compared to pre-CPB, there was a 26% increase in the median blood enflurane *concentration* (not partial pressure) upon cooling to 28 °C. The blood enflurane concentration returned to within the pre-CPB range after separation from CPB, suggesting that body cooling increased the enflurane concentration during CPB.

Benzodiazepines

The plasma concentration of benzodiazepines falls after the initiation of CPB but tend to rise after separation from CPB. This may be explained on the basis of the prolonged elimination half-life, redistribution and haemoconcentration in the post-CPB period.

Opioids

The effect of CPB on opioids depends on the mode of administration. It has been demonstrated that, following administration of a single bolus dose, plasma concentrations of fentanyl and sufentanil decreased by 53% and 34%, respectively, upon initiation of CPB. The extracorporeal and pulmonary sequestration of opiates is directly proportional to lipid solubility. Like benzodiazepines, the elimination half-life of opioids may be prolonged after CPB.

Opiate infusions during hypothermic CPB may lead to a significant accumulation due to reduced hepatic clearance. A near constant remifentanil concentration can be achieved by reducing the infusion rate by 30% for every 5 °C decrease in temperature.

Muscle Relaxants

Plasma concentrations of these typically polar drugs would be expected to fall, as a result of haemodilution, at the onset of CPB. However, an altered organ blood flow and hypothermic CPB decrease the metabolism and elimination. The net effect is that muscle-relaxant requirements fall during CPB. Because of significant inter-patient variability, it is suggested that neuromuscular monitoring be used if early tracheal extubation is contemplated.

Key Points

- A number of physical and chemical factors account for the alteration of drug pharmacokinetics during CPB.
- Changes in the plasma concentration of drugs, secondary to an increased volume of distribution, are often balanced by a reduction in PPB.
- Hypothermia and altered regional blood flow reduce drug metabolism and elimination.
- Hypothermia increases the solubility of volatile anaesthetic agents in the blood. This simultaneously increases the concentration of the agent, while reducing its partial pressure.
- Hypothermia reduces the MAC of anaesthetic agents.
- Hypothermia may significantly increase the time required to achieve a therapeutic partial pressure when a volatile agent is first administered after the onset of CPB.

Further Reading

Goucke CR, Hackett LP, Barrett PH, Ilett KF. Blood concentrations of enflurane before, during, and after hypothermic cardiopulmonary bypass. *J Cardiothorac Vasc Anesth* 2007; 21: 218–23.

Mets B, Reich NT, Mellas N, Beck J, Park S. Desflurane pharmacokinetics during cardiopulmonary bypass. *J Cardiothorac Vasc Anesth* 2001; 15: 179–82.

Mets B. The pharmacokinetics of anesthetic drugs and adjuvants during cardiopulmonary bypass. *Acta Anaesthesiol Scand* 2000; 44: 261–73.

Nussmeier NA, Lambert ML, Moskowitz GJ, *et al.* Washin and washout of isoflurane administered via bubble oxygenators during hypothermic cardiopulmonary bypass. *Anesthesiology* 1989; 71: 519–25.

Sherwin J, Heath T, Watt K. Pharmacokinetics and dosing of anti-infective drugs in patients on extracorporeal membrane oxygenation: a review of the current literature. *Clin Ther* 2016; 38: 1976–94.

Takizawa E., Hiraoka H., Takizawa D., Goto F. Changes in the effect of propofol in response to altered plasma protein binding during normothermic cardiopulmonary bypass. *Br J Anaesth* 2006; 96: 179–85.

van Saet A, de Wildt SN, Knibbe CA, *et al.* The effect of adult and pediatric cardiopulmonary bypass on pharmacokinetic and pharmacodynamic parameters. *Curr Clin Pharmacol* 2013; 8: 297–318.

Controversies in Cardiopulmonary Bypass

Will Tosh and Christiana Burt

Despite more than six decades of clinical experience and considerable research, the characteristics of 'optimal' CPB remain imprecisely defined. This chapter discusses the main areas of controversy (Box 26.1).

Pressure versus Flow

Prolonged periods of hypotension and hypoperfusion are deleterious, with the brain being the organ most at risk. Despite the fact that routine CPB perfusion pressures of 40–60 mmHg represents deliberate hypotension, the majority of patients appear to survive without evidence of significant injury. When the pressure falls below this range, an increase in either pump flow rate or administration of a vasoconstrictor to increase the SVR is the usual response. The question of whether perfusion pressure or flow rate is more important for organ preservation remains unanswered. The proposed advantages and disadvantages of higher and lower CPB perfusion pressure are summarized in Table 26.1.

At normocarbia, cerebral autoregulation maintains the cerebral blood flow (CBF) over a range of perfusion pressures (50–150 mmHg). During hypothermic CPB, the lower limit of cerebral autoregulation falls to as low as 30 mmHg. In the absence of significant cerebrovascular disease, cerebral hypoperfusion will be unlikely with a MAP higher than 40 mmHg and this remains the lowest acceptable

Box 26.1 Controversies in CPB management

CPB perfusion characteristics	Optimum perfusion pressure Pressure versus flow Pulsatile versus non-pulsatile
Temperature	Normothermia versus hypothermia
Acid–base management	pH-stat versus α-stat
Hb	Minimum haematocrit on CPB
CPB equipment	Pump characteristics Circuit surface modification Reservoir characteristics Processing cardiotomy blood
Mini CPB	Reduced RBC transfusion to correct haemodilution versus logistic challenges
Ventilation and oxygenation	Optimal target for oxygenation To ventilate or not to ventilate the lungs?

Table 26.1 Proposed advantages and disadvantages of low and high CPB perfusion pressure

Perfusion pressure	Advantages	Disadvantages
Lower (<60 mmHg)	↓ Incidence of emboli ↓ Haematological trauma ↓ Collateral warming of the heart Less blood in operative field ↑ Myocardial protection ↓ Cardiotomy suction	Cerebral and renal hypoperfusion
Higher (>80 mmHg)	Vital organ perfusion maintained In event of cerebral injury secondary to emboli, collateral flow is said to be pressure-dependent	↑ Haematological trauma ↑ Risk of emboli ↑ Bleeding complications ↑ Suture line stress ↑ Collateral flow to heart ↓ Reduced duration of cardioplegia

203

pressure in adult practice. There is general agreement that a target of perfusion pressure of 50–60 mmHg is safe in the majority of cases.

Cerebral autoregulation is altered by a number of disease processes (e.g. hypertension, DM) and, to a lesser extent, by volatile anaesthetic agents and vasodilators. It has been argued that two groups of patients might benefit from an increased perfusion pressure (i.e. 70–80 mmHg) during CPB – those with altered cerebral autoregulation and those with cerebrovascular disease (Box 26.2).

In 1995, a randomized trial of higher (80–100 mmHg) versus lower (50–60 mmHg) CPB perfusion pressures in 248 CABG patients showed that *combined* neurological and cardiac outcomes, 6 months after surgery, were significantly better in the higher-pressure group. The study was criticized for analyzing combined outcomes, for using multiple comparisons, for the finding of a greater stroke rate (7.2%) in the lower-pressure (control) group and for being insufficiently powered to detect a 50% reduction in stroke rate. The following year, TOE findings in 75% of these patients were published and it became apparent that the incidence of high-grade aortic atheroma was greater in the lower-pressure group (~30% versus 40%). It can be tentatively concluded that higher perfusion pressures may reduce the risk of stroke in patients with severe aortic atheroma (Box 26.2).

By contrast, a retrospective study of ~3,000 patients undergoing CABG surgery demonstrated a significant association between lower CPB perfusion pressure and increased postoperative stroke or coma. This finding might indicate that patients deemed to be at higher risk were managed using higher perfusion pressures. Alternatively, it might be concluded that a higher perfusion pressure during CPB is not without risk.

Multiple variables, including blood viscosity, flow rate, depth of anaesthesia and vasoactive drug use, affect the MAP. The effect of these variables on clinical outcomes makes the interpretation of studies assessing the MAP difficult and, as such, there is currently insufficient evidence to recommend an optimal MAP for patients undergoing cardiac surgery.

Studies examining the influence of the CPB flow rate on the CBF and metabolism have produced conflicting results – the principal study design flaw being the failure to control for the haematocrit. The only conclusion that can be drawn is that, within the bounds of usual clinical practice, modest

---

Box 26.2   Patient groups which may benefit from a higher CPB perfusion pressure

Advanced atherosclerosis
Severe (grade IV and V) atheromatous disease of the descending thoracic aorta (visible on TOE) is a good marker of atheromatous disease near the aortic cannulation site, which is not well visualized with TOE

Chronic hypertension
In patients with chronic, poorly controlled hypertension the pressure–flow autoregulation curve is shifted to the right, therefore a mean perfusion pressure > 50 mmHg is required to maintain the flow

Cerebrovascular disease
Patients with cerebrovascular disease and those with a history of stroke may have impaired regional cerebral autoregulation and are at a greater risk of a neurological injury

DM
These patients appear to have an impaired metabolism–flow coupling during CPB, with possibly some loss of pressure–flow regulation. It has therefore been postulated, but not proven, that a higher perfusion pressure is required during rewarming or during normothermic CPB.

Age > 70 years
Increasing age does not affect cerebral autoregulation per se. However, there may be slower vasodilatation of cerebral resistance vessels during rewarming, leading to transient episodes of metabolism–flow mismatch, with resultant ischaemia. Unless there is coexisting atherosclerotic or hypertensive disease there is, as yet, no evidence that age per se is a reason for using high perfusion pressures.

---

changes in flow rate have little impact on the CBF at normocarbia.

It should be borne in mind that:

- Tissue oxygen delivery is a function of the pump flow rate, SaO_2 and haematocrit
- The pump flow rate gives no indication of regional organ perfusion

The only organ amenable to flow modification at a constant pressure is the brain (by changing the $PaCO_2$). Evidence of inadequate tissue perfusion includes a reduced SvO_2, metabolic acidosis and hyperlactataemia. Assuming a normal Hb

Box 26.3 Reasons for failure to demonstrate hypothermic neuroprotection

- Normothermic CPB in many cases meant a temperature of 35.5 °C, which may have conferred a degree of neuroprotection
- Inadvertent cerebral hyperthermia during the rewarming phase of hypothermic CPB
- Patients in both hypothermic and normothermic CPB groups were relatively normothermic at times of greatest cerebral vulnerability – aortic cannulation/decannulation and onset/offset of CPB

Box 26.4 Putative benefits of pulsatile and non-pulsatile CPB

Pulsatile

↑ Myocardial (subendocardial) perfusion, oxygenation and contractility

↑ Renal (cortical) blood flow and urine output

↑ Cerebral perfusion

↓ Catecholamine, renin, angiotensin, aldosterone and lactate levels

Preserved baroreceptor function

Maintenance of pancreatic β-cell function

Non-pulsatile

↓ Haemolysis

↓ Platelet damage

Less complex CPB system

concentration, the recommended pump flow rate at normothermia is 2.2 l min^{-1} m^{-2}. The reduction in metabolic rate that accompanies hypothermia (50% for every 7 °C) permits flow rates to be reduced.

In a recent study, TCD was used to monitor cerebral autoregulation and to tailor the perfusion pressure during non-pulsatile CPB in 617 patients undergoing cardiac surgery. Interestingly, the lower and upper limits of autoregulation were reported as 65±12 mmHg and 84±11 mmHg, and the 'optimal' MAP was 78±11 mmHg.

Normothermia versus Hypothermia

Hypothermic CPB was widely practised until the mid 1990s. Studies suggesting that normothermic cardioplegia and CPB may improve myocardial protection during cardiac surgery led to the adoption of so-called 'warm-heart' or normothermic techniques. The principal concern is that an improved myocardial outcome is achieved at the expense of decreasing the margin of safety afforded by hypothermia and increasing the risk of neurological injury.

The Toronto Warm Heart Investigators reported no increase in adverse neurological outcomes in patients maintained at normothermia (33–37 °C versus 25–30 °C) during CPB, whereas the Atlanta Group (Mora *et al.*) reported a marked increase in neurological injury. Based on patient numbers, however, the evidence accumulated in subsequent studies suggests that the avoidance of hypothermia during CPB does not increase the risk of adverse neurological outcomes (Box 26.3).

Published in 2001, a Cochrane review of 17 studies (Rees *et al.*) revealed that hypothermia was associated with a *trend* towards a reduction in non-fatal strokes and a *trend* towards an increase in non-stroke-related perioperative deaths. In addition, hypothermia was associated with a higher incidence of myocardial damage and low CO syndrome, although the temperature management strategy appeared to have no impact on the incidence of non-fatal MI. The authors concluded that there was no definite advantage of hypothermia over normothermia in the incidence of clinical events.

Pulsatile versus Non-Pulsatile Flow

It has long been thought that pulsatile CPB is physiological and therefore beneficial. The extra kinetic energy applied to blood during pulsatile flow appears to improve RBC transit, capillary perfusion and microvascular flow, and to enhance lymphatic drainage. In patients undergoing prolonged periods of CPB using non-pulsatile flow, increases in catecholamines and activation of the renin–angiotensin system leads to systemic vasoconstriction, reduced organ perfusion and a predisposition to low CO syndrome following separation from CPB. Generation of pulsatile flow can be achieved with programmable roller pumps, ventricular blood pumps, compression plate pumps and with an IABP during non-pulsatile flow. Most modern CPB machines can deliver pulsatile flow without additional equipment or expense (Box 26.4). The contradictory conclusions of clinical studies may in part be explained by differences in the pressure–flow characteristics of pulsatile CPB employed.

In patients with pre-existing renal insufficiency, pulsatile CPB appears to be associated with improved postoperative renal function. The application of an

AXC abolishes any potential benefit to the ischaemic heart during pulsatile CPB. Published in 1995, a Canadian study of 316 CABG patients demonstrated that pulsatile CPB was associated with a lower mortality and cardiovascular morbidity but there was no improvement in neurological and cognitive outcomes (Murkin *et al*). One reason why subsequent investigations may have failed to replicate these findings is the lack of definition of what constitutes pulsatile flow, how to quantify it and whether or not a certain period of bypass time is required before a difference is seen. In addition, the amount of haemodynamic energy delivered by different pulsatile pumps can vary widely and the pressure waveform can be affected by other components of the bypass system. A recent review called for future investigators to standardize CPB systems and conduct when investigating this question.

Alpha-Stat versus pH-Stat

The solubility of a gas in a liquid is inversely proportional to temperature. As the temperature falls, the total gas content remains unchanged but the partial pressure exerted by the gas will fall as a result of increased solubility. In a hypothermic patient, blood-gas analysis performed at 37 °C will mask a fall in the PaO_2 and $PaCO_2$. The $PaCO_2$ is reduced by 4.4% for every 1 °C decrease in temperature, roughly 2 mmHg for each degree less than 37 °C. If temperature-corrected blood-gas analysis is performed, hypothermic patients will appear hypocapnic and alkalotic. Two blood-gas management strategies have emerged to maintain normal physiology, α-stat and pH-stat blood-gas management (Table 26.2).

During hypothermic CPB, blood vessels maintain their responsiveness to $PaCO_2$ and modulate organ blood flow accordingly. The impact of the blood-gas management strategy on neurological, cardiac and renal outcomes following hypothermic CPB has generated considerable debate (Table 26.3).

Based on results of laboratory and clinical studies, the α-stat strategy is recommended for adults undergoing uninterrupted hypothermic CPB, while pH-stat should probably be used during hypothermic CPB prior to deep hypothermic circulatory arrest (DHCA). The risk of neurological injury during DHCA appears, in part, to be due to incomplete brain cooling and insufficient metabolic rate reduction in the early part of cooling. As cerebral autoregulation is

Table 26.2 The differences between the clinical applications of α-stat and pH-stat blood-gas management strategies

α-stat	pH-stat
Derives its name from the ionization state of enzymatic α-histidine-imidazole groups, which is maintained constant Blood-gas analysis results are *not* corrected for temperature Target is 'normal' blood gases at 37 °C Temperature-corrected hypocarbia and alkalosis tolerated No additional CO_2 administered to patient	So-called because pH is maintained at ~7.4 regardless of blood temperature Blood-gas analysis results are corrected for temperature Target is 'normal' blood gases at *blood temperature* Temperature-uncorrected hypercarbia and acidosis tolerated Additional CO_2 administered to patient

Table 26.3 Putative advantages and disadvantages of α-stat and pH-stat blood-gas management strategies

	Advantages	Disadvantages
α-stat	Cerebral autoregulation preserved ↓ Cerebral microembolization Improved neurological outcomes ↓ Cerebral injury post DHCA Improved myocardial function	Risk of cerebral hypoperfusion
pH-stat	More uniform cerebral cooling ↑ H$^+$ reduces organ metabolism HbO$_2$ dissociation curve right shifted	Pressure-passive CBF ↑ Cerebral microembolization ↑ Free-radical-induced tissue damage

lost as temperature falls, the blood-gas management strategy has progressively less influence on the CBF. A randomized trial of α-stat versus pH-stat demonstrated the CBF in both groups to be dependent on arterial BP rather than CPB flow.

The reduction in organ metabolism (O_2 consumption) that is associated with an increased H$^+$ concentration during pH-stat is attributed to acidosis-induced intracellular enzyme dysfunction and impaired O_2 utilization.

Haematocrit

Blood viscosity is inversely related to temperature and is a positive exponential function of the haematocrit. Hypothermia increases the overall blood viscosity – plasma viscosity increases and red-cell membrane plasticity decreases. It was believed that the reduction in blood viscosity that is associated with haemodilution improved tissue perfusion during hypothermic CPB – counteracting the negative impact of anaemia. Consequently, profound anaemia (haematocrit < 20%) during CPB was commonplace until the end of the 1990s.

While the majority of patients undergoing hypothermic CPB tolerate dilutional anaemia, the use of normothermic perfusion techniques has forced a reconsideration of the minimum acceptable haematocrit during CPB. Early observational studies suggested that the severity of anaemia during CPB correlated with a failure to wean from CPB, IABP use and mortality. One prospective study (Mathew *et al.*) in which patients were randomized to a minimum haematocrit of either 27% or ~16%, was halted because of the excess adverse events in the lower haematocrit group. Other investigators have demonstrated a similar relationship between lowest haematocrit during CPB and early (in-hospital) mortality, late mortality, stroke, low CO syndrome, cardiac arrest, pulmonary dysfunction, renal dysfunction and sepsis. The cut-off value for the lowest acceptable haematocrit on CPB is often dictated by the use of hypothermia, and appears to be in the range of 21–25%.

Blood Transfusion during CPB

Inadequate tissue oxygen delivery during CPB – evidenced by metabolic acidosis and a low SvO_2 – in the presence of an SaO_2 that is greater than 95% and a low haematocrit should prompt consideration of RBC transfusion. In 2011, the STS and the SCA jointly released an updated clinical practice guideline, addressing the issue of perioperative blood transfusion and blood conservation in cardiac surgery. Within these guidelines, specific reference is made to the indications for transfusion during CPB (Table 26.4). It is now acknowledged that recognition and treatment of anaemia preoperatively, the

Table 26.4 STS and SCA practice guidelines for blood transfusion during CPB

Indication class	LOE	Indication
IIa	C	Trigger Hb = 6 g dl^{-1} unless patient is at risk for decreased cerebral O_2 delivery (previous CVA, DM, carotid stenosis, cerebrovascular disease)
IIa	C	Transfusion above Hb 6 g dl^{-1} needs to be guided by • Patient factors (age, severity of illness, cardiac function, risk of critical end-organ ischaemia) • Laboratory parameters such as haematocrit or SvO_2
IIb	C	It is not unreasonable to keep patients at risk for critical end-organ injury at Hb > 7 g dl^{-1}

LOE, level of evidence.

cessation of platelet-inhibiting drugs and the use of cell salvage intraoperatively all play a major role in reducing perioperative blood transfusion in cardiac surgery.

Mini CPB

Over the last 10 years there has been a drive to reduce CPB priming solutions, the inflammatory response generated by CPB and the use of blood products. This has led to the development of the mini CPB circuit. Advantages and disadvantages of the mini CPB circuit are shown in Table 26.5

The use of mini CPB is specifically mentioned in the 2011 STS/SCA guidance on blood conservation where it is a class 1A recommendation for blood conservation, particularly in patients at high risk for adverse effects from haemodilution (Jehovah's witnesses, paediatric patients). The majority of published data are in low-risk elective CABG surgery where the mini circuit has been shown to be associated with reduced RBC transfusion without an increase in major adverse outcomes. A recent retrospective review of over 45,000 cases has suggested, however, that there is a limit to 'how low can you go?' in terms of circuit size and prime volume. In addition, the use of the mini circuit has considerable logistic challenges relating to physical space, increased vigilance and a

Table 26.5 Advantages and disadvantages of the mini CPB circuit

Advantages	Disadvantages
Reduced priming volumes – 500 ml compared to 2,000 ml Higher Hb and haematocrit on CPB leading to reduced transfusion Absence of a venous reservoir – reduced blood–air interface and a reduced inflammatory response to CPB	Removal of venous reservoir – loss of safety margin, if venous drainage falls or becomes obstructed, mini-CPB stops Air-bubble trap easily overwhelmed – air can potentially reach arterial side of circuit Increased labour intensity for perfusionist, surgeon and anaesthetist

decrease in ease of positioning the heart. All of these factors may limit the increase in the use of mini CPB.

Ventilation and Oxygenation

Mechanical ventilation of the lungs during CPB does not contribute to patient oxygenation as long as the pulmonary circulation is effectively isolated, but it is proposed to improve lung function after separation from CPB. A recent meta-analysis concluded that ventilation during CPB was associated with improved oxygenation and an improved shunt fraction in the immediate postoperative period, but that it was not associated with a significant difference in postoperative pulmonary complications or hospital stay. CPBVENT, an ongoing randomized controlled trial, comparing different ventilation strategies during CPB, aims to determine whether or not the ventilation strategy improves pulmonary function and reduces postoperative complications (ClinicalTrials. gov. ID: NCT02090205).

The optimum targets for oxygenation during CPB are unknown. A high PaO_2 hastens the absorption of air emboli and may reduce the incidence of wound infection, but potentially worsens end-organ function secondary to oxidative stress and vasoconstriction. There is currently no clear evidence to support a particular target for oxygenation during CPB.

Conclusions

The number of unanswered questions in the conduct of CPB is a reflection of the increasing willingness of cardiac teams to challenge established practice. A recent global CPB survey highlighted the differences in worldwide CPB management practice. It is likely that CPB will continue to be an expanding area of research for the foreseeable future.

Key Points

- Higher perfusion pressures may reduce the risk of stroke in patients with DM, chronic hypertension or severe aortic atheroma.
- The α-stat management strategy is recommended for adults undergoing uninterrupted hypothermic CPB.
- The minimum acceptable haematocrit during CPB should be dictated by the adequacy of tissue oxygenation.

Further Reading

Alsatli RA. Mini cardiopulmonary bypass: anesthetic considerations. *Anesth Essays Res* 2012; 6: 10–13.

Chi D, Chen C, Shi Y, *et al.* Ventilation during cardiopulmonary bypass for prevention of respiratory insufficiency: a meta-analysis of randomized controlled trials. *Medicine (Baltimore)* 2017; 96: e6454.

Gold JP, Charlson ME, Williams-Russo P, *et al.* Improvement of outcomes after coronary artery bypass. A randomized trial comparing intraoperative high versus low mean arterial pressure. *J Thorac Cardiovasc Surg* 1995; 110: 1302–11.

Grigore AM, Mathew J, Grocott HP, *et al.* Prospective randomized trial of normothermic versus hypothermic cardiopulmonary bypass on cognitive function after coronary artery bypass graft surgery. *Anesthesiology* 2001; 95: 1110–19.

Hori D, Nomura Y, Ono M, *et al.* Optimal blood pressure during cardiopulmonary bypass defined by cerebral autoregulation monitoring. *J Thorac Cardiovasc Surg* 2017; 154: 1590–8.

Martin TD, Craver JM, Gott JP, *et al.* Prospective, randomized trial of retrograde warm blood cardioplegia: myocardial benefit and neurologic threat. *Ann Thorac Surg* 1994; 57: 298–302.

Mathew JP, Mackensen GB, Phillips-Bute B, *et al.* Effects of extreme hemodilution during cardiac surgery on cognitive function in the elderly. *Anesthesiology* 2007; 107: 577–84.

Miles LF, Coulson TG, Galhardo C, Falter F. Pump priming practices and anticoagulation in cardiac surgery: results from the global cardiopulmonary bypass survey. *Anesth Analg* 2017; 125: 1871–7.

Mora CT, Henson MB, Weintraub WS, *et al.* The effect of temperature management during cardiopulmonary bypass on neurologic and neuropsychologic outcomes in patients undergoing coronary revascularization. *J Thorac Cardiovasc Surg* 1996; 112: 514–22.

Murkin JM, Martzke JS, Buchan AM, Bentley C, Wong CJ. A randomized study of the influence of perfusion technique and pH management strategy in 316 patients undergoing coronary artery bypass surgery. II. Neurologic and cognitive outcomes. *J Thorac Cardiovasc Surg* 1995; 110: 349–62.

O'Dwyer C, Prough DS, Johnston WE. Determinants of cerebral perfusion during cardiopulmonary bypass. *J Cardiothorac Vasc Anesth* 1996; 10: 54–64.

Patel RL, Turtle MR, Chambers DJ, *et al.* Alpha-stat acid–base regulation during cardiopulmonary bypass improves neuropsychologic outcome in patients undergoing coronary artery bypass grafting. *J Thorac Cardiovasc Surg* 1996; 111: 1267–79.

Rees K, Beranek-Stanley M, Burke M, Ebrahim S. Hypothermia to reduce neurological damage following coronary artery bypass surgery. *Cochrane Database Syst Rev* 2001; 1: CD002138.

Rogers AT, Prough DS, Roy RC, *et al.* Cerebrovascular and cerebral metabolic effects of alterations in perfusion flow rate during hypothermic cardiopulmonary bypass in man. *J Thorac Cardiovasc Surg* 1992; 103: 363–8.

Society of Thoracic Surgeons Blood Conservation Guideline Task Force, Society of Cardiovascular Anesthesiologists, International Consortium for Evidence Based Perfusion. 2011 update to the Society of Thoracic Surgeons and the Society of Cardiovascular Anesthesiologists blood conservation clinical practice guidelines. *Ann Thorac Surg* 2011; 91: 944–82.

Sun BC, Dickinson TA, Tesdahl EA, *et al.* The unintended consequences of over-reducing cardiopulmonary bypass circuit prime volume. *Ann Thorac Surg* 2017; 103: 1842–8.

The Warm Heart Investigators: Randomised trial of normothermic versus hypothermic coronary bypass surgery. *Lancet* 1994; 343: 559–63.

van Wermeskerken GK, Lardenoye JW, Hill SE, *et al.* Intraoperative physiologic variables and outcome in cardiac surgery: part II. Neurologic outcome. *Ann Thorac Surg* 2000; 69: 1077–83.

Chapter

27

Cardiopulmonary Bypass Emergencies

David J. Daly

Failure of tissue oxygenation represents an emergency during CPB. The principal causes are gaseous embolism, inadequate oxygenation and inadequate CPB flow.

Massive Air Embolism

Massive air embolism (AE) is defined as the witnessed or likely entry of air into the circulation. The quoted incidence is 1:1,000 cases, which is probably an underestimate. In 25% of recorded cases, massive AE leads to permanent injury or death.

Air can enter the circulation from the surgical field, from the CPB circuit and via indwelling venous and arterial cannulae. A degree of venous AE probably occurs in all patients undergoing CPB and appears to have few obvious consequences.

Surgical Field Entrainment

This is by far the most common source of significant AE. Air enters the circulation when the heart is opened or when a loose suture allows air to be entrained via the venous cannula. The inadvertent delivery of air with cardioplegia solutions may lead to coronary embolism. An aortic root or pulmonary vein venting at high negative pressure can draw air into the ventricle via a coronary arteriotomy. Valveless centrifugal pumps may allow retrograde siphoning of arterial blood and air entrainment via the arterial cannula.

Cardiopulmonary Bypass Air

The maintenance of an adequate volume in the CPB venous reservoir is a fundamental principle of perfusion. Advances in CPB circuit design, monitoring and alarm systems have dramatically reduced the likelihood of this event. Nowadays, CPB equipment includes venous- and arterial-line bubble detectors, and a system that automatically shuts off the pump when the reservoir volume falls below a critical level.

The transition from bubble to membrane oxygenators has significantly reduced the amount of gas deliberately added to the circulation during oxygenation. Punctured or misconnected lines and the loss of membrane integrity may, however, lead to significant gas embolism.

Anaesthetic Sources

Unprimed monitoring and IV infusion lines, and the use of pressurized infusion devices, may result in the inadvertent delivery of significant quantities of air. The practice of re-connecting partially used infusion bags greatly increases the risk of AE and should be avoided.

Physical Principles

An understanding of the gas laws and the properties of air bubbles within the circulation are the keys to successful management (Box 27.1). Nitrogen and oxygen are the main constituents of air. As oxygen is readily absorbed, the challenge is the enhancement of nitrogen elimination. Hypothermia tends to reduce

Box 27.1	The gas laws
Charles' law	States that at a constant pressure the volume of a given mass of gas varies directly with the absolute temperature
Boyle's law	States that at constant temperature the volume of a given mass varies inversely with the absolute pressure
Henry's law	States that at a particular temperature the amount of a given gas dissolved in a given liquid is directly proportional to the partial pressure of the gas in equilibrium with the liquid

the bubble size (Charles' law) and increase blood nitrogen solubility (Henry's law). Barometric and hydrostatic pressures (Boyle's law) prevent dissolved nitrogen leaving solution, while the partial pressure dictates any tendency to bubble formation (Henry's law). Self-contained underwater breathing apparatus ('scuba') divers know that too rapid an ascent can lead to the formation of nitrogen bubbles, causing decompression illness (the bends).

The institution of hyperoxia ($PaO_2 \gg 13$ kPa) gradually leads to nitrogen displacement (denitrogenation). The arteriovenous oxygen difference (i.e. $PaO_2 - PvO_2$) reflects the gradient favouring nitrogen absorption. A nitrogen bubble, 4 mm in diameter (i.e. 0.025 ml), takes more than 10 hours to be absorbed while breathing air, but less than 1 hour while breathing 100% oxygen. As with anaesthetic gas elimination, the rate of denitrogenation is CO dependent.

Box 27.2 Basic principles of the management of massive AE during CPB

- Make the diagnosis
- Communicate the diagnosis
- Prevent further AE
- Identify the source of the AE
- Limit organ damage
- Clear the CPB circuit of air
- Expel air from the major arteries
- Re-establish circulation

Management

As massive AE is rare, it is essential that anaesthetists are aware of the possibility and the goals of management *before* they encounter the problem for the first time. For this reason, many centres have developed their own management protocols, with action plans for the anaesthetist, surgeon and perfusionist. Such plans should be developed after consideration of local practice (e.g. whether or not retrograde coronary sinus cardiac protection is practised). The clinical scenario also lends itself well to simulation (Box 27.2 and Table 27.1). The fundamental principles of good management are early diagnosis, good communication and rapid institution of measures of proven or likely benefit.

Most management plans include retrograde cerebral perfusion (RCP) on the grounds that cerebral AE will have occurred. After the CPB pump is stopped and the line clamped, the surgeon will usually clamp the aortic cannula, cut the arterial line close to the cannula and assist the perfusionist in refilling the line. This practice reduces the risk of aortic injury caused by decannulation and subsequent recannulation. The primed arterial line is then inserted into the RA or SVC, retrograde perfusion commenced at 1–$2 \; l \; min^{-1}$ and the 'stump' of the cut aortic cannula unclamped to allow air to be vented from the aorta. Ideally, the IVC should be compressed or occluded to encourage cephalad blood flow and to maximize the effectiveness of RCP. RCP is continued until no more bubbles are seen emerging in the aortic cannula. De-airing the

Table 27.1 The roles of surgeon, perfusionist and anaesthetist in the management of massive AE during CPB

Perfusionist	Surgeon	Anaesthetist
Stop CPB pump and clamp lines	Clamp aortic cannula Cut aortic cannula	Carotid compression Steep head-down position Ventilate with 100% O_2
Add cold fluid to reservoir	Prevent cardiac ejection	Cerebroprotectants?
Refill arterial line	Connect arterial line to RA	
RCP at 1–$2 \; l \; min^{-1}$	Initiate RCP at 20 °C Vent air from aortic cannula	
Stop RCP	Reconnect arterial line to aorta	
Restart CPB and cool	Complete surgery	Maintain MAP $\sim$ 80 mmHg
Slow partial rewarm		Consider hyperbaric O_2

> **Box 27.3** Putative neuroprotectants used after cerebral AE
>
> - Therapeutic hypothermia
> - Corticosteroids
> - Antioxidants
> - Free radical scavengers
> - General anaesthetic agents
> - Local anaesthetics

> **Box 27.4** Checklist for inadequate oxygenation during CPB
>
> | | |
> |---|---|
> | **Gas supply** | Gas delivery circuit not compromised |
> | | Gas source connected to gas inlet port of oxygenator |
> | | Gas flow > 0.5 l min^{-1} (visual and by back-pressure in line) |
> | | No leak from vaporizer manifold |
> | | Ensure adequate F_iO_2 via in-line oxygen analyzer |
> | | Gas scavenging system (if used) not obstructed |
> | **Blood flow** | Ensure adequate blood flow through oxygenator |
> | | Ensure adequate anticoagulation |
> | **Patient factors** | Ensure depth of anaesthesia is adequate (vaporizer leak) |
> | | Check for hyperthermia ($\uparrow$CMRO$_2$) |
> | | Cold agglutinins |
> | | Anaphylaxis |
> | **Surgical factors** | Severe AR |
> | | Over-venting the heart without adequate forward flow |
> | | Unsecured cava snares without lung ventilation (creates an effective right-to-left shunt) |

ascending aorta and aortic arch may be monitored with TOE.

Gross AE occurring during atrio-femoral CPB can be managed in a similar manner, although de-airing the aorta will require insertion of a vent into the ascending aorta or aortic arch – typically, a cardioplegia administration cannula.

If a coronary sinus catheter is being used, it can be removed from the RA and inserted into the SVC, and directed cranially to facilitate RCP. The aorta can be vented from the aortic cardioplegia cannula. The CPB circuit can be reprimed during RCP.

The theoretical benefits of intermittent carotid compression (to reduce antegrade cerebral air delivery and encourage air-flushing from the vertebral arteries during RCP) have to be balanced against the small risk of plaque fissuring and embolization.

The role of pharmacological neuroprotectants remains controversial. Although a number of agents are used in this setting, none have demonstrated unequivocal efficacy and none are licensed for this specific indication (Box 27.3).

Inadequate Oxygenation

Inadequate oxygenation of blood during CPB can occur as a result of failure of the gas delivery system or the oxygenator. The presenting features are darkening of arterial blood and a reduced SvO_2, which may be associated with a rising transmembrane pressure gradient. ABG analysis is used to confirm the clinical diagnosis. As a temporization measure the pump flow rate can be increased and some of the arterial flow can be diverted (i.e. shunted) back to the venous reservoir, thus increasing the SvO_2. The sequence of checks given in Box 27.4 is suggested.

The use of point-of-care anticoagulation monitors means that oxygenator failure due to coagulation is exceedingly rare. In addition to a falling PaO_2 and a rising $PaCO_2$, the presence of 'frothy' pink fluid in the gas exit port (the result of protein and water entering the gas phase of membrane) may signal impending oxygenator failure. Changing an oxygenator during CPB requires at least two perfusionists and a period of circulatory arrest; it should therefore be considered an intervention of last resort. A discussion of this unusual procedure is shown below.

Oxygenator Changeout during CPB

Changing the core components of the CPB system during the course of CPB is a major undertaking (Table 27.2). Ideally, this should be performed as a planned 'urgent' procedure under hypothermia. The perfusionist must alert both the surgeon and the anaesthetist of impending CPB system failure.

Inadequate Flow

Inadequate flow can result from electrical or mechanical pump failure, a venous 'air lock', cannula obstruction (e.g. kinking, malposition and clamping), covert

Table 27.2 Abbreviated example of an oxygenator changeout protocol

Perfusionist 1	Perfusionist 2
Shouts 'coming off bypass' Stops pump and clamps venous and arterial lines Starts timer	
Cuts venous line from reservoir Removes pump boot and level sensor	Divides arterial line with sterile shears between two clamps Disconnects heat exchanger water pipes Removes old oxygenator Installs new oxygenator
Connects venous line	Connects arterial line and de-airs tubing Reservoir level sensor reattached
Installs pump boot in roller pump Recirculates reservoir contents through arterial line filter Shouts 'back on bypass' Starts pump Stops timer	Connects heat-exchanger water pipes to oxygenator Reconnects cardiotomy suckers to cardiotomy reservoir Complete and file critical incident report

Box 27.5 Causes of inadequate CPB flow

Electrical pump failure	Impact minimized by: Uninterruptible Power Supply Backup generators and Emergency backup batteries incorporated in pump
Mechanical pump failure	Roller head under occlusion
Venous return	Air locks, lifting heart
Cannula problem	Total obstruction: Retained clamp Partial obstruction: Small size, kinking
Aortic dissection	↑ Line pressure and ↓ patient arterial pressure

circulating volume loss and aortic dissection (Box 27.5).

By its very nature, electrical power failure during CPB is a rare and unpredictable event. An uninterruptible power supply combined with an on-site backup generator should make total electrical failure in the operating room an extremely rare occurrence. Modern CPB pumps have emergency battery backup, which can be used to drive the pump and critical monitors. Although roller pump heads can be manually cranked during total power loss, this procedure is tiring and requires two individuals if undertaken for more than 5 minutes. Total power loss causes heater unit failure, which makes rewarming virtually impossible.

As air entrainment interferes with a siphon, venous return to the reservoir may be halted by the presence of a sufficiently large volume of air – an 'air lock'. If elevation of the tubing in sections fails to rectify the problem, the venous cannula is clamped, and the venous line disconnected and back-filled.

The cannula size determines the flow rate within the venous line. An inappropriately small cannula or kinks in the line will lead to decreased venous return, necessitating a reduction in the pump flow. Obstruction to the flow in the arterial line or oxygenator is confirmed by finding a high CPB flow line pressure and a low patient arterial pressure.

Aortic dissection is generally noticed when CPB is first commenced. The CPB arterial line pressure is elevated while the patient arterial pressure is low. The aorta may be flaccid on palpation with an obvious expanding mural haematoma. Unrecognized aortic dissection is associated with significant morbidity and mortality. The extent and impact of aortic dissection can be minimized by prompt diagnosis, discontinuation of CPB and repositioning of the aortic cannula. Despite this approach, many surgeons will opt for formal ascending aortic repair (e.g. an interposition graft).

Key Points

- Emergencies during CPB are uncommon but potentially catastrophic.
- All staff should be familiar with the management of massive AE during CPB.
- RCP is used in the management of AE during CPB on the grounds that cerebral AE will have occurred.
- Therapeutic postoperative hypothermia (24–48 hours) and hyperbaric oxygen therapy should be considered after significant AE during CPB.

Further Reading

Jones NC, Howell CW. Massive arterial air embolism during cardiopulmonary bypass: antegrade blood cardioplegia delivered by the pump – an accident waiting to happen. *Perfusion* 1996; 11: 157–61.

Mills NL, Ochsner JL. Massive air embolism during cardiopulmonary bypass. Causes, prevention, and management. *J Thorac Cardiovasc Surg* 1980; 80: 708–17.

Tovar EA, Del Campo C, Borsari A, *et al.* Postoperative management of cerebral air embolism: gas physiology for surgeons. *Ann Thorac Surg* 1995; 60: 1138–42.

von Segesser LK. Unusual problems in cardiopulmonary bypass. In Gravlee GP, Davis RF, Stammers AH, Ungerleider RM (eds), *Cardiopulmonary Bypass: Principles and Practice*. 3rd edn. London: Lippincott Williams & Wilkins; 2008, pp. 608–13.

Chapter

28

Non-Cardiac Applications of Cardiopulmonary Bypass

Joseph E. Arrowsmith and Jonathan H. Mackay

Since its introduction into clinical practice in the early 1950s, the indications for CPB have broadened, from operations on or within the heart, to include non-cardiac thoracic, abdominal and neurological procedures. The indications for CPB for non-cardiac surgery are shown in Box 28.1.

Anaesthetic Considerations

Similar principles apply to the application of CPB in both cardiac and non-cardiac surgery. In practice, however, there are a number of important factors that must be considered. With the exception of thoracic aortic surgery, non-cardiac CPB procedures are performed rarely and frequently involve staff who have little or no regular experience of CPB. Moreover, non-cardiac surgeons do not routinely operate on fully anticoagulated patients. Published case series and

---

Box 28.1 Non-cardiac surgical applications of CPB

Thoracic	Surgery of the great vessels Pulmonary embolectomy/ endarterectomy Tracheobronchial reconstruction Resection of mediastinal tumours Lung transplantation
Abdominal	Resection of renal tumours with IVC extension Liver transplantation
Neurological	Arteriovenous malformations Basilar artery aneurysm
Resuscitation	Accidental hypothermia Trauma care CPR Respiratory failure (ECMO) Patient transfer

---

experience gained in previous cases should form the basis of detailed protocols for future reference.

The use of femoro-femoral CPB, which avoids the need for sternotomy or thoracotomy, is often employed in procedures that do not routinely involve chest opening. In this situation, there is retrograde perfusion of the aorta. Although the size of the femoral arterial cannula has a minimal impact on CPB flow rates, a small femoral venous cannula may significantly reduce venous return. For this reason, the maximal achievable flow rate may be insufficient at normothermia. To circumvent this problem, partial or incomplete CPB is initiated and lung ventilation continued until the degree of hypothermia is compatible with CPB at reduced flow rates. It is essential that hypothermia-induced VF does not occur before reaching this level of hypothermia.

The risk of CPB-related adverse events is the same, regardless of the clinical application. The basic principles of adequate anticoagulation, avoidance of air embolism and maintenance of vital organ perfusion are no less important. Femoral cannulation may result in lower limb ischaemia or neurological injury (Chapter 29). In difficult cases, it should be borne in mind that femoro-femoral CPB can be established under local anaesthesia prior to the induction of general anaesthesia.

Thoracic Surgery

CPB for surgery on the ascending aorta and aortic arch is discussed in Chapter 13. Pulmonary embolectomy and (thrombo)endarterectomy, performed for acute and chronic pulmonary thromboembolic disease, respectively, typically requires CPB with or without deep hypothermic circulatory arrest (DHCA).

In the past, resection of tracheal and carinal tumours was routinely performed with CPB. Advances in endoluminal intervention (e.g. stents, cryotherapy, lasers, etc.) have limited the indications for CPB to:

- Patients at high risk of airway obstruction following induction of anaesthesia
- Repair of tracheal dehiscence following heart–lung transplantation
- Resuscitation of patients suffering massive haemorrhage after pulmonary resection

Mediastinal Surgery

Patients with large anterior mediastinal tumours (e.g. teratoma, lymphoma or seminoma) may develop airway collapse and great vessel compression following induction of anaesthesia. In addition, initiation of intermittent positive-pressure ventilation (IPPV) may cause distal air trapping. Although an inhalational induction and maintenance of spontaneous respiration is theoretically attractive, induction, even with sevoflurane, may be slow and hazardous. The left lateral position may be preferable as placing the patient in the supine position may lead to cardiac arrest from PA or SVC obstruction. Neither inhalational induction nor awake-intubation completely avoid the risk of airway obstruction distal to the endotracheal tube. If there is any doubt, the groins should be prepared for femoral cannulation prior to induction of anaesthesia.

Transplantation Surgery

Although the majority of single- and double-lung transplants can be accomplished using standard thoracic anaesthetic techniques without CPB, a perfusionist should always be immediately available. Induction of anaesthesia and initiation of IPPV in patients with end-stage emphysema commonly results in severe hypotension. Air trapping and breath 'stacking' have been likened to a tourniquet being applied to the right heart. If in doubt, the patient should be deliberately disconnected from the ventilator to let the trapped gas out. The patient with emphysematous lungs will *expire* if given insufficient time to *exhale*!

Intolerance of one-lung anaesthesia, due to haemodynamic instability, severe hypercarbia or hypoxia, is the principal indication for CPB. Severe gas trapping in the dependent lung or, more rarely, a dependent pneumothorax may produce rapid decompensation. The choice of cannulation site is largely dictated by the surgical approach (i.e. lateral thoracotomy, sternotomy or 'clam shell') and expediency.

CPB is occasionally used during liver transplantation to decompress the portal circulation or to support a haemodynamically unstable patient.

Urological Surgery

The principal indication for CPB in this setting is resection of renal tumours (e.g. renal cell carcinoma or hypernephroma, nephroblastoma) with IVC extension. The aim of surgery is radical, curative resection with the operative approach being largely determined by the superior limit of caval extension. In advanced cases, the tumour may prolapse through the TV and produce haemodynamic compromise. In this situation, sternotomy is required to establish CPB (i.e. the SVC to the ascending aorta) as IVC obstruction precludes femoro-femoral CPB. A short period of DHCA may be required for removal of the tumour from the RA.

The anaesthetist should be aware of the potential for massive haemorrhage, tumour fragmentation/embolism and paraneoplastic phenomena (e.g. hyperglycaemia, hypertension, hypercalcaemia and hypokalaemia). Short central venous cannulae and TOE should be used, and PAFCs avoided.

Neurosurgery

First used in the late 1950s, DHCA was widely used for intracranial aneurysm surgery until the late 1960s. Extrathoracic cannulation techniques largely overcame the need for simultaneous thoracotomy and craniotomy. Subsequent advances in neurosurgery led to the abandonment of DHCA for all but the most technically demanding cases, for example posterior fossa haemangioblastomas and giant basilar aneurysms.

Resuscitation

In the setting of cardiac surgery, surgical re-exploration and re-institution of CPB is a common means of dealing with cardiovascular collapse in the early postoperative period. CPB may also be of use in major trauma, particularly in the presence of airway disruption. The benefits of heparinization and CPB have to be carefully weighed against the risk of exsanguination or intracranial haemorrhage. Less commonly, CPB has been successfully used to treat accidental hypothermia and drug overdose (e.g. flecainide, bupivacaine). In practice, the logistical difficulties of moving a patient to a centre that offers CPB, the high mortality and low chance of full neurological recovery limit its application.

The use of CPB in the resuscitation of patients without a spontaneous circulation should be reserved for those who have suffered a *witnessed* cardiac arrest, for example during percutaneous interventions in the cardiac catheter laboratory. Use of CPB following *unwitnessed* cardiac arrest is associated with unacceptably high mortality and cerebral morbidity.

The development of compact membrane oxygenators and disposable centrifugal blood pumps provides a means by which patients with acute cardiorespiratory failure can be sufficiently stabilized for transfer to a centre offering ECMO support.

In practice, however, veno-venous (rather than veno-arterial) ECMO is used for respiratory patients with preserved cardiac function.

Key Points

- Induction of anaesthesia and initiation of IPPV is hazardous in patients with large anterior mediastinal tumours.
- Maximal achievable flow rates during femoro-femoral bypass may be insufficient at normothermia.
- The use of CPB in the resuscitation of patients without a spontaneous circulation should be reserved for those who have suffered a *witnessed* cardiac arrest.

Further Reading

Chen Z, Liu C, Huang J, *et al.* Clinical efficacy of extracorporeal cardiopulmonary resuscitation for adults with cardiac arrest: meta-analysis with trial sequential analysis. *Biomed Res Int* 2019; 2019: 6414673.

Conacher ID. Dynamic hyperinflation – the anaesthetist applying a tourniquet to the right heart. *Br J Anaesth* 1998; 81: 116–17.

Ong LP, Nair SK. Non-cardiac surgery functions of cardiopulmonary bypass: In Ghosh S, Falter F, Perrino AC (eds), *Cardiopulmonary Bypass,* 2nd edn. Cambridge: Cambridge University Press; 2015, pp. 239–53.

Chapter

29

Extracorporeal Membrane Oxygenation

Simon Colah

ECMO can either provide total cardiopulmonary support (veno-arterial or VA-ECMO) or pulmonary support (veno-venous or VV-ECMO). The technique effectively enables the use of CPB in an ICU setting. In adult practice, ECMO was initially reserved for patients with severe respiratory failure secondary to ARDS. ECMO in adults fell out of favour, largely because of poor outcomes. In paediatric practice, where outcomes are generally better, ECMO has remained in routine use for over three decades. Recent H1N1 ('swine flu') epidemics have led to a re-examination of the role of ECMO in adults with respiratory failure and a re-emergence of VV-ECMO.

The eighth Interagency Registry for Mechanical Circulatory Support (INTERMACS) annual report revealed that more than 20,000 patients from over 180 centres were included in their database. Disposable, durable extracorporeal versions of mechanical support technology are particularly suited to short- and medium-term ECMO. These devices are associated with significantly improved survival, fewer malfunctions, reduced bleeding during implantation and a reduced infection rate. These factors may explain the trend from VAD to ECMO therapy in patients requiring short-term, post-cardiotomy cardiopulmonary support.

Indications

The broad indications for instituting ECMO are shown in Box 29.1. A number of scoring systems have been developed to assist prediction of outcome following VA-ECMO, for example the Survival After Veno-arterial ECMO (SAVE) score developed jointly by the Extracorporeal Life Support Organization (ELSO) and the Alfred Hospital, Melbourne (save-score.com).

Contraindications

The decision to initiate ECMO is often difficult (Box 29.2). Not infrequently, the decision is clouded by emotion – the frustrated surgeon faced with

---

Box 29.1   Indications for ECMO

- Acute MI
- Dilated cardiomyopathy
- Fulminant myocarditis
- Post-cardiotomy low CO state
- Persistent PHT (post pulmonary thromboendarterectomy)
- Intractable ventricular arrhythmias
- Perioperative cardiac arrest
- Primary graft failure after heart transplantation
- Fulminant respiratory failure

Box 29.2   Contraindications for ECMO

- Severe AR
- Aortic dissection
- Contraindications to anticoagulation – e.g. intracerebral haemorrhage
- Established multi-organ failure
- Mechanical ventilation > 10 days

---

intractable cardiac failure in an elderly patient at the end of long and complex surgery, or the intensivist managing a young mother with fulminant post-viral respiratory failure.

Equipment

A typical ECMO system comprises three principal components – a pump, an oxygenator and a heat exchanger – connected by polyvinyl chloride or silicone tubing to inflow and outflow cannulae (Figure 29.1). Unlike conventional CPB systems, ECMO systems are closed, have no venous reservoir or arterial line filter and can be operated at lower levels of anticoagulation.

Oxygenator

Three types of so-called 'membrane lungs' are used to oxygenate blood and remove CO_2. The original

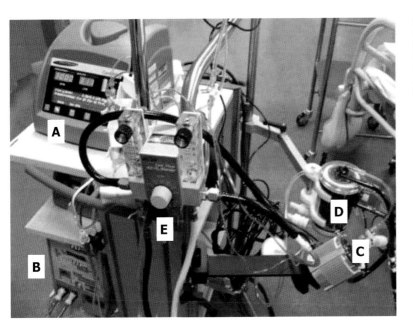

Figure 29.1 An example of an ECMO system employing a Levitronix Centrimag blood pump. (A) Pump control console. (B) Hot water supply for heat exchanger. (C) Disposable pump head mounted on pump motor. (D) Oxygenator with inbuilt heat exchanger. (E) Sweep gas blender.

silicone spiral coil oxygenators have been largely superseded by polymethylpentene oxygenators.

Cannulation

Cannulation for VA-ECMO may be either central or peripheral.

Central ECMO

Failure to wean from CPB is an indication for central VA-ECMO; with the (RA-to-aorta) CPB cannulae being used for up to 72 hours. If longer-term support is required, the patient will typically require VAD or peripheral ECMO support. Larger cannulae allow increased flow rates and maximum haemodynamic support. The main problems are bleeding and infection.

Peripheral ECMO

Peripheral VA-ECMO usually involves cannulation of a femoral or internal jugular vein and a femoral artery. Peripheral (femoro-jugular) cannulation is usually used for VV-ECMO. The availability of specialized cannulae (e.g. the Avalon Elite™ bicaval dual-lumen catheter) in a range of sizes (e.g. 16–31 Fr) has made peripheral cannulation a relatively straightforward bedside procedure. The distal (inlet) end is placed in the IVC, the proximal (inlet) is placed in the SVC and the outlet in the lower RA – typically

under TOE and fluoroscopic guidance. Femoral arterial cannulation carries two significant risks.

1. The risk of *distal limb ischaemia* may be reduced by inserting a small antegrade perfusion line distal to the perfusion cannula.
2. Differential cyanosis ('Harlequin syndrome') occurs when deoxygenated blood that is ejected from the LV encounters oxygenated blood flowing from the femoral cannula. This may result in significantly reduced PaO_2 in blood entering the head and right arm. The problem may only be resolved by proximal reinsertion of the arterial inflow cannula.

Management

The overall goals of management are $SaO_2 > 90\%$, $SvO_2 > 70\%$, and adequate tissue perfusion (normal lactate concentration). Low-dose inotropic support is often used to prevent ventricular distention and stasis-induced ventricular thrombosis. Frequent TOE examination is required to exclude these complications. LV decompression may be achieved by increasing the inotropic support, insertion of an apical LV vent or the addition of ventricular assist device support. Use of an IABP may reduce pulmonary oedema.

Anticoagulation

Unless contraindicated, an infusion of unfractionated heparin is used for anticoagulation. The ACT is

219

maintained at 180–240 s. Thrombocytopenia and haemolysis are inevitable consequences of extracorporeal support. Erythrocytes and platelet transfusion are required to maintain a haematocrit of 40–45% and a platelet count of $>80 \times 10^9 \, l^{-1}$.

Prevention of Air Entrainment

The very real and ever-present risk of air entrainment during ECMO support dictates the need for both emergency protocols and ongoing staff training. It should be borne in mind that indwelling venous catheters and haemofilters connected to the ECMO system are potential sources of air entrainment. The management of air entrainment is presented in Box 29.3.

Mechanical Ventilation

Low low tidal volume (<5 ml kg^{-1}), low RR (10 min^{-1}) and low FiO$_2$ (<0.6) ventilation with PEEP (5–10 cmH$_2$O) are usually continued during ECMO support. This reduces the risk of barotrauma, volutrauma and pulmonary atelectasis.

Weaning

The timing of weaning from ECMO is largely dictated by the patient's clinical state. Weaning VA-ECMO support removes both respiratory and cardiac support. The patient should be haemodynamically stable with a MAP greater than 60 mmHg on minimal inotropic support and have adequate tissue perfusion (i.e. normal lactate, SvO$_2$ > 60%). After a bolus of heparin (5,000 IU), the pump flow rate is reduced in steps while TOE is used to assess the cardiac function. Decannulation may be considered if the patient remains stable for a period of 60 minutes.

The effects of weaning from VV-ECMO can be replicated by simply reducing the 'sweep' gas flow to the ECMO oxygenator. In adults, stable haemodynamics and acceptable oxygenation on sweep gas (FiO$_2$ = 0.3) are a prerequisite for considering weaning. Minimal acceptable ABGs without VV-ECMO on an FiO$_2$ of 0.6 and at an RR of 15 bpm are: PaO$_2$ > 8 kPa (60 mmHg) and PaCO$_2$ < 6.5 kPa (50 mmHg).

Outcomes

Survival to hospital discharge or transfer to an intermediate care facility after VA-ECMO is reported to be as high as 50% in some series. The significantly lower survival rates seen in some centres probably reflects poor patient selection rather than poor intensive care.

Chronic renal failure, a longer duration of mechanical ventilation prior to ECMO initiation, pre-ECMO organ failure, pre-ECMO cardiac arrest, congenital heart disease, low pulse pressure and low serum bicarbonate are factors associated with mortality. Factors associated with improved outcome include: younger age, lower body weight, acute myocarditis, cardiac transplantation, refractory ventricular dysrhythmia, higher diastolic BP and lower peak inspiratory pressure.

For patients on established VA-ECMO, the 6-hour PREDICT VA-ECMO score (based on lactate, pH and standard bicarbonate concentration) is highly predictive of outcome.

Key Points

- Femoro-femoral CPB can be established under LA *before* the induction of anaesthesia.
- The use of ECMO to manage low CO state post-cardiac surgery is increasing.
- More detailed evaluation of quality of life in survivors of ECMO is required to refine current indications and patient selection.

Further Reading

Charlesworth M, Venkateswaran R, Barker JM, Feddy L. Postcardiotomy VA-ECMO for refractory cardiogenic shock. *J Cardiothorac Surg* 2017; 12: 116.

Grecu L. Extracorporeal membrane oxygenation. In Ghosh S, Falter F, Perrino AC (eds), *Cardiopulmonary Bypass*, 2nd edn. Cambridge: Cambridge University Press; 2015, pp. 121–8.

Khorsandi M, Dougherty S, Bouamra O, *et al.* Extra-corporeal membrane oxygenation for refractory cardiogenic shock after adult cardiac surgery: a systematic review and meta-analysis. *J Cardiothorac Surg* 2017; 12: 55.

Kirklin JK, Pagani FD, Kormos RL, *et al.* Eighth annual INTERMACS report: special focus on framing the impact of adverse events. *J Heart Lung Transplant* 2017; 36: 1080–6.

Schmidt M, Burrell A, Roberts L, *et al.* Predicting survival after ECMO for refractory cardiogenic shock: the survival after veno-arterial-ECMO (SAVE)-score. *Eur Heart J* 2015; 36: 2246–56.

Wengenmayer T, Duerschmied D, Graf E, *et al.* Development and validation of a prognostic model for survival in patients treated with venoarterial extracorporeal membrane oxygenation: the PREDICT VA-ECMO score. *Eur Heart J Acute Cardiovasc Care* 2018 Jul 1:2048872618789052. doi: 10.1177/ 2048872618789052.

Cardiovascular Monitoring

Arturo Suarez and Jonathan B. Mark

Arterial Blood Pressure Monitoring

When the rapid detection of haemodynamic change is imperative, the 'gold standard' is direct arterial pressure monitoring. Other indications for invasive arterial pressure monitoring include severe underlying cardiovascular disease, the inability to obtain indirect measurements and the need for frequent blood sampling. While the radial artery is the most frequently used site, other commonly used arterial cannulation sites include the femoral, brachial, axillary and dorsalis pedis arteries. Complications of arterial cannulation include haemorrhage, thrombosis, vasospasm, distal ischaemia, dissection, infection, unintentional arterial drug administration, pseudoaneurysm and arteriovenous fistula formation.

The MAP is nearly constant throughout the arterial tree and provides the most accurate single measure of the pressure driving the blood flow to the organs. In contrast, the values for the systolic and diastolic BP vary throughout the arterial tree (Figure 30.1). As the monitoring site moves more distally, the arterial pressure waveform changes – the sharper systolic upstroke, the higher systolic peak, the delayed and less distinct dicrotic notch, more prominent diastolic wave and lower end-diastolic pressure (Figure 30.2).

As a result, peripherally recorded arterial pressure waveforms have a wider pulse pressure than central aortic pressure. However, in contrast to the normal distal pulse pressure amplification seen in peripheral arterial pressure traces, pressure waveforms recorded during hypothermic CPB often underestimate both the systolic and the mean central aortic pressure.

For accurate pressure measurements, the monitoring transducer should be referenced to the level of the heart, which is typically chosen to be the mid-axillary level. Patient or bed movement without adjustment of the transducer height yields inaccurate pressure values.

An *underdamped* system (Figure 30.3A) can lead to falsely high systolic, falsely low diastolic or an exaggerated pulse pressure. Conversely, an *overdamped* system (Figure 30.3B) will cause a slurred arterial systolic upstroke and narrowed pulse pressure, which result in an underestimation of the systolic pressure and an overestimation of the diastolic pressure. The most common causes are blood clots, air bubbles, compliant or kinked tubing, loose connections or low flush bag pressure.

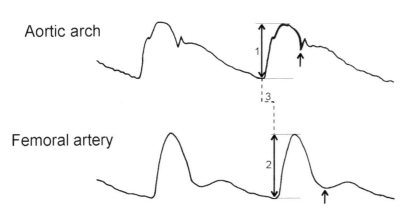

Aortic arch

Femoral artery

Figure 30.1 The effect of monitoring site on arterial pressure waveform – aortic arch versus femoral artery. Although the mean pressure remains unchanged, the systolic and pulse pressure are both amplified as the monitoring site moves peripherally in the arterial tree. (Reproduced with permission from Mark JB. *Atlas of Cardiovascular Monitoring.* New York, NY: Churchill Livingstone, 1998; Figure 8.4.)

223

Central Venous Pressure Monitoring

The CVP, an estimate of the RA pressure, is dependent upon intravascular volume, RV function and venous tone. Common sites for central venous cannulation include the internal jugular veins (IJVs), the subclavian veins (SCVs) and the femoral veins. Complications include bleeding, haematoma, arterial

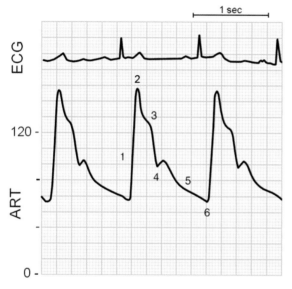

Figure 30.2 Normal arterial BP waveform components include (1) systolic upstroke, (2) systolic peak pressure, (3) systolic decline, (4) dicrotic notch, (5) diastolic runoff and (6) end-diastolic pressure. (Reproduced with permission from Mark JB. *Atlas of Cardiovascular Monitoring.* New York, NY: Churchill Livingstone, 1998; Figure 8.1.)

puncture, nerve injury, arrhythmias, infection, pneumothorax, thrombosis, airway compromise, air embolism and cardiac tamponade.

Arrhythmias encountered while advancing the guidewire can be avoided by limiting its insertion depth to a point above the superior cavo-atrial junction (CAJ). The right IJV–CAJ distance is the shortest (16 cm) and the left SCV–CAJ is the longest (21 cm). Right SCV–CAJ and left IJV–CAJ distances are intermediate (18 and 19 cm, respectively). The use of the SCV is associated with the lowest infection rate and is preferred for long-term use. However, the SCV is not easily compressible and its use is relatively contraindicated in coagulopathic patients. Although the femoral veins are more compressible and associated with fewer mechanical complications, this site is associated with a greater infection risk. Multiple clinical studies have shown that the use of ultrasound decreases both the rate of failed cannulation and the incidence of complications.

Although the CVP is often used as a surrogate for intravascular volume, its measurement is influenced by patient positioning, positive-pressure ventilation, TV integrity, RV dysfunction, and pulmonary and pericardial disease. Consequently, trends in the CVP provide a better guide to fluid management compared with isolated absolute values.

Analysis of the RA pressure or CVP waveform reveals three systolic components (c-wave, x-descent, v-wave) and two diastolic components (y-descent, a-wave). The a-wave represents atrial contraction and the c-wave, closure of the TV at the beginning of systole. During the ensuing x-descent, rapid atrial filling begins

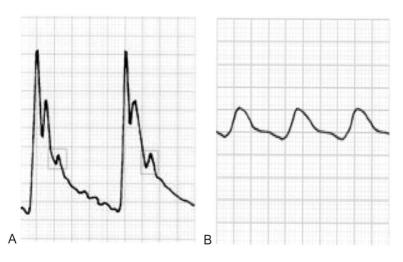

Figure 30.3 (A) Underdamped arterial BP waveform. Note that the dicrotic notch follows the second systolic peak. (B) Overdamped arterial BP waveform. (Reproduced with permission from Mark JB. *Atlas of Cardiovascular Monitoring.* New York, NY: Churchill Livingstone, 1998; Figures 9.3 & 9.4.)

A   B

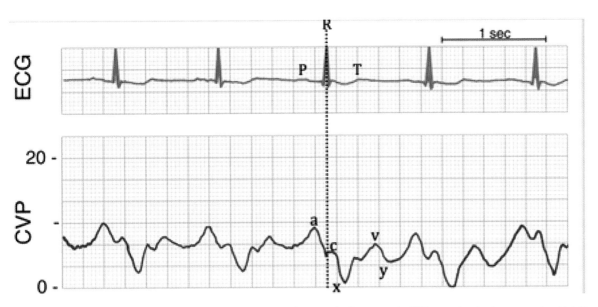

Figure 30.4 Normal CVP tracing. Note the timing of the waves in relation to the R-wave on the ECG. (Reproduced with permission from Mark JB. *Atlas of Cardiovascular Monitoring.* New York, NY: Churchill Livingstone, 1998; Figure 2.4.)

as the ventricle contracts and ejects, resulting in the v-wave at the end of systole. As the TV opens during diastole, the CVP falls as blood rapidly flows into the RV during the y-descent. The blood flow from the vena cavae into the RA is maximal during the x- and y-pressure descents (Figure 30.4).

Several diagnostic clues to cardiac rhythm abnormalities can be gleaned from careful observation of the CVP waveform. In AF, the absence of synchronized atrial contraction eliminates the a-wave. Atrial flutter may produce saw-tooth waves on the pressure tracing, known as f-waves. Junctional rhythm, complete heart block and VT are all forms of atrioventricular dissociation in which cannon a-waves may be evident. These result from atrial contraction against a closed TV during ventricular systole.

The normal CVP (RA pressure) ranges between 0 mmHg and 8 mmHg, and it is typically lower than the PAWP. However, in cardiac tamponade, the CVP and PAWP are both markedly increased and of similar value, with diastolic right and left heart pressure equalization being a characteristic haemodynamic finding.

Pulmonary Artery Catheterization

The PAFC has been used to manage cardiac and critically ill patients since the 1970s. To date, however, no randomized trial or meta-analysis has been able to definitively demonstrate an improved patient outcome attributable to PAFC monitoring. Some studies even suggest that PAFC use increases complications, length of stay and hospital costs. The PAFC allows direct measurement of the RA, PA and PA wedge pressures. Additionally, the SvO_2 and the RV CO can be measured (Figure 30.5).

Complications of PAFC use include those associated with central venous cannulation (see above) as well as serious complications such as catheter knotting, pulmonary infarction and PA rupture. Although rare (reported incidence 0.1–1%), PA rupture carries a mortality approaching 50%. To reduce the risk of this complication, the PAFC should never be left in the wedged position, nor should the balloon remain inflated for prolonged periods of time, as this may cause pulmonary ischaemia and infarction. Any attempt to inflate the balloon while the catheter is 'wedged' can result in PA rupture. In addition, the PAFC should be withdrawn a few centimetres following PAWP measurement, because the catheter may subsequently migrate distally. Likewise, the balloon must always be deflated when withdrawing the catheter, to minimize the risk of damaging the PV and TV.

PAFC placement is achieved by 'floatation' through the right heart chambers, facilitated by a small (1.5 ml) balloon, located at the catheter tip. The right IJV is the preferred site for PAFC insertion

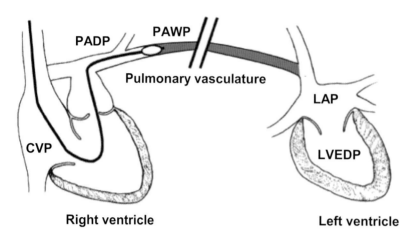

Figure 30.5 Estimating cardiac filling with the PAFC. The schematic shows the PAFC wedging in a proximal PA to measure indirectly the downstream left heart filling pressures. The PA diastolic pressure provides an estimate of the left atrial pressure (LAP) and the LVEDP. LV compliance, HR, MV disease, PVR and alveolar pressure are key factors that influence the relationship between upstream pressures (such as the CVP and PA diastolic pressure) and their relationship to downstream pressures (LAP and LVEDP). The PAWP overestimates the LVEDP when the alveolar pressure exceeds the pulmonary intravascular pressure, and also in MS, PHT and in the presence of tachycardia. (Modified and reproduced with permission from Mark JB. *Atlas of Cardiovascular Monitoring*. New York, NY: Churchill Livingstone, 1998; Figure 4.1.)

because it offers a direct route to the RV. From this site, the RA pressure tracing is typically acquired at a depth of 20–25 cm, the RV pressure at a depth of 25–35 cm, and the PA pressure at a depth of 35–45 cm. The PAWP is usually acquired at a depth of 50–60 cm. Manoeuvres that aid PAFC placement include head-down tilt (during passage from the RA to the RV) and head-up and right lateral tilt (during passage from the RV to the PA).

Observation of the pressure waveforms is essential to ensure correct PAFC placement (Figure 30.6). After wedging the PAFC in a distal PA, a *static* column of blood connects the catheter tip and the LV during diastole. This is the physiological basis for using the PAWP as an estimate of the LVEDP. The PAWP is also an indirect measure of the LA pressure. It should be borne in mind that the LA pressure waveform will be delayed and damped by transmission through the pulmonary vasculature. The PAWP waveform closely resembles that of the RA, although it is delayed in relation to the ECG tracing.

The PAFC has a thermistor at its tip to measure the PA blood temperature and facilitate CO measurement using the thermodilution technique. Knowledge of the CO, CVP and MAP allows calculation of the SVR:

$$SVR = \frac{MAP - CVP}{CO}$$

Multiplying by 80 converts traditional Wood units to dyne s cm^{-5}.

Venous Oximetry

The process of oxygen transport includes loading oxygen into RBC, binding to Hb, delivering it to the peripheral tissues by the heart (via CO), utilization of the oxygen in the periphery and return of deoxygenated blood to the right side of the heart.

The following are important physiological concepts:

1. Arterial oxygen content (CaO_2) is the amount of oxygen (ml) in 100 ml of arterial blood:
   $CaO_2 = (Hb \times 1.36$ ml O_2 g$^{-1} \times SaO_2) + (0.0031 \times PaO_2)$.
2. Mixed venous oxygen content (CvO_2) is the amount of oxygen (ml) in 100 ml of mixed venous blood:
   $CvO_2 = (Hb \times 1.36$ ml O_2 g$^{-1} \times SvO_2) + (0.0031 \times PvO_2)$.
3. DO_2 is the volume of oxygen delivered (ml min^{-1}) from the LV to the tissues each minute:
   $DO_2 = CO \times CaO_2 \times 10$.
4. Oxygen demand is the minimal cellular oxygen requirement to avoid anaerobic metabolism.
5. VO_2 is the amount of oxygen consumed by the tissues:
   $VO_2 = (CaO_2 - CvO_2) \times CO \times 10$.
6. Oxygen extraction ratio (O_2 ER) is the fraction of delivered oxygen that is consumed:
   O_2 ER $= VO_2/DO_2$.

The four determinants of SvO_2 are CO, Hb, CaO_2, and VO_2 (Figure 30.7).

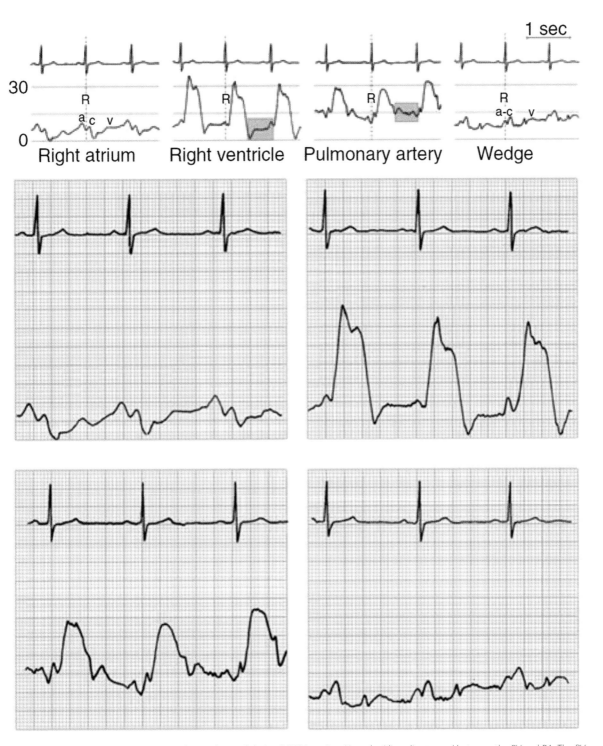

Figure 30.6 Characteristic pressure waveforms observed during PAFC insertion. Note the 'diastolic step-up' between the RV and PA. The RV waveform lacks a dicrotic notch, and pressure *increases* steadily during diastole. In contrast, the PA waveform has a notch and the pressure *decreases* during diastole. (Modified and reproduced with permission from Mark JB. *Atlas of Cardiovascular Monitoring*. New York, NY: Churchill Livingstone, 1998; Figure 3.1.)

Table 30.1 Haemodynamic parameters in shock

	CVP	PAWP	CO	SVR	SvO$_2$
Hypovolaemic	↓↓	↓↓	↓↓	↑	↓
Cardiogenic					
LV MI	N or ↑	↑	↓↓	↑	↓
RV MI	↑↑	N or ↑	↓↓	↑	↓
Obstructive					
Pericardial tamponade	↑↑	↑↑	↓ or ↓↓	↑	↓
Massive PE	↑↑↑↑	N or ↓	↓↓	↑	↓
Distributive					
Early	N or ↑	N	↓ or N or ↑	↓ or N or ↑	N or ↓
Early after fluid administration	N or ↑	N or ↑	↑	↓	↓ or N or ↑
Late	N	N	↓	↑	↓ or ↑

N, normal. From Todd SR, Turner KL, Moore FA. Shock. In Civetta JM, Taylor RW, Kirby RR (eds). *Civetta, Taylor & Kirby's Critical Care*, 4th edn. Philadelphia, PA: Lippincott Williams & Wilkins; 2009.

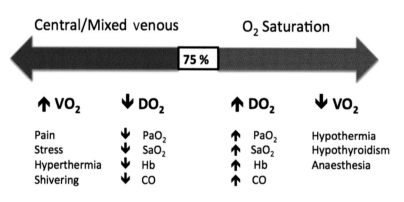

Central/Mixed venous O$_2$ Saturation

75 %

↑ VO$_2$ ↓ DO$_2$ ↑ DO$_2$ ↓ VO$_2$

Pain   ↓ PaO$_2$ ↑ PaO$_2$ Hypothermia
Stress   ↓ SaO$_2$ ↑ SaO$_2$ Hypothyroidism
Hyperthermia ↓ Hb   ↑ Hb   Anaesthesia
Shivering   ↓ CO   ↑ CO

Figure 30.7 Variables that affect the SvO$_2$. (Modified From: Rivers EP, Otero RM, Garcia JA, Reinhart K, Suarez, A. Venous oximetry. In Civetta JM, Taylor RW, Kirby RR (eds). *Civetta, Taylor & Kirby's Critical Care*, 4th edn. Philadelphia, PA: Lippincott Williams & Wilkins; 2009.)

The SvO$_2$ is determined by the admixture of all blood from the capillary tissues of the body and is measured from a PA blood sample. In contrast, central venous oxygen saturation (ScvO$_2$) reflects the venous blood returned from the upper body and is measured from a central venous blood sample. The normal SvO$_2$ range is 65–75%. When values in this range are present, this suggests that the oxygen supply to the body is meeting the demands of the tissues. In contrast, SvO$_2$ values below 50% are considered critically low and are generally associated with metabolic acidosis. In general, ScvO$_2$ values are approximately 5–6 % higher than their simultaneously measured

SvO$_2$ values, and ScvO$_2$ values below 65% have been associated with increased lactate levels. Despite the fact that these alternative measures of venous oxygen saturation may be slightly different, changes in ScvO$_2$ values closely parallel changes in SvO$_2$ values and might be used as a trend measure of the adequacy of systemic oxygen transport.

Putting it All Together

Using the information gathered from cardiovascular monitoring allows the characterization of the underlying pathology and guides intervention (Table 30.1).

Further Reading

Gelman S. Venous function and central venous pressure: a physiologic story. *Anesthesiology* 2008; 108: 735-48.

Michard F, Boussat S, Chemla D, *et al.* Relation between respiratory changes in arterial pulse pressure and fluid responsiveness in septic patients with acute circulatory failure. *Am J Respir Crit Care Med* 2000; 162: 134-8.

Michard F, Teboul J. Predicting fluid responsiveness in ICU patients: a critical analysis of the evidence. *Chest* 2002; 121: 2000–8.

Rivers EP, Otero R, Garcia JA, Reinhart K, Suarez A. Venous oximetry. In Civetta JM, Taylor RW, Kirby RR (eds.), *Civetta, Taylor & Kirby's Critical Care,* 4th edn. Philadelphia, PA: Lippincott Williams & Wilkins; 2009, pp. 296–315.

Schroeder RA, Barbeito A, Bar-Yosef S, Mark JB. Cardiovascular monitoring. In Miller RD (ed), *Miller's Anesthesia,* 8th edn. Philadelphia, PA: Churchill Livingstone Elsevier; 2015, pp. 1345–95.

Chapter 31

Neurological Monitoring

Brian D. Gregson and Hilary P. Grocott

Monitors of neurological function have been available since the 1950s. Until recently, however, many have remained in the hands of enthusiasts at academic centres. Many laboratory methods are not readily adaptable for intraoperative use or cannot be practically used routinely because of cost or the need for expert interpretation. The invasive nature of other monitors (e.g. cerebral microdialysis) precludes their use in the setting of systemic anticoagulation. Emerging evidence suggests that modern neuromonitoring technologies – particularly when used together – can be used both to predict and to modify clinical outcome.

Currently available technologies can be broadly classified as either monitors of the physiological milieu (cerebral perfusion and oxygen delivery) or monitors of neuronal function (Table 31.1). It should be borne in mind that neurological monitors complement, rather than replace, routine clinical monitoring of the MAP, CVP, SaO_2, $PaCO_2$, temperature, pupil size and the concentrations of Hb and glucose.

Neuronal Function

Neuronal function can be assessed using EEG (raw and processed) and evoked potential (sensory and motor) monitoring.

Electroencephalography

Measurement of cerebral cortical electrical activity is one of the oldest methods of neurophysiological monitoring. The EEG signal represents summated post-synaptic potentials (20–200 μV) of pyramidal neurones, typically measured simultaneously between several pairs of scalp electrodes (Figure 31.1).

The EEG is described in terms of location, amplitude and frequency. Frequency is conventionally grouped into four bands: δ, θ, α and β (Table 31.2). A normal awake adult has a posteriorly located,

Table 31.1 Neurological monitoring during cardiac surgery

Physiological milieu (O₂ delivery)	Neuronal function
Cerebral blood flow	*Electroencephalography*
TCD	Raw EEG
Angiography/retinal fluoroscopy	Processed EEG
	Evoked potentials
Perfusion-based imaging	Somatosensory
Xenon wash-in/wash-out	Motor
Thermal diffusion probe	Auditory
Oxygen delivery/ utilization	*Visual*
NIRS (rSO₂)	
Jugular venous O₂ saturation $P_{Ti}O_2$	
Brain tissue chemistry	
Cerebral microdialysis	

rSO₂, regional cerebral oxygen saturation; $P_{Ti}O_2$, partial pressure of oxygen in brain tissue. *Italics* indicate research modalities not available for routine clinical use.

symmetrical EEG frequency of around 9 Hz (i.e. α rhythm). Opioids and most anaesthetic agents produce a dose-dependent EEG slowing ($\downarrow \alpha$ and $\uparrow \delta$ and θ) culminating in periods of very low EEG amplitude and burst suppression (periods of high-voltage electrical activity alternating with periods of silence). N_2O induces high-frequency frontal activity and decreased amplitude. Ketamine increases the EEG amplitude at low doses and slows the EEG at higher doses.

The EEG has long been regarded as the 'gold standard' for the detection of cerebral ischaemia. At constant temperature and depth of anaesthesia (DOA), progressive ischaemia produces a reduction in total power and slowing – decreased α and β power and increased δ and θ power. These changes only become apparent when the cerebral blood flow (CBF) halves (i.e. <50 ml 100 g^{-1} min^{-1}). An EEG

Table 31.2 EEG waveforms

Waveform	Frequency (Hz)		Amplitude (µV)	Comments
Delta (δ)	1.5–3.5		>50	Normal during sleep and deep anaesthesia, indication of neuronal dysfunction
Theta (θ)	3.6–7.5		20–50	Normal in children and elderly, normal adults during sleep, produced by hypothermia
Alpha (α)	7.6–12.5		20–50	Awake, relaxed, eyes open, mainly over occiput
Beta (β)	12.6–25		<20	Awake, alert, eyes open, mainly in parietal cortex, produced by barbiturates, benzodiazepines, phenytoin, alcohol
Gamma (γ)	25.1–50		<20	

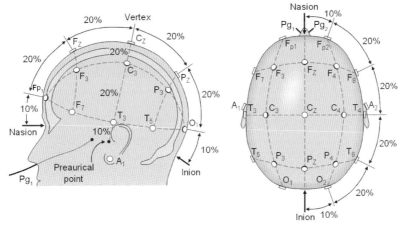

Figure 31.1 The internationally standardized *10-20 system* of EEG electrode placement. Four bony landmarks – the nasion, inion and preauricular points – act as a reference and the cranium is then apportioned into 10% or 20% segments between these landmarks, as originally described by Jasper. F, frontal; Fp, frontal polar; C, central; O, occipital; P, parietal; T, temporal; A, ear lobe; Pg, nasopharyngeal. Right-sided placements are indicated by even numbers, left-sided placements by odd numbers and midline placements by Z. Auricular (A₁ and A₂) positions complete the standard 21-electrode positions. The figure also identifies the anticipated locations of the Rolandic and Sylvian fissures, and commonly used additional Pg and cerebellar (Cb) electrodes. The location and nomenclature of these electrodes is standardized by the American Clinical Neurophysiology Society, formerly the American Electroencephalographic Society. (Adapted with permission from Malmivuo J, Plonsey R. *Bioelectromagnetism – Principles and Applications of Bioelectric and Biomagnetic Fields.* New York: Oxford University Press; 1995)

amplitude attenuation of <50% or increased δ power is regarded as being indicative of mild ischaemia, whereas >50% attenuation or a doubling in δ power is regarded as being indicative of severe ischaemia. An isoelectric or 'silent' EEG is seen when CBF < 7–15 ml 100 g^{-1} min^{-1}. EEG changes are not specific for pathology.

Under conditions of constant DOA and autoregulated cerebral perfusion, the effects of hypothermia on the EEG can be used to guide temperature management in cases requiring deep hypothermic circulatory arrest (DHCA). The wide range of temperatures at which patients reach burst suppression (15.7–33.0 °C) and EEG silence (12.5–27.2 °C) suggests that the use of arbitrary DHCA temperatures (e.g. 20 °C) may be inappropriate for many patients (Figure 31.2). Temperature-induced EEG changes are not predicted by age, isoflurane concentration, $PaCO_2$, or other physiological factors.

Individualized temperature management may allow safe DHCA at higher temperatures, reducing the physiological burden of extreme hypothermia and CPB duration.

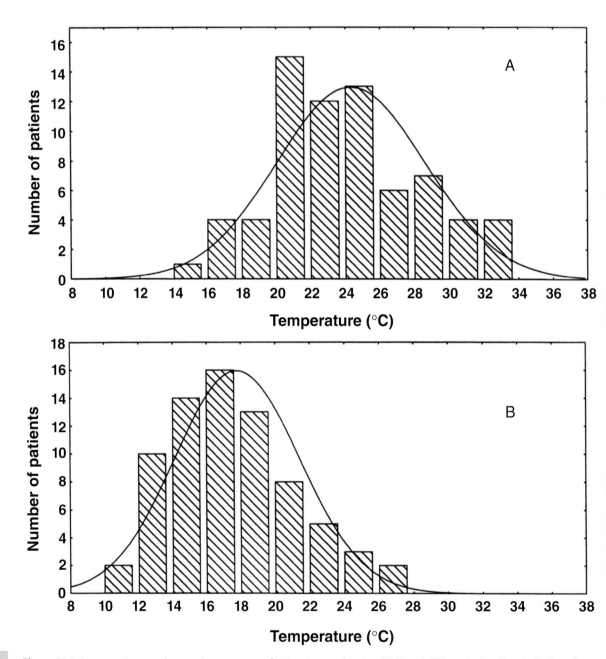

Figure 31.2 Intraoperative nasopharyngeal temperatures of 109 patients undergoing DHCA with EEG monitoring. The distribution of temperatures at which burst suppression (A) and EEG silence (B) were achieved. From Stecker *et al., Ann Thorac Surg* 2001; 71(1): 14–21.

Depth of Anaesthesia

Although ubiquitous, routine clinical monitoring (e.g. MAP, HR, respiratory pattern, diaphoresis and pupil size) is a crude and imprecise measure of DOA. The use of more reliable monitors of DOA has been driven, at least in part, by the recognition that:

- Pharmacological suppression of EEG activity does not mitigate against cerebral ischaemic injury
- Anaesthetic agents may themselves be neurotoxic
- There is a correlation between DOA and mortality
- There may be a link between DOA and postoperative cognitive dysfunction

Using a 16-channel EEG montage to monitor DOA is fraught with problems:

- Interpreting the EEG requires training and is time-consuming
- There is no 'gold standard' for wakefulness, sedation, anaesthesia and deep anaesthesia
- The EEG is altered by ischaemia, temperature and metabolism – as well as drugs

Currently available DOA monitors process the raw EEG obtained from electrodes placed on the forehead, to produce a time-averaged, proprietary number: typically, a dimensionless integer (e.g. 0 to 100). For the reasons stated above, both ketamine and N_2O may paradoxically increase this index, suggesting an apparent decrease in DOA.

Evoked Potential Monitoring

Sensory evoked potentials (SEPs) are the electrical responses of the CNS to peripheral stimulation. Typically, a stimulus is delivered at regular intervals and an averaged evoked response is extracted from background electrical activity. In clinical practice, the stimulus may be visual (VEPs), auditory (AEPs; Figure 31.3) or somatosensory (SSEPs; Figure 31.4). In contrast, motor evoked potential (MEP) monitoring employs transcutaneous transcranial electrical stimulation of the motor cortex and measurement of the evoked electromyography. Use of the MEP technique is precluded by dense neuromuscular blockade. Lower limb SSEPs and, more recently, MEPs have been be used in spinal and major vascular surgery to monitor spinal cord function and prevent postoperative paraplegia (Chapter 13).

Cerebral Perfusion Monitoring

Monitors of the adequacy of cerebral perfusion and oxygenation include TCD, jugular venous oxygen saturation monitoring and cerebral near-infrared spectroscopy (NIRS).

Transcranial Doppler Sonography

Although the intact adult skull is impervious to the transmission of conventional ultrasound (5–10 MHz), insonation of the basal cerebral arteries is possible

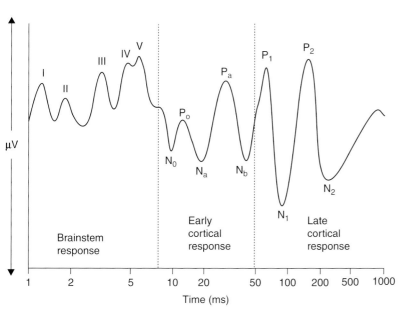

Figure 31.3 AEPs. An auditory stimulus or 'click' is repeated at regular intervals and signal averaging over several cycles used to extract the AEP from background EEG activity. Short-latency (<10 ms) brainstem auditory evoked responses (BAERs) reflect neural activity between the cochlear nucleus (I) and the inferior colliculus (V). BAERs are unaffected by anaesthesia but are temperature-sensitive, making them useful for monitoring the effects of cooling and rewarming. Mid-latency (10–100 ms) AEPs represent cortical processing – necessary for awareness and recall of auditory events. Analysis of early cortical AEPs form the basis of DOA monitors such as the bispectral index (BIS) monitor. P, peak; N, nadir.

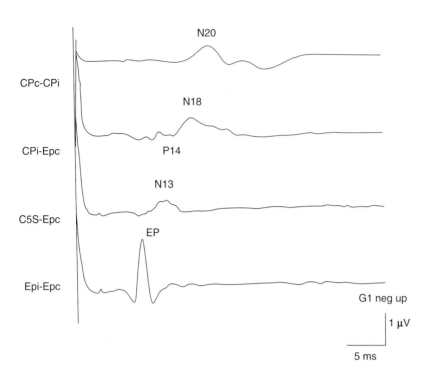

CPc-CPi

N20

N18

CPi-Epc

P14

N13

C5S-Epc

EP

Epi-Epc

G1 neg up

1 µV

5 ms

Figure 31.4 Normal median nerve SSEPs, using minimum recommended montage. Electrode CPi denotes either CP3 or CP4, whichever is ipsilateral to the stimulated limb; CPc is the contralateral centroparietal scalp electrode. Epi and Epc refer to electrodes sited at Erb's point (brachial plexus) on the ipsilateral and contralateral sides, respectively. The C5S electrode is placed over the body of the fifth cervical vertebra.

using low frequency ultrasound (2 MHz) directed through regions of the skull where bone is thinnest (the temporal bones) or absent (the orbit and foramen magnum; Figure 31.5). Insonation of the MCA, via the temporal window, is most commonly used in the setting of cardiac surgery. Pulsed-wave TCD provides a non-invasive means of measuring cerebral artery blood flow velocity – an indirect measure of the CBF. In addition, TCD can detect microemboli.

Jugular Bulb Oxygen Monitoring

Oxygen saturation monitoring in the jugular venous bulb, either by intermittent blood-gas sampling or using a continuous catheter oximeter, has been used as a measure of the balance between global cerebral metabolism ($CMRO_2$) and cerebral oxygenation during cardiac surgery, neurosurgery and in the neurosurgical ICU. Retrograde advancement of a catheter to the jugular bulb, a focal dilatation of the vein near the skull base, minimizes extracranial contamination of sampled blood (Figure 31.6). Measurement of the jugular venous oxygen saturation ($SjvO_2$), normally 55–75%, can be used as a monitor of cerebral oxygen delivery.

The technique has the following limitations:

- Optimal positioning is required to minimize extracerebral contamination

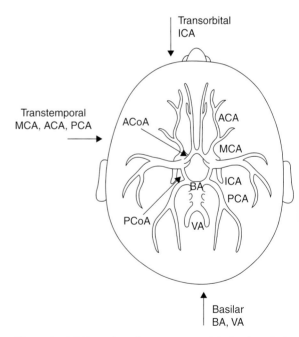

Transorbital
ICA

Transtemporal
MCA, ACA, PCA

ACoA

ACA

MCA

BA

ICA

PCA

PCoA

VA

Basilar
BA, VA

Figure 31.5 TCD windows for examination of the basal cerebral arteries (the circle of Willis) – submandibular approach not shown. ACA, anterior cerebral artery; AcoA, anterior communicating artery; MCA, middle cerebral artery; ICA, internal carotid artery; PCoA, posterior communicating artery; BA, basilar artery; PCA, posterior cerebral artery; VA, vertebral arteries.

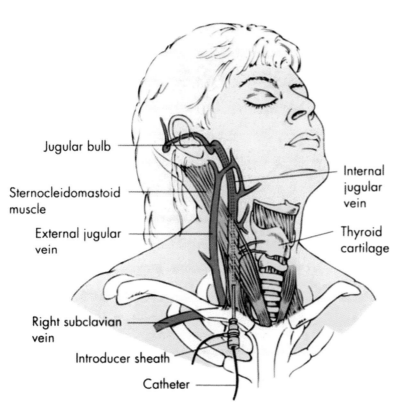

Figure 31.6 Position of a jugular bulb catheter for oxygen saturation monitoring. Precise placement of the tip is essential to facilitate accurate monitoring, to minimize extracerebral contamination, and to minimize the risk of complications. From Schell *et al.*, *Anesth Analg* 2000; 90: 559–66.

- Unilateral sampling from the jugular bulb does not always reflect the status of all brain regions
- It may be insensitive to significant focal areas of ischaemia or infarction

Jugular bulb saturation monitoring now has a relatively limited role in perioperative cardiac care.

Near-Infrared Spectroscopic Cerebral Oximetry

Similar to pulse oximeters, NIRS systems typically employ self-adhesive sensors, applied to the forehead. Photodiodes emit up to four frequencies of near-infrared light (690–950 nm) and light emerging from the scalp is detected by optodes. Differential absorption by several important chromophores (mainly oxy- and deoxyhaemoglobin and cytochrome c oxidase) allows the calculation of the rSO_2. The figure obtained is dependent on the ratio of venous to arterial blood in the brain regions sampled.

Given the dependence of the signal on reflectance by both brain and other tissues, the potential exists for significant contamination by extracranial tissue. Several manufacturers minimize this effect by using multiple wavelengths and two sensors – one with a longer transmission path to penetrate deeper tissue, including the brain, and one with a shorter path to selectively measure scalp and bone absorption and to allow subtraction of this component (Figure 31.7). The normal range of rSO_2 is device-dependent, but is frequently reported to be 60–75%. Clinically significant desaturation is commonly considered to be an absolute rSO_2 of less than 50%, or a relative decrease of 20% from the baseline.

Because NIRS is non-invasive, it has been increasingly embraced as a clinically useful tool in cardiac surgery. It offers the ability to recognize abnormal oxygen delivery and utilization resulting from systemic compromise, as well as alterations in the regional CBF and venous drainage during CPB. Several studies have correlated the 'burden' of intraoperative cerebral desaturation with adverse events such as postoperative cognitive decline, prolonged length of stay and major morbidity. In addition, preoperative rSO_2 has been reported to predict postoperative morbidity and mortality. When used as part of an algorithmic intervention protocol, NIRS has the potential to improve clinical outcomes (Figure 31.8).

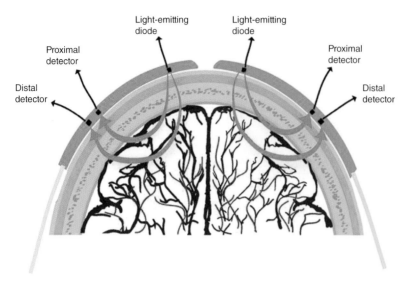

Figure 31.7 A NIRS device is typically fixed to the forehead where bilateral monitoring strips overlie the frontal lobes. Each strip emits light, which may be reflected towards one of several ipsilateral detectors. The amount of light arriving at a detector depends on the light intensity, the position of detectors and the degree of reflection and absorption by the tissue. Although there are differences in light wavelength, detector configuration, and processing algorithms, most manufacturers incorporate a method of selectively measuring superficial (mainly extracranial) tissue oxygenation in order to exclude this portion of the signal and focus on deeper (brain) tissue. From Zheng et al, 2013.

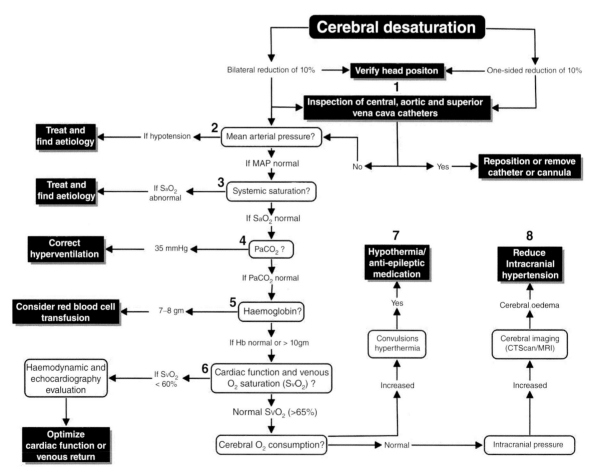

Figure 31.8 Algorithmic approach to reverse cerebral oxygen desaturation. From Deschamps et al., 2016.

Key Points

- The risk of neurological injury is reduced by early detection and intervention.
- At normothermia, the EEG is a sensitive measure of cerebral ischaemia.
- TCD measures the CBF velocity – not the CBF rate.
- NIRS monitoring during CABG surgery has been shown to be predictive of adverse outcome.

Further Reading

Arrowsmith JE, Ganugapenta MSSR. Intraoperative brain monitoring in cardiac surgery. In Bonser R, Pagano D, Haverich A (eds.), *Brain Protection in Cardiac Surgery*. London: Springer-Verlag; 2011, pp. 83–112.

Colak Z, Borojevic M, Bogovic A, *et al.* Influence of intraoperative cerebral oximetry monitoring on neurocognitive function after coronary artery bypass surgery: a randomized, prospective study? *Eur J Cardio-Thorac Surg* 2015; 47: 447–54.

Deschamps A, Hall R, Grocott HP, Mazer CD. Cerebral oximetry monitoring to maintain normal cerebral oxygen saturation during high-risk cardiac surgery. *Anesthesiology* 2016; 124: 826–36.

Fritz BA, Kalarickal PL, Maybrier HR, *et al.* Intraoperative electroencephalogram suppression predicts postoperative delirium. *Anesth Analg* 2016; 122: 234–42.

Grocott HP, Thiele RH. Brain tissue oximetry: what are we really measuring? *Anesth Analg* 2017; 124: 2091–2.

Stecker MM, Cheung AT, Pochettino A, *et al.* Deep hypothermic circulatory arrest: I. Effects of cooling on electroencephalogram and evoked potentials. *Ann Thorac Surg* 2001; 71: 14–21.

Stecker MM, Cheung AT, Pochettino A, *et al.* Deep hypothermic circulatory arrest: II. Changes in electroencephalogram and evoked potentials during rewarming. *Ann Thorac Surg* 2001; 71: 22–8.

Subramanian B, Nyman C, Fritock M, *et al.* A multicenter pilot study assessing regional cerebral oxygen desaturation frequency during cardiopulmonary bypass and responsiveness to an intervention algorithm. *Anesth Analg* 2016; 122: 1786–93.

Wildes TS, Mickle AM, Ben Abdallah A, *et al.* Effect of electroencephalography-guided anesthetic administration on postoperative delirium among older adults undergoing major surgery: the ENGAGES Randomized Clinical Trial. *JAMA* 2019; 321: 473–83.

Zheng F, Sheinberg R, Yee MS, *et al.* Cerebral near-infrared spectroscopy monitoring and neurologic outcomes in adult cardiac surgery patients: a systematic review. *Anesth Analg* 2013; 116: 663–76.

Comprehensive TOE Examination

Justiaan Swanevelder and Andrew Roscoe

TOE is now commonplace in the cardiac operating theatre and critical care setting. The practising cardiac anaesthetist must be fully trained and proficient at performing TOE, both as a haemodynamic monitor and as a diagnostic tool. This chapter will cover the basic physics of ultrasound and Doppler, the indications and contraindications of TOE and the format of a comprehensive TOE examination.

Physics of Ultrasound

Sound is a longitudinal, mechanical wave, with alternating regions of high pressure (compressions) and low pressure (rarefactions). Ultrasound has a frequency greater than 20 kHz. TOE probes typically emit ultrasound at a frequency of 4–8 MHz. Higher-frequency probes produce improved image resolution but have lower tissue penetration. The speed of ultrasound in the heart is approximately 1,540 m s^{-1}. Reflections occur at a tissue boundary, where there is a change in acoustic impedance, and the returning signal is processed by the machine to create an image.

Doppler

The frequency of a sound wave reflected by a moving object is different from the frequency emitted: this change of frequency is the Doppler frequency. This principle is used to calculate the velocity of RBCs and myocardial tissue. Once the peak velocity (V) of blood flow is known, the pressure gradient (PG) between two chambers can be estimated using the simplified Bernoulli equation:

$$PG = 4V^2$$

Doppler modalities include pulse wave (PWD), continuous wave (CWD) and colour flow Doppler (CFD). CWD measures velocities along the entire ultrasound path and is capable of measuring high velocities.

However, it is not possible to determine from where the peak velocity has arisen, known as the range ambiguity artefact. PWD is utilized to measure blood flow in a specific region but is restricted by artefacts at higher velocities. CFD is based on PWD and displays 'real-time' blood flow on the 2D image.

Indications

In cardiac surgery, intraoperative TOE is a standard of care for all open-heart procedures and thoracic aortic operations. It is also indicated in selected patients undergoing CABG surgery, although in many centres it has become routine practice in *all* adult cardiac surgery. In the critical care setting, TOE is invaluable in managing haemodynamic instability where the diagnosis cannot be obtained by TTE. In the cardiac catheter laboratory, TOE is indicated in guiding catheter-based intracardiac procedures, such as septal defect closure.

Absolute contraindications to TOE include oesophagectomy, recent upper GI surgery and significant oesophageal or gastric pathology, such as perforation and active bleeding. In the presence of a relative contraindication, TOE may be performed if the expected benefits outweigh the potential risks.

Complications

Although TOE is generally considered to be safe, it is a semi-invasive procedure and is not without its complications. Injuries may occur anywhere from the oropharynx to the stomach. The most common complications include oral injuries, hoarseness and dysphagia. Major morbidity occurs in approximately 0.2% and the incidence of oesophageal perforation ranges from 0.01–0.1%. The reported mortality is less than 0.01%.

Basic TOE Views

There are four levels for image acquisition (Figure 32.1): upper oesophageal, mid-oesophageal, transgastric and deep transgastric. The TOE probe may be anteflexed or retroflexed, turned left or right, and the plane can be rotated from 0° to 180°.

Guidelines recommend performing a comprehensive intraoperative TOE examination, comprising 28 basic 2D views (Figure 32.2) and appropriate use of Doppler modalities. It is prudent to perform the study in a systematic manner and to allow sufficient time, in order to confirm the preoperative diagnosis and to optimize the ability to identify important pathologies that were not detected in the preoperative investigations. Management-changing unexpected intraoperative TOE findings can occur in up to 4% of patients. However, it is important to recognize the effect of anaesthesia on the patient's pathophysiology and how this influences the TOE assessment.

In the critical care setting a more focused examination may be employed to rapidly evaluate the haemodynamically unstable patient, or as a follow-up study to assess ventricular recovery in a patient requiring mechanical circulatory support.

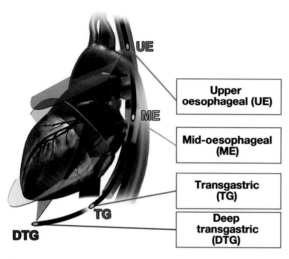

Figure 32.1 Standard TOE probe levels. Adapted from Hahn RT *et al.*, *J Am Soc Echocardiogr* 2013; 26: 921–64.

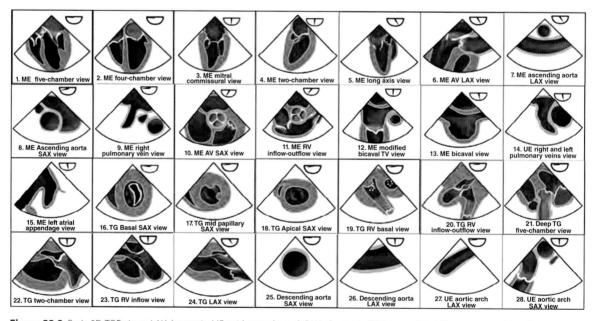

Figure 32.2 Basic 2D TOE views. LAX, long axis; ME, mid-oesophageal; SAX, short axis; TG, transgastric; UE, upper oesophageal. Adapted from Hahn RT *et al.*, *J Am Soc Echocardiogr* 2013; 26: 921–64.

Key Points

- TOE is standard of care for all open-heart and thoracic aortic surgical procedures.

- TOE is a semi-invasive procedure with a low rate of major complications.

- An intraoperative TOE study should be comprehensive, with a formal report.

Further Reading

Feneck R, Kneeshaw J, Fox K, *et al.* Recommendations for reporting perioperative transoesophageal echo studies. *Eur J Echocardiogr* 2010; 11: 387–93.

Feneck RO, Kneeshaw J, Ranucci M (eds.). *Core Topics in Transesophageal Echocardiography.* Cambridge: Cambridge University Press; 2010.

Hahn RT, Abraham T, Adams MS, *et al.* Guidelines for performing a comprehensive transesophageal echocardiographic examination: recommendations from the American Society of Echocardiography and the Society of Cardiovascular Anesthesiologists. *J Am Soc Echocardiogr* 2013; 26: 921–64.

Hilberath JN, Oakes DA, Shernan SK, *et al.* Safety of transesophageal echocardiography. *J Am Soc Echocardiogr* 2010; 23: 1115–27.

Skinner HJ, Mahmoud A, Uddin A, *et al.* An investigation into the causes of unexpected intra-operative transoesophageal echocardiography findings. *Anaesthesia* 2012; 67: 355–60.

Wheeler R, Steeds R, Rana B, *et al.* A minimum dataset for a standard transoesophageal echocardiogram: a guideline protocol from the British Society of Echocardiography. *Echo Res Pract* 2015; 2: G29–45.

Chapter

33

Assessment of Ventricular Function

Catherine M. Ashes and Andrew Roscoe

Ventricular dysfunction is associated with increased cardiovascular morbidity and mortality after both cardiac and non-cardiac surgery. Traditionally, invasive pressure monitoring has been used to make inferences regarding ventricular function. However, the relationship between pressure and organ perfusion may be affected by many variables in the dynamic intraoperative environment. TOE has the advantage of real-time visualization of ventricular filling, contractility and ischaemia. As such, TOE is now considered to be the 'gold standard' intraoperative monitor of ventricular function.

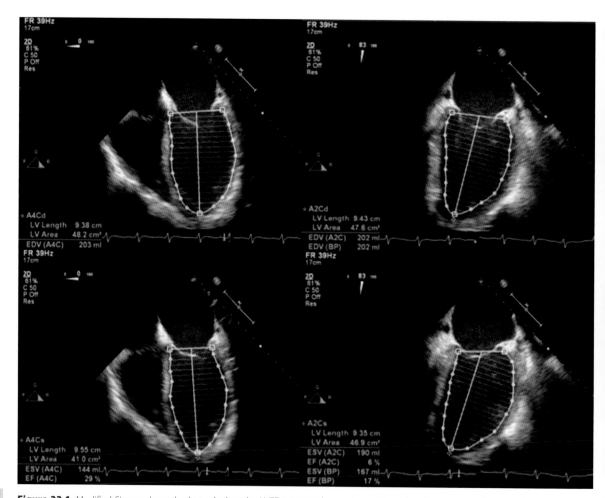

Figure 33.1 Modified Simpson's method to calculate the LVEF using mid-oesophageal four-chamber and two-chamber views.

Left Ventricular Systolic Function

Fractional Shortening

Fractional shortening (FS) can be measured using either M-mode or 2D imaging. Measurements of internal LV dimensions are taken at end-diastole (LVIDd) and end-systole (LVIDs) from the transgastric two-chamber view at a level of the tips of the papillary muscles. The FS is then calculated as:

$$FS = \frac{LVIDd - LVIDs}{LVIDd}$$

A normal value is 25–42%. However, as the FS is derived from linear measurements, it becomes inaccurate in the presence of regional wall motion abnormalities (RWMAs).

Ejection Fraction

The LV ejection fraction (LVEF) is derived from measurements of the LV end-diastolic volume (LVEDV) and end-systolic volume (LVESV):

$$LVEF = \frac{LVEDV - LVESV}{LVEDV}$$

The LVEDV and LVESV may be obtained from 2D images, using the biplane method of discs (modified Simpson's method, Figure 33.1) or from reconstruction of 3D imaging. A normal LVEF is 52–74%.

Strain Imaging

Strain is defined as the change in length of an object (L_1) compared to its baseline (L_0):

$$Strain\ (\%) = \frac{100(L_1 - L_0)}{L_0}$$

Myocardial deformation analysis typically utilizes speckle-tracking echocardiography to assess the change of LV myocardial length from end-diastole to end-systole to derive the global longitudinal strain (GLS, Figure 33.2). A normal LV GLS is –20%.

Regional Systolic Function

TOE is a highly sensitive tool for detecting myocardial ischaemia: RWMAs are usually present prior to ECG evidence of ischaemia. The 17-segment model is used to assess the regional LV function (Figure 33.3). Each myocardial segment is analyzed and scored

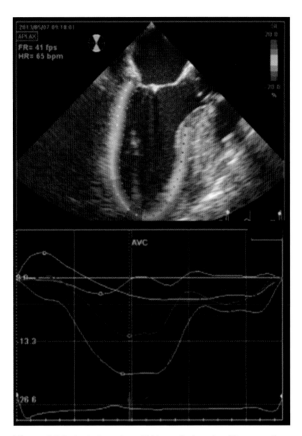

Figure 33.2 Strain imaging of LV systolic function. The wavy lines at bottom represent strain from different LV regions (walls).

according to both wall motion and thickening – see Table 33.1.

Strain imaging is also utilized to detect more subtle degrees of regional dysfunction.

Left Ventricular Diastolic Function

Diastolic dysfunction is associated with poor outcomes for patients with congestive heart failure. In cardiac surgical patients, it is predictive of the difficulty in separating from CPB and of increased postoperative morbidity.

The approach to assessing the LV diastolic function is based on the transmitral flow pattern (E/A ratio and E velocity), tissue Doppler imaging of MV annular motion (e' velocity), the LA size and the presence of secondary PHT (Table 33.2.). LV diastolic function can be graded into normal, grade I dysfunction (impaired relaxation), grade II dysfunction (pseudonormalization) and grade III dysfunction (restrictive filling).

243

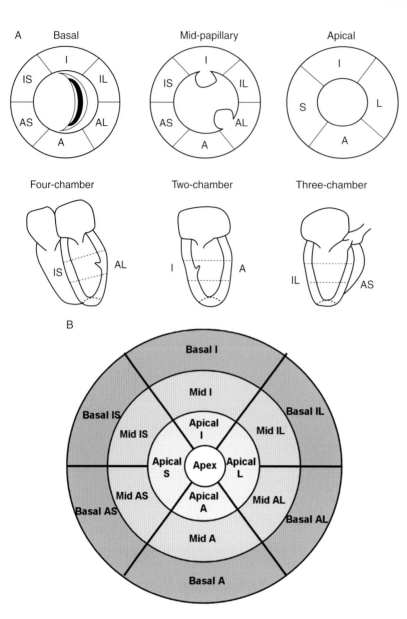

Figure 33.3 The 17-LV-segment model: (A) mid-oesophageal and TG views at basal, mid-papillary and apical levels, with anterior (A), anteroseptal (AS), inferoseptal (IS), inferior (I), inferolateral (IL) and anterolateral (AL) walls. (B) 17-segment model. Adapted from Lang RM et al., *J Am Soc Echocardiogr* 2015; 28: 1–39.

Right Ventricular Function

Echocardiographic assessment of the RV function can be challenging, due to its complex geometrical shape. RV dimensions are measured in an RV-focused mid-oesophageal four-chamber view at end-diastole. RV volumes are difficult to measure accurately with 2D echocardiography, although disc summation methods have been described. 3D imaging may provide a more accurate measure of the RV ejection fraction (RVEF) than 2D imaging.

TAPSE

Tricuspid annular plane systolic excursion (TAPSE) is the distance the lateral TV annulus moves from base to apex during the cardiac cycle. It is typically measured using M-mode imaging, although optimal alignment is challenging and may require the use of anatomical M-mode modality or a modified transgastric RV inflow view. A value of <17 mm indicates RV dysfunction.

Table 33.1 Ventricular RWMA scoring

Score	Wall motion	Endocardial movement	Endocardial thickening
1	Normokinesia	Normal	Normal (30%)
2	Hypokinesia	Reduced	Reduced
3	Akinesia	Absent	Negligible
4	Dyskinesia	Outward	Thinning/aneurysmal

Table 33.2 LV diastolic dysfunction parameters

Parameter	Normal	Grade I	Grade II	Grade III
E/A	0.8–2.0	< 0.8	0.8–2.0	> 2.0
E velocity (cm s^{-1})	50–80	< 50	> 50	> 50
E/e'	< 10	< 10	10–14	> 14
LA size	Normal	Normal	Dilated	Dilated
LA pressure	Normal	Normal	Increased	Increased
Secondary PHT	No	No	Yes	Yes

S' Velocity

Tissue Doppler imaging of the motion of the lateral TV annulus can be used to measure the peak velocity (S') of the annulus as it moves from base to apex in systole. A value of <9.5 cm s^{-1} reflects RV systolic dysfunction.

Fractional Area Change

The RV fractional area change (RVFAC) provides a simple and validated method to assess the RV contractility. Using an RV-focused mid-oesophageal four-chamber view, the RV end-diastolic area (RVEDA) and end-systolic area (RVESA) are traced (Figure 33.4). The RVFAC is then calculated:

$$RVFAC = \frac{RVEDA - RVESA}{RVEDA}$$

An RVAFC of <35% indicates reduced RV systolic function. RV dysfunction may be graded according to the RVFAC – see Table 33.3.

Strain

Using an RV-focused mid-oesophageal four-chamber view, speckle-tracking echocardiography strain of the RV free wall (Figure 33.5) provides a reproducible and objective measure of the RV function. A normal value for RV strain is –20%.

3D RV Ejection Fraction

Due to the shape of the RV, 3D echocardiography has been shown to provide more accurate measures of RV volumes. However, good-quality 2D imaging is still required to allow tracking of the RV cavity throughout the cardiac cycle, and reconstruction of the RV may be time-consuming. In addition, the RVEF is significantly dependent on preload and afterload. An RVEF of less than 45% suggests RV dysfunction.

Assessment in the perioperative setting of cardiac surgery is further complicated by the effect of pericardial opening, which causes a reduction in the longitudinal measures of the RV function (TAPSE and S'), rendering them no longer representative of the overall RV function. This precludes comparison of the pre-CPB to the post-CPB TAPSE as an accurate measurement of change in the RV systolic function. The RVFAC and 3D imaging may provide a better comparison.

Table 33.3 Grading of RV dysfunction

RVFAC	RV function
>35%	Normal
25–35%	Mild dysfunction
18–25%	Moderate dysfunction
<18%	Severe dysfunction

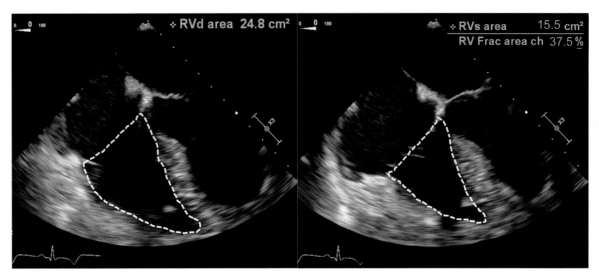

Figure 33.4 Measurement of the RVFAC

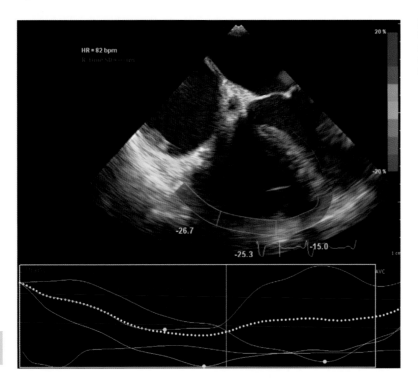

Figure 33.5 RV free wall strain measurement. The wavy dotted white line represents the overall RV free wall strain; other coloured wavy lines represent strain from different RV regions.

Key Points

- TOE is the 'gold standard' intraoperative monitor of biventricular function.
- TOE is a sensitive marker of myocardial ischaemia.
- The RV function is best assessed by the RVFAC in the intraoperative setting.
- Strain imaging provides a reproducible method of assessing both the LV and RV systolic function.

Further Reading

Lang RM, Badano LP, Mor-Avi V, *et al.* Recommendations for cardiac chamber quantification by echocardiography in adults. *J Am Soc Echocardiogr* 2015; 28: 1–39.

Mor-Avi V, Lang RM, Badano LP, *et al.* Current and evolving echocardiographic techniques for the quantitative evaluation of cardiac mechanics. *J Am Soc Echocardiogr* 2011; 24: 277–313.

Nagueh SF, Smiseth OA, Appleton CP, *et al.* Recommendations for the evaluation of left ventricular diastolic function by echocardiography. *J Am Soc Echocardiogr* 2016; 29: 277–314.

Silverton N, Meineri M. Speckle tracking strain of the right ventricle: an emerging tool for intraoperative echocardiography. *Anesth Analg* 2017; 125: 1475–8.

Chapter

34

Assessment of Valvular Heart Disease

Massimiliano Meineri and Andrew Roscoe

TTE evaluation of the heart valves requires both quantification of the severity of the pathology and identification of the underlying mechanism. This information will determine if surgical intervention is warranted and will guide the surgical decision as whether to repair or replace the diseased valve.

Aortic Valve

The normal AV is composed of three leaflets: right, left and non-coronary cusps. The normal AV area is 2.5–4.0 cm^2. It is evaluated by TOE using long- and short-axis mid-oesophageal views and with Doppler in the deep transgastric view.

Aortic Stenosis

The most common aetiologies for AS are trileaflet AV calcification, bicuspid AV with calcific changes and rheumatic valve disease. A bicuspid AV is present in 1–2% of the general population and typically results from fusion of the right and left coronary cusps (80%) or the right and non-coronary cusps (20%). Rheumatic AS typically displays commissural fusion.

TOE assessment of severity (Table 34.1) involves measuring velocities across the valve to calculate mean and peak pressure gradients. The AV area

(AVA) can be derived using the continuity equation once the LVOT area and peak velocity (LVOT$_{VEL}$) have been determined:

$$AVA = \frac{LVOT_{AREA} \times LVOT_{VEL}}{AV_{VEL}}$$

The dimensionless index (DI) is more frequently used to grade the severity of AS, as it removes errors introduced during the LVOT area calculation (Figure 34.1):

$$DI = \frac{LVOT_{VEL}}{AV_{VEL}}$$

Aortic Regurgitation

AR can be classified according to its mechanism (Figure 34.2), which determines surgical repair or replacement. The severity of AR is based on qualitative and quantitative methods (Table 34.2). Under general anaesthesia, with reduced LV afterload, the severity of AR is often underestimated when determined by qualitative methods; quantitative techniques are largely unaffected by the changes in loading conditions.

Mitral Valve

The MV complex is comprised of the anterior and posterior valve leaflets, the annulus, the chordae tendinae and the papillary muscles. The LV myocardium also plays an important role in normal MV function. The MV is assessed in the mid-oesophageal views from 0° to 130° and in the transgastric basal views. 3D imaging of the MV is now standard for complex lesions (Figure 34.3).

Mitral Regurgitation

The mechanism of MR is divided into primary MR, where there is a leaflet abnormality, and secondary MR, due to annular dilatation or LV dysfunction, and is based on the Carpentier classification (Figure 34.4).

Table 34.1 Grading severity of AV stenosis

	Mild	Moderate	Severe
Mean gradient (mmHg)	<20	20–40	>40
Peak gradient (mmHg)	<36	36–64	>64
AV area (cm^2)	>1.5	1.0–1.5	<1.0
Indexed AV area (cm^2 m^{-2})	>0.85	0.6–0.85	<0.6
DI	>0.5	0.25–0.5	<0.25

Table 34.2 Grading severity of AV regurgitation

	Mild	Moderate	Severe
Qualitative			
Pressure half-time (ms)	>500	200–500	<200
PWD aortic diastolic flow reversal	Brief	Intermediate	Holodiastolic
Semi-quantitative			
Jet width/LVOT diameter (%)	<25	25 – 65	>65
Vena contracta width (mm)	<3	3 – 6	>6
Quantitative			
EROA (cm^2)	<0.1	0.1 – 0.3	>0.3
Regurgitant volume (ml)	<30	30 – 60	>60
Regurgitant fraction (%)	<30	30 – 50	>50

EROA, effective regurgitant orifice area.

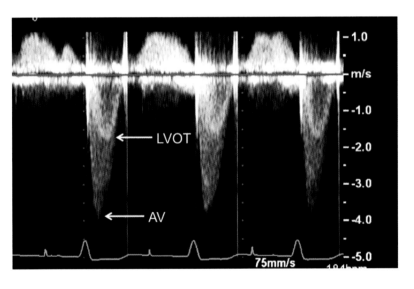

Figure 34.1 CMD spectral display, showing a double envelope, used to calculate the DI

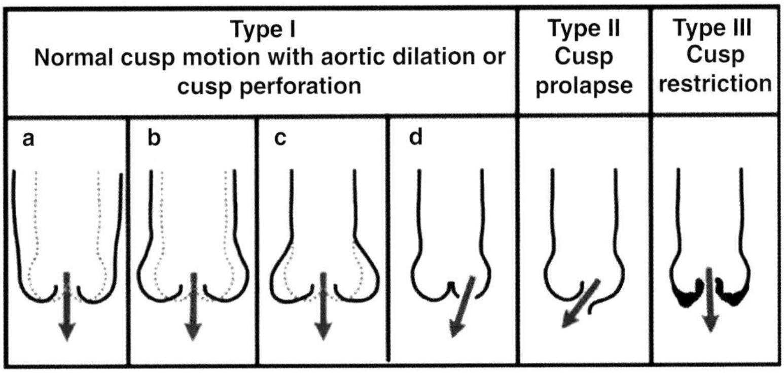

Figure 34.2 Mechanisms of AR. Adapted from Boodhwani *et al.*, 2009.

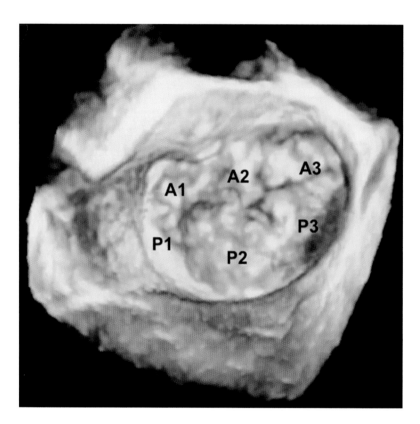

Figure 34.3 3D en-face view of the MV, showing prolapse of segments P2 and P3. A: anterior; P: posterior.

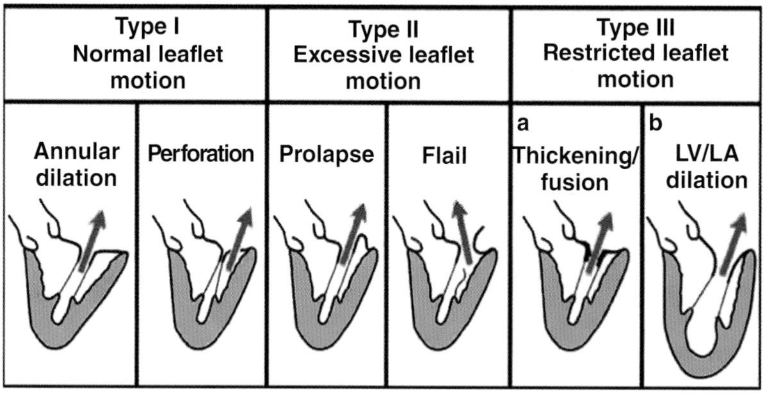

Type I Normal leaflet motion		Type II Excessive leaflet motion		Type III Restricted leaflet motion	
Annular dilation	Perforation	Prolapse	Flail	a Thickening/ fusion	b LV/LA dilation

Figure 34.4 Carpentier classification of the mechanisms of MR. Adapted from Zoghbi *et al.*, 2017.

Primary causes include myxomatous degeneration, fibroelastic deficiency, endocarditis, rheumatic disease and congenital abnormalities. Elucidating the mechanism will influence the surgical management and determine if valve repair is feasible and the type of repair technique.

Qualitative and quantitative methods are available to assess the severity of MR (Table 34.3). Quantitative methods are less affected by loading conditions and are recommended whenever feasible.

Mitral Stenosis

Rheumatic heart disease remains the leading cause of MS worldwide. Others include congenital, inflammatory, infiltrative and drug-induced causes.

Table 34.3 Grading severity of MR

	Mild	Moderate	Severe
Qualitative			
CFD jet area	Small and narrow	Variable	Large (>50% of LA)
Semi-quantitative			
Vena contracta width (mm)	<3	3–7	>7
PWD pulmonary vein flow	S-wave dominance	S-wave blunting	S-wave reversal
Quantitative			
EROA (cm^2)	<0.2	0.2–0.4	>0.4
Regurgitant volume (ml)	<30	30–60	>60
Regurgitant fraction (%)	<30	30 – 50	>50

EROA, effective regurgitant orifice area; S, systolic.

Table 34.4 Grading severity of MS

	Mild	Moderate	Severe
Mean gradient (mmHg)	<5	5–10	>10
Pressure half-time (ms)	<150	150–220	>220
MV area (cm^2)	>1.5	1.0–1.5	<1.0

Rheumatic MS typically presents with commissural fusion, leaflet thickening starting at the tips and chordal shortening. Assessment of the MS severity is based on Doppler interrogation of flow through the MV, to calculate pressure gradients and the MV area (Table 34.4). Percutaneous balloon commissurotomy or surgical intervention are usually indicated when the MV area is <1.5 cm^2.

Tricuspid Valve

The TV is comprised of the anterior, septal and posterior leaflets; the TV annulus, chordae tendinae and papillary muscles. It is the most apical of the four cardiac valves.

Tricuspid Regurgitation

Trace-to-mild TR is present in many normal individuals. Significant TR (Figure 34.5) is most commonly functional, secondary to RV and TV annulus dilatation and subsequent leaflet tethering. Primary causes include myxomatous degeneration, endocarditis, rheumatic disease, congenital abnormalities and carcinoid disease.

Qualitative and quantitative methods are used to assess the severity of TR (Table 34.5). In assessing TV annulus dilatation, the annulus should be measured in the mid-oesophageal four-chamber view, at the beginning of diastole. Surgical intervention is recommended when there is severe TR or moderate TR with annular dilatation (TV annulus > 40 mm).

Tricuspid Stenosis

TS is typically due to rheumatic heart disease, but other causes include carcinoid disease, lupus valvulitis and adhesions secondary to pacemaker leads. The severity is based on Doppler interrogation (Box 34.1).

Pulmonary Valve

The PV is the most anterior of the cardiac valves, making it often difficult to assess with TOE. It is comprised of anterior, left posterior and right posterior leaflets.

Pulmonary Stenosis

PS is usually congenital in origin, but may occur secondary to carcinoid disease. Assessment of the severity of PS is based on Doppler interrogation (Table 34.6).

Table 34.5 Grading severity of TR

	Mild	Moderate	Severe
Qualitative			
CWD waveform	Faint, parabolic	Dense, parabolic	Dense, triangular
Semi-quantitative			
CFD jet area (cm^2)	—	—	>10
Vena contracta width (mm)	<3	3–7	>7
PWD hepatic vein flow	S-wave dominance	S-wave blunting	S-wave reversal
Quantitative			
EROA (cm^2)	<0.2	0.2 – 0.4	>0.4
Regurgitant volume (ml)	<30	30 – 45	>45

EROA, effective regurgitant orifice area; S, systolic.

Box 34.1 Criteria for haemodynamically significant TS

Mean gradient (mmHg)	>5
TV area (cm^2)	<1.0
Pressure half-time (ms)	>190
Velocity–time integral (cm)	>60

Table 34.6 Grading severity of PS

	Mild	Moderate	Severe
Peak gradient (mmHg)	<36	36–64	>64

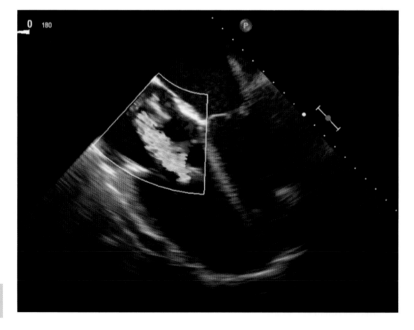

Figure 34.5 Mid-oesophageal four-chamber view showing TR

Table 34.7 Grading severity of PR

	Mild	Moderate	Severe
PR jet width/PV annulus	–	–	>0.7
Pressure half-time (ms)	–	–	<100
PR deceleration time (ms)	–	–	<260

Table 34.8 Grading severity of prosthetic paravalvular leaks

	Mild	Moderate	Severe
Aortic valve			
Pressure half-time (ms)	>500	200–500	<200
Regurgitant volume (ml)	<30	30 – 60	>60
Mitral valve			
CFD jet area (cm^2)	<4	4–8	>8
Vena contracta (mm)	<3	3–6	>6
EROA (cm^2)	<0.2	0.2–0.4	>0.4
Tricuspid valve			
CFD jet area (cm^2)	<5	5–10	>10
Vena contracta (mm)	—	<7	>7

EROA, effective regurgitant orifice area.

Pulmonary Regurgitation

Mild PR is a common finding in normal individuals. Significant PR can be caused by PHT, endocarditis, carcinoid disease and congenital abnormalities. Assessment of the severity of PR is based on limited data (Table 34.7).

Assessment of Prosthetic Valves

TOE assessment of prosthetic valves is often challenging. Valve structures can cause acoustic shadowing and limit visualization; regurgitation jets may be physiological and part of the design of the valve or they may be pathological.

Comprehensive evaluation of prosthetic valves is important and involves looking for manifestations of malfunction: paravalvular leaks, thrombosis, pannus formation, defective leaflet motion, valve degeneration, evidence of endocarditis and patient–prosthesis mismatch. The calculation of the effective orifice area (EOA) provides a better measure of valvular function than the pressure gradient, which is influenced by haemodynamics. Quantification of paravalvular leaks is often difficult due to the irregular shape of the regurgitant orifice and the eccentricity of the jet. Recommended parameters for assessing the severity are listed in Table 34.8.

Further Reading

Baumgartner H, Hung J, Bermejo J, *et al.* Echocardiographic assessment of valve stenosis: EAE/ASE recommendations for clinical practice. *J Am Soc Echocardiogr* 2009; 22: 1–23.

Boodhwani M, de Kerchove L, Glineur D, *et al.* Repair-oriented classification of aortic insufficiency: impact on surgical techniques and clinical outcomes. *J Thorac Cardiovasc Surg* 2009; 137: 286–94.

Cremer PC, Rodriguez LL, Griffin BP, *et al.* Early bioprosthetic valve failure: mechanistic insights via correlation between echocardiographic and operative findings. *J Am Soc Echocardiogr* 2015; 28: 1131–48.

Lancellotti P, Moura L, Pierard LA, *et al.* EAE recommendations for the assessment of valvular regurgitation. Part 2: mitral and tricuspid regurgitation. *Eur J Echocardiogr* 2010; 11: 307–32.

Lancellotti P, Tribouilloy C, Hagendorff A, *et al.* EAE recommendations for the assessment of valvular regurgitation. Part 1: aortic and pulmonary regurgitation. *Eur J Echocardiogr* 2010; 11: 223-44.

Nishimura RA, Otto CM, Bonow RO, *et al.* 2014 AHA/ACC guideline for the management of patients with valvular heart disease. *J Am Coll Cardiol* 2014; 63: e57–185.

Sidebotham DA, Allen SJ, Gerber IL, *et al.* Intraoperative transesophageal echocardiography for surgical repair of mitral regurgitation. *J Am Soc Echocardiogr* 2014; 27: 345–66.

Vegas A. *Perioperative Two-Dimensional Transesophageal Echocardiography: A Practical Handbook*, 2nd edn. New York, NY: Springer; 2018.

Zoghbi WA, Adams D, Bonow RO, *et al.* Recommendations for noninvasive evaluation of native valvular regurgitation. *J Am Soc Echocardiogr* 2017; 30: 303–71.

Zoghbi WA, Chambers JB, Dumesnil JG, *et al.* Recommendations for evaluation of prosthetic valves with echocardiography and Doppler ultrasound. *J Am Soc Echocardiogr* 2009; 22: 975–1014.

Chapter

TOE for Miscellaneous Conditions

Lachlan F. Miles and Andrew Roscoe

Introduction

The utility of TOE in cardiac surgery extends beyond the assessment of ventricular and valvular function. A comprehensive study reveals much about the structural abnormalities of the heart and associated vessels. This chapter will cover some ancillary topics, including:

- *Congenital heart disease* – ASDs
- *Cardiac masses* – thrombus, tumours and vegetations
- *Pericardial disease* – tamponade and constrictive pericarditis
- *Aortic disease* – aortic dissection

Atrial Septal Defects

An ASD is a common congenital cardiac lesion, comprising 6–10% of such anomalies at birth, although diagnosis may not occur until adulthood. The lesion may present as an atrial arrhythmia, paradoxical embolic stroke or exercise limitation secondary to RV volume overload. ASDs may be single or multiple and are associated with additional cardiac lesions in 30% of cases.

A PFO is not, by the strictest definition, an ASD, as there is no deficiency of septal tissue. The prevalence of a PFO at autopsy is approximately 25%. The PFO is associated with atrial septal aneurysm and Chiari networks.

ASDs are anatomically classified into:

- Secundum ASD – 80%
- Primum ASD – 15%
- Sinus venosus ASD – 4–5%
- Coronary sinus ASD – <1%

Secundum ASDs occur in the fossa ovalis area of the interatrial septum (Figure 35.1A). Primum ASDs are best viewed in the mid-oesophageal 4-chamber view, with the defect occurring just above the crux of the heart (Figure 35.1B) and are often associated with atrioventricular (A-V) valve abnormalities. Sinus

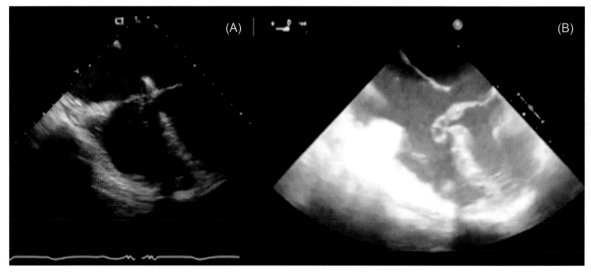

Figure 35.1 Mid-oesophageal four-chamber view showing (A) secundum ASD and (B) primum ASD

venosus ASDs are visualized in the mid-oesophageal bicaval view, occurring at the SVC–RA junction (superior sinus venosus ASD) or the IVC-RA junction (inferior SV ASD). They are typically associated with partial anomalous pulmonary venous drainage. Coronary sinus ASDs involve an unroofed coronary sinus and are usually associated with a persistent left-sided SVC.

Many secundum ASDs are amenable to percutaneous device closure and the goal of the echocardiographer is to determine the size, location and number of defects.

Cardiac Masses

Intracardiac masses are a common source of embolism and can be categorized into thrombi, tumours and vegetations.

Cardiac Thrombus

The pathogenic continuum begins with a low-flow state within a cardiac chamber, visible as spontaneous echo contrast or 'smoke'. This eventually leads to the deposition of thrombus in areas of stasis. In AF, the left atrial appendage (LAA) is particularly vulnerable to clot formation. Due to its position adjacent to the oesophagus, the LA and LAA are well suited to interrogation by TOE. Prominent pectinate muscles in the LAA may create difficulty in the diagnosis of thrombus. The use of CFD and PWD can provide additional information: an absence of blood flow in the LAA on CFD and an ejection velocity below 40 cm s^{-1} on PWD are suggestive of thrombus.

Ventricular thrombus formation occurs in areas of stasis, typically in akinetic or aneurysmal regions following infarction. When evaluating a potential thrombus, diagnosis requires visualization of the lesion in orthogonal planes and the lesion must be differentiated from artefact, false tendons and prominent trabeculations. Right-sided thrombi are often attached to foreign material, such as central venous catheters or pacemaker leads.

Tumours

The vast majority of cardiac tumours are caused by secondary malignant disease, with spread to the heart via direct tumour extension and venous or lymphatic metastasis. Typical primary malignancies with secondary cardiac involvement include lung, oesophagus, breast, kidney and melanoma.

Of the primary cardiac neoplasms, approximately 90% are benign, of which most are myxomas. Other benign tumours include papillary fibroelastoma, lipoma and fibroma.

Most myxomas occur in the LA, arising from the fossa ovalis (Figure 35.2.). They are more common in females and 7% are associated with Carney complex. They may be an incidental finding; they can present with systemic embolization; or they can cause

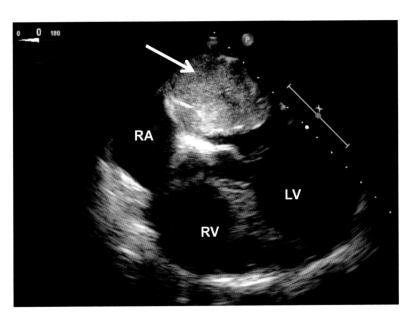

Figure 35.2 Mid-oesophageal four-chamber view showing a myxoma (arrow) filling most of the LA

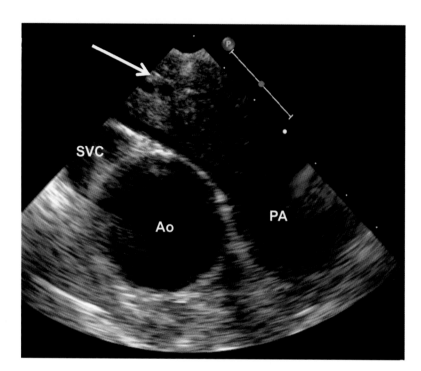

Figure 35.3 Upper oesophageal view showing a sarcoma (arrow) occluding the right PA. Ao, ascending aorta

complications due to the mass effect, often causing functional MS due to MV orifice obstruction.

Papillary fibroelastomas are the second most common benign cardiac tumour. They are typically seen adherent to valves, on the aortic side of the AV and the ventricular side of the MV. They are well-circumscribed, attached to the valve by a stalk and often highly mobile.

Approximately 95% of primary cardiac malignant tumours are sarcomas. They are more common in the right side of the heart. Sarcomas occurring in the PA (Figure 35.3) are typically poorly differentiated with an unfavourable prognosis.

Vegetations

TOE has an important role in the assessment of infective endocarditis. Surgical intervention can be guided by intraoperative TOE findings: size, location and mobility of vegetations; extension of infection into surrounding structures; mechanism and severity of valvular defects; assessment of prosthetic valve function; and the haemodynamic consequences of the various lesions.

Vegetations typically colonize the low-pressure side of valves: the atrial side of the A-V valves (Figure 35.4.) and the ventricular side of the semilunar valves. Right-sided lesions are associated with IV drug use. The embolic risk is proportional to vegetation size and more common when occurring on the anterior leaflet of the MV.

Pericardial Disease

Cardiac Tamponade

A life-threatening condition, cardiac tamponade is most commonly encountered in the early postoperative period due to bleeding within the pericardial sac. An acute rise in pericardial pressure compresses the cardiac chambers, preventing normal filling. As the pressure continues to rise, the pericardial pressure exceeds the intracavity pressure, leading to an elevated CVP, reduced SV, a low CO state, pulsus paradoxus and eventual cardiac arrest.

A circumferential effusion is normally easily diagnosed on TOE. The classical echocardiographic sign is collapse of the RA during ventricular systole and RV collapse during diastole. However, a localized clot following cardiac surgery can impede the blood flow into a single chamber (Figure 35.5) and may not present with classical signs.

Constrictive Pericarditis

Constrictive pericarditis is the result of scarring of the pericardium, leading to a non-compliant and calcified structure that resists cardiac filling. It is important to

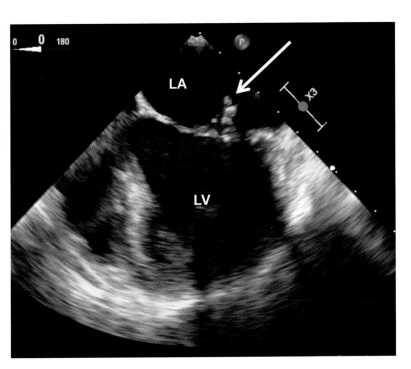

Figure 35.4 Mid-oesophageal four-chamber view showing a vegetation (arrow) on the MV

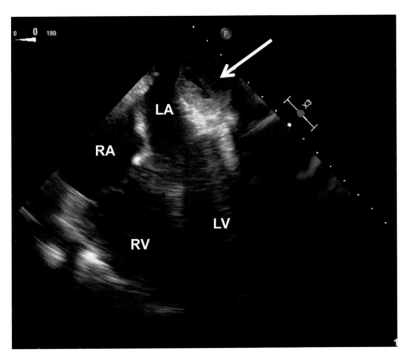

Figure 35.5 Mid-oesophageal four-chamber view showing a thrombus (arrow) compressing the LA

differentiate constrictive pathophysiology from restrictive disease. Echocardiographic features of constrictive pericarditis include a thickened, hyperechogenic pericardium (Figure 35.6), dilated atria, a septal 'bounce' and diastolic flattening of the LV inferolateral endocardium.

Doppler interrogation is essential to establish the diagnosis. Transmitral flow typically shows a

257

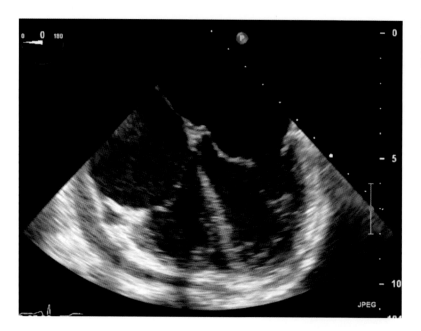

Figure 35.6 Mid-oesophageal four-chamber view showing a hyperechogenic pericardium, dilated atria and a small pericardial effusion

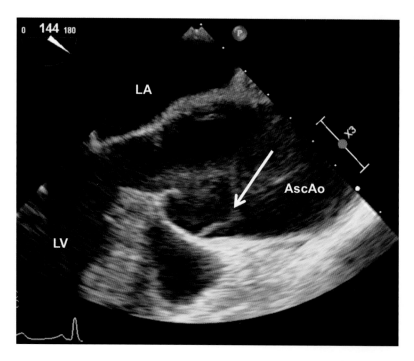

Figure 35.7 Mid-oesophageal long-axis view of a dissection flap (arrow) in the ascending aorta (AscAo)

restrictive filling pattern with a decreased E-wave deceleration time, and significant variation in E-wave velocity with respiration. Tissue Doppler imaging of mitral annular velocities reveals annulus reversus (medial e' velocity > lateral e' velocity).

Aortic Disease

Aortic Dissection

Stanford type A dissection involves an intimal tear in the ascending aorta, forcing blood between the intima and media to form a dissection flap. Rapid diagnosis is essential to expedite emergency surgery. This is based on the presence of an intimal flap that divides the aorta into a true and false lumen (Figure 35.7). A TOE examination should also attempt to determine the proximal and distal extent of the lesion, as well as detect any complications of dissection: pericardial collection, coronary ostia involvement and AV regurgitation (AR). Type A dissection is frequently associated with ascending aorta dilatation, so close interrogation of the mechanism of any AR is important to facilitate the appropriate surgical repair.

Key Points

- TOE is well suited to diagnose LAA thrombus.
- TOE is useful in infective endocarditis to guide the surgical intervention.
- It is important to differentiate constrictive pathophysiology from restrictive disease.
- In type A dissection, TOE is useful to detect any complications.

Further Reading

Bruce CJ. Cardiac tumours: diagnosis and management. *Heart* 2011; 97: 151–60.

Goldstein SA, Evangelista A, Abbara S, *et al.* Multimodality imaging of diseases of the thoracic aorta in adults. *J Am Soc Echocardiogr* 2015; 28: 119–82.

Hara H, Virmani R, Ladich E, *et al.* Patent foramen ovale: current pathology, pathophysiology, and clinical status. *J Am Coll Cardiol* 2005; 46: 1768–76.

Klein AL, Abbara S, Agler DA, *et al.* American Society of Echocardiography clinical recommendations for multimodality cardiovascular imaging of patients with pericardial disease. *J Am Soc Echocardiogr* 2013; 26: 965–1012.

Mankad R, Herrmann J. Cardiac tumors: echo assessment. *Echo Res Pract* 2016; 3: R65–77.

Methangkool E, Howard-Quijano K, Ho JK, *et al.* Infective endocarditis: the importance of intraoperative transesophageal echocardiography. *Anesth Analg* 2014; 119: 35–40.

Saric M, Armour AC, Arnaout MS, *et al.* Guidelines for the use of echocardiography in the evaluation of a cardiac source of embolism. *J Am Soc Echocardiogr* 2016; 29: 1–42.

Silvestry FE, Cohen MS, Armsby LB, *et al.* Guidelines for the echocardiographic assessment of atrial septal defect and patent foramen ovale. *J Am Soc Echocardiogr* 2015; 28: 910–58.

Haematology

Martin W. Besser and Kiran M. P. Salaunkey

Over the last decade, there have been three major developments in perioperative blood management. Firstly, the recognition of preoperative anaemia and perioperative transfusion as risk factors for perioperative morbidity and mortality. Secondly, there is much greater involvement of haematologists in preoperative planning and perioperative care. Thirdly, there has been a widespread introduction of point-of-care testing and aggressive, protocol-driven blood component use in the management of perioperative bleeding.

Preoperative Considerations

Over 36,000 cardiac surgical procedures a year are undertaken in the UK. Cardiac surgery accounts for 10% of UK blood supply consumption. Approximately a third of cardiac surgical patients are anaemic at admission. As a consequence, cardiac surgery is associated with a transfusion rate of approximately 45%. Transfusion has a dose-related impact on the length of stay and complication rates.

Anaemia

Where possible, anaemia should be corrected before elective surgery. UK national guidance advocates the identification of preoperative iron deficiency before planned surgery and has stated that iron-deficient patients should not have planned surgery without preoperative intervention.

Clinical pathways for dealing with iron-deficient patients have the potential to significantly reduce transfusions. In addition, perioperative measures such as cell salvage and low volume blood sampling reduce transfusion requirements.

Preoperative autologous blood donation is discouraged in the UK because of concerns about sterility, storage and short shelf-life (<6 weeks).

Abnormalities of Haemostasis

It is important to identify patients with a bleeding history. A tool such as the International Society of Thrombosis and Hemostasis Bleeding Assessment Tool (ISTH BAT) questionnaire is more sensitive and specific than laboratory tests (i.e. PT, APTT, platelet count).

Patients taking anticoagulants and antiplatelet agents should be given explicit instructions regarding cessation before surgery.

Mild thrombocytopenia is common in elderly patients. More marked thrombocytopenia may be secondary to immune thrombocytopenia, right heart failure, hepatic impairment, drug therapy, haematinic deficiency or myelodysplasia. Where time allows, a platelet count of $<75 \times 10^9 \, l^{-1}$ should prompt haematology referral to establish if the cause is reversible.

The minimum platelet count required for cardiac surgery is debated. The question is confounded by antiplatelet and anticoagulant drug therapy. In most centres, a platelet count of $100 \times 10^9 \, l^{-1}$ is regarded as the minimum necessary for elective cardiac surgery. In life-threatening situations, a platelet count of $\sim 35 \times 10^9 \, l^{-1}$ may be tolerated, albeit with a greater risk of bleeding and transfusion.

A prednisolone 'challenge' ($1 \, mg \, kg^{-1}$) may temporarily increase the platelet count in the perioperative period. A positive response is not absolutely indicative of steroid-responsive immune thrombocytopenia as some patients with myelodysplasia may show a transient response.

In the setting of urgent or emergent surgery, platelet administration at the start of surgery should be considered in patients with a platelet count of $<70 \times 10^9 \, l^{-1}$ and post CPB-transfusion in patients with a platelet count $70–90 \times 10^9 \, l^{-1}$. Earlier platelet transfusion is not recommended because of the risk of human leucocyte antigen sensitization.

Antiplatelet Agents

Virtually all cardiac surgery patients take aspirin. Aspirin irreversibly blocks cyclooxygenase, leading to permanent platelet inactivation (Box 36.1). Upon cessation, normal platelet production restores platelet function in 8 days, meaning that patients exhibit 10% platelet recovery per day. For this reason, many centres no longer advocate stopping aspirin before surgery (Box 36.1).

Around 30% of patients exhibit a degree of *in vitro* resistance to clopidogrel. By contrast, there is little resistance to prasugrel and ticagrelor. Patients undergoing cardiac surgery within 5 days of discontinuing clopidogrel, ticagrelor or prasugrel have greater perioperative blood loss. In unstable patients, the decision to discontinue adenosine diphosphate (ADP) receptor blockers must balance the risks of bleeding and coronary ischaemia.

Box 36.1 Characteristics of commonly used antiplatelet drugs	
Aspirin	Impairs ability of platelets to synthesis and release thromboxane
Clopidogrel **Plavix**®	Irreversibly inhibits ADP-induced platelet aggregation Half-life of main metabolite 8 hours Excreted in urine and faeces Platelet function normalizes ~5 days after discontinuation
Prasugrel **Effient**® **Efient**®	A prodrug; irreversibly inhibits ADP-induced platelet aggregation Half-life of main metabolite 7 hours Platelet function normalizes 5–9 days after discontinuation
Abciximab **Reopro**®	Non-selective monoclonal antibody Duration of platelet inhibition 24–48 hours
Eptifibatide **Integrilin**®	Cyclic heptapeptide Duration of platelet inhibition 2–4 hours Renal excretion; no active metabolites
Tirofiban **Aggrastat**®	Synthetic non-peptide Duration of platelet inhibition 4–8 hours Renal excretion; no active metabolites

Congenital Haemolytic Anaemia and Haemoglobinopathy

With the exception of sickle cell disease (HbAS, HbSS), no special precautions are necessary. There is general agreement that moderate and deep hypothermia should be avoiding in patients with sickle cell trait.

Case series from Ghana and India have demonstrated that patients with sickle cell disease (HbSS) can successfully undergo cardiac surgery without additional precautions. In the UK however, patients with sickle cell disease invariably undergo preoperative red cell exchange to achieve HbS 25–30% and Hb concentration 100 g l^{-1}. Allogenic blood should be Rhesus and Kell matched and ideally less than 10 days old.

Hereditary spherocytosis requires no special precautions. Where it is suspected, a preoperative haematology opinion should be sought to exclude rarer congenital red cell membrane disease. Some patients who have undergone splenectomy for congenital haemolytic anaemia may have abnormal blood films that can be confused with hereditary spherocytosis.

Patients with cryohydrocytosis, a subtype of hereditary stomatocytosis, may develop hyperkalaemia during cooling followed by hypokalaemia on rewarming.

Cold Agglutinins

Most patients will show a degree of autoagglutination if their blood is cooled to 4 °C. A number of elderly patients may have significant cold agglutination. This may be idiopathic or associated with low-grade lymphoma. Clinically relevant cold agglutinins are evident at room temperature or even at 37 °C.

The incidental finding of autoagglutination is typically followed by a direct antiglobulin test (DAT). If this proves positive for complement immunoglobulin M (IgM) or IgG a thermal range of agglutination (4–37 °C) is obtained.

Treatment ranges from plasma exchange, immunosuppression, avoidance of cold cardioplegia, maintenance of normothermia to avoidance of surgery altogether. Where lymphoma is thought to be the cause, targeted chemo/immune therapy may induce agglutinin remission sufficient to permit surgery.

Anticoagulants

The management of patients on warfarin is largely governed by the original indication for anticoagulation.

Patients who have AF without high-risk features can usually stop their warfarin 5 days before surgery without bridging. Similarly, patients on direct-acting oral anticoagulants (DOACs) for AF can stop their DOAC at the recommended time point and have prophylactic low-molecular-weight heparin (LMWH) from the time of admission. Higher-risk patients typically require bridging with an infusion of unfractionated heparin (UFH).

High-risk patients typically restart anticoagulation 6–8 h after the surgery with UFH or LMWH, whereas in low-risk patients, prophylactic LMWH can be used.

Dabigatran and other alternatives to UFH may have an increased role because of the availability of reversal agents. Idarucizumab (Praxbind®) is licensed for dabigatran reversal and andexanet alfa (Andexxa®) has recently been FDA-approved for reversal of rivaroxaban and apixaban.

Where interruption of thrombotic therapy is considered within 6 weeks of a venous thromboembolic (VTE) event the insertion of a removable embolus filter should be considered in discussion with a haematologist. If one is placed, it is absolutely paramount that a removal date is agreed prior to insertion as any filter that remains in situ becomes an indication for long-term anticoagulation in its own right.

In patients with a known thrombophilia (e.g. factor V Leiden, antiphospholipid syndrome), extended thromboprophylaxis should be considered. The decision to anticoagulate should be based on actual past thrombotic events rather than perceived risk.

Thrombolytic Agents

These drugs are currently indicated in the early management of acute MI. On rare occasions, a patient presenting with stroke in association with an, as yet, undiagnosed acute type A aortic dissection may receive thrombolytic therapy. It is not uncommon therefore, for the anaesthetist to be presented with a patient who has recently received drugs such as streptokinase or recombinant tissue plasminogen activators (t-PA; alteplase, reteplase). The surgical team needs to be aware of the half-lives of individual drugs and appreciate that their effects may persist for several days.

Intraoperative Considerations

Despite the administration of a large dose of UFH, thrombin generation and platelet activation are not completely inhibited during CPB. Thrombin levels are elevated, the concentration of coagulation factors is reduced, the platelet count is reduced, and leucocytes and fibrinolysis are activated.

In addition to triggering the intrinsic coagulation cascade, CPB induces factor XII-mediated complement activation and pathological clot formation. Exposure of leucocytes to the extracorporeal circuit induces adhesion molecular expression and platelet degranulation, and activation of the classical and alternative complement pathways leading to cytokine generation.

Factor VIII or IX deficiency requires factor replacement to achieve therapeutic levels. To reduce prothrombotic risk, patients with factor XI deficiency should have factor replacement to achieve a concentration of ~70%. Repeat doses will be necessary. Tranexamic acid (TXA) is useful in factor VIII deficiency.

Lupus anticoagulant is a misnomer – it is actually a procoagulant. It spuriously prolongs the APTT and ACT, exposing patients to the risk of inadequate anticoagulation during CPB. This can be circumvented by using a higher target ACT or monitoring anti-Xa levels.

Heparin Resistance

In patients requiring therapeutic anticoagulation, heparin resistance is widely defined as the need for greater than 35,000 IU UFH per day to achieve a therapeutic APTT. In the setting of cardiac surgery with CPB, failure to achieve an ACT of >450 s after UFH 350 IU kg^{-1} is usually considered as representing heparin resistance. Causes include: antithrombin deficiency, elevated concentrations of factor VIII, fibrinogen or heparin binding protein; and increased heparin clearance. In addition, patients with a chronic aortic dissection and chronic obstructive pulmonary disease are reported to be at a greater risk of heparin resistance. It should be borne in mind that heparin itself may produce antithrombin deficiency.

Antithrombin deficiency can usually be treated with either antithrombin concentrate or FFP. In patients with elevated clotting factor concentrations an anti-Xa assay may be used as an alternative to ACT or APTT monitoring. In patients with increased heparin binding or heparin clearance, an alternative anticoagulation strategy may be required.

Alternatives to Heparin

A number of agents have been used as alternatives to UFH. These include argatroban, prostacyclin and bivalirudin. Dosing, monitoring and reversal of these infrequently used drugs are challenging. The use of these drugs should be preceded by a current literature search and a haematology consult. The short half-life of some of these drugs means that stasis of blood with the extracorporeal circuit must be avoided to prevent clotting. When used to avoid patient exposure to UFH, it is important to ensure that heparin-coated equipment is not inadvertently used.

Aprotinin

Aprotinin is a serine protease inhibitor that reduces blood loss and transfusion requirements during cardiac surgery. It exerts its antifibrinolytic effects by inhibiting t-PA, kallikrein and fibrinolysin. In 2007, it was withdrawn from the market after a clinical study was halted because of concerns about increased risk of perioperative renal failure, MI and stroke. In 2008, Royston questioned this interpretation and the decision to terminate the study. After re-stratifying patients according to the risk of adverse outcome, he found no increase in the relative risk of these complications. Aprotinin is currently available for use in Europe on a named-patient basis. It remains licensed only for primary CABG surgery with CPB.

Lysine Analogues

TXA and ε-aminocaproic acid bind to plasminogen, preventing its conversion to plasmin and reducing fibrinolysis (Figure 36.1). In comparative studies with aprotinin in cardiac surgery, these agents have been shown to reduce perioperative bleeding, but not to reduce blood donor exposure. The use of TXA in the UK increased considerably following the withdrawal of aprotinin. It soon became apparent that high-dose TXA was associated with early postoperative seizures.

Monitoring Coagulation

In many centres, this consists of intraoperative measurement of ACT, standard laboratory coagulation studies and point-of-care tests of whole blood clotting and platelet function. Viscoelastic tests (e.g. thromboelastography (TEG) and rotational thromboelastometry (ROTEM); Figure 36.2), allow characterization of clotting abnormalities and guide therapeutic intervention (Figure 36.3).

Blood Product Replacement

Available blood products include RBCs, FFP, cryoprecipitate, platelets, prothrombin complex concentrate (PCC), fibrinogen concentrate and individual clotting factors.

Having corrected anaemia (Hb >80 g l^{-1}), first-line therapy in coagulopathic bleeding is FFP (15 ml kg^{-1}), cryoprecipitate (two pools) or fibrinogen (3–4 g) to maintain fibrinogen >1.5 g dl^{-1} and PCC (15 IU kg^{-1}) where warfarin was given preoperatively. PCC may be useful in DOAC-induced bleeding. Despite the risks of spontaneous thrombosis, recombinant factor VIIa (90 μg kg^{-1}) may be used as a measure of last resort in patients with severe postoperative bleeding despite correction of coagulopathy. A smaller dose (0.3 μg kg^{-1}) has been shown to release endogenous von Willebrand's factor and improve platelet function.

Reducing Systemic Inflammation

A number of strategies have been proposed to reduce the systemic inflammatory response as a means to reduce the perioperative morbidity and mortality associated with cardiac surgery (Figure 36.4):

Pharmacological:

Antioxidant, anticomplement, antiplatelet and anti-protease inhibitors

Corticosteroids and antifibrinolytics (class IIa evidence)

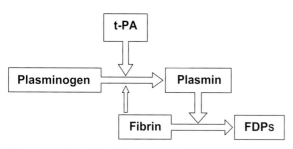

Figure 36.1 Fibrinolysis. The conversion of plasminogen to plasmin is catalyzed by activators such as tissue and urokinase plasminogen activators (t-PA and u-PA, respectively). The rate of conversion is increased 500-fold in the presence of fibrin. FDPs, fibrin degradation (split) products.

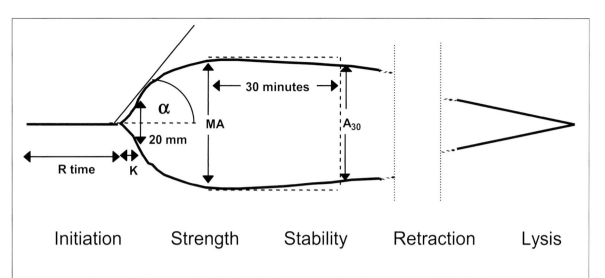

| Initiation | Strength | Stability | Retraction | Lysis |

Parameter	Comments	Normal values
R	Reaction time – time from start of the trace until oscillatory amplitude reaches 1 mm Analogous to whole blood clotting time ↑ by anticoagulants and clotting factor deficiencies	6–8 minutes
K	The time from initiation of oscillatory movement to until oscillatory amplitude reaches 20 mm – a measure of the speed of clot formation Prolonged by ↓platelets and ↓fibrinogen	4–6 minutes
α angle	The angle of the tangent from R to K Reduced by ↓platelets and ↓fibrinogen	50–60°
R + K	Sum of R time and K time represents the coagulation time	10–14 minutes
MA	Maximum amplitude – the point at which rotational torque is greatest Represents strength of clot formation Reduced by platelet dysfunction, ↓fibrinogen and heparin	50–60 mm
A_{30} & A_{60}	The rotational torque amplitude 30 minutes and 60 minutes after maximum amplitude reached – a measure of clot stability and lysis	
MA/A_{60}	Whole blood clot lysis index Reduced by fibrinolysis	>0.85

Figure 36.2 The thromboelastogram and derived parameters

Circuit modification:

Reducing circuit volume/eliminating reservoir

Low volume priming

Use of biocompatible surfaces - heparin-coated or bonded circuits

Use of centrifugal pump heads instead of roller pumps

Arterial line leucocyte depleting filters

Care of the aorta:

Intraoperative TOE and epiaortic ultrasound to guide aortic cannulation

Avoidance of repeated application of an AXC

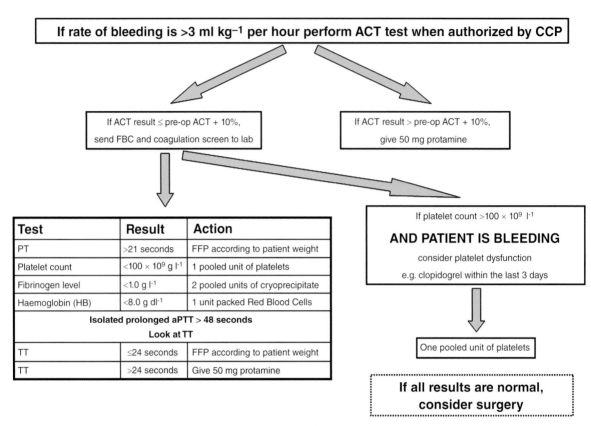

If rate of bleeding is >3 ml kg⁻¹ per hour perform ACT test when authorized by CCP

If ACT result ≤ pre-op ACT + 10%, send FBC and coagulation screen to lab

If ACT result > pre-op ACT + 10%, give 50 mg protamine

Test	Result	Action
PT	>21 seconds	FFP according to patient weight
Platelet count	<100 × 10⁹ g⁻¹	1 pooled unit of platelets
Fibrinogen level	<1.0 g l⁻¹	2 pooled units of cryoprecipitate
Haemoglobin (HB)	<8.0 g dl⁻¹	1 unit packed Red Blood Cells
Isolated prolonged aPTT > 48 seconds		
Look at TT		
TT	≤24 seconds	FFP according to patient weight
TT	>24 seconds	Give 50 mg protamine

If platelet count >100 × 10⁹ l⁻¹

AND PATIENT IS BLEEDING

consider platelet dysfunction

e.g. clopidogrel within the last 3 days

One pooled unit of platelets

If all results are normal, consider surgery

Figure 36.3 Protocol for using laboratory and point-of-care coagulation testing to guide blood component therapy. CCP, critical care (nurse) practitioner.

Care of conduits:

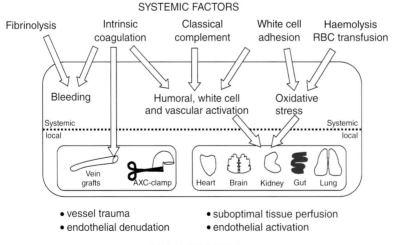

SYSTEMIC FACTORS

Fibrinolysis   Intrinsic coagulation   Classical complement   White cell adhesion   Haemolysis RBC transfusion

Bleeding   Humoral, white cell and vascular activation   Oxidative stress

Systemic
local

Vein grafts   AXC-clamp   Heart   Brain   Kidney   Gut   Lung

Systemic
local

• vessel trauma
• endothelial denudation

• suboptimal tissue perfusion
• endothelial activation

LOCAL TRIGGERS

Figure 36.4 The interaction with systemic and local pathways and their effect on organ dysfunction

Box 36.2 Causes of coagulopathy after cardiac surgery

Quantitative platelet problem	Destruction, haemodilution, sequestration, activation, consumption, use of cell salvage
Qualitative platelet problem	Damage, heparin, aspirin, clopidogrel, glycoprotein-IIb/IIIa inhibitors, NSAIDs, uraemia, hypothermia, hypofibrinogenaemia
Coagulation factor deficiency	Haemodilution, consumption, liver disease, congenital
Altered enzyme kinetics	Hypothermia
Anaemia	Haemorrhage, haemodilution, haemolysis
Anticoagulants	Residual heparin, excessive protamine
Altered factor clearance	Hepatic and renal hypoperfusion, hypothermia

Avoid repeated/excessive distension of vein grafts

Managing CPB:

Maintaining adequate organ blood flow

Postoperative Problems

Common problems include haemorrhage, anaemia and thrombocytopenia. Less common are non-overt DIC and heparin-induced thrombocytopenia. The risk of coagulopathic bleeding is increased by endocarditis and prolonged CPB (Box 36.2).

Anaemia

Preoperative iron-deficiency anaemia or anaemia of chronic disease aggravated by perioperative bleeding are the commonest causes of postoperative anaemia. Haemolytic transfusions are rare and may occur after discharge. Persistent haemolysis following AV replacement should raise the suspicion of paravalvular leak.

Heparin-Induced Thrombosis

Heparin-induced thrombosis (HIT) is an IgM- or IgG-mediated phenomenon that results in venous and arterial thrombosis. The antibodies bind to heparin–platelet factor 4 (PF4) complexes on the surface of monocytes and platelets. These complexes then activate platelet FcγIIa receptors, inducing degranulation. The likelihood of HIT is determined by the type heparin, the duration of the heparin–PF4 antibody titre and the type of surgery. Patients receiving UFH during cardiac or orthopaedic surgery have a 5–10 times greater risk of HIT than medical or obstetric patients. Women have twice the risk of developing HIT than men. The initial diagnosis is clinical, and a laboratory confirmation is often delayed. The most widely used pre-test probability score is the Warkentin score.

The management of suspected or proven HIT consists of stopping *all* heparin and starting an alternative, such as bivalirudin, argatroban or danaparoid. LMWH should not be used because of UFH cross-reactivity. If cardiac surgery with CPB is required, this should be delayed until the heparin–PF4 antibody titre falls. Alternatively, plasmapheresis or an alternative anticoagulant may be considered.

Key Points

- Anaemia and transfusion are risk factors for perioperative morbidity and mortality.
- Acquired antithrombin deficiency is a common sequel of heparin administration.
- Heparin-induced thrombosis and the lupus anticoagulant both produce paradoxical procoagulant states.

Further Reading

Besser MW, Klein AA. The coagulopathy of cardiopulmonary bypass. *Crit Rev Clin Lab Sci* 2010; 47: 197–212.

Besser MW, Ortmann E, Klein AA. Haemostatic management of cardiac surgical haemorrhage. *Anaesthesia* 2015; 70 Suppl 1: 87–95.

Choxi AA, Patel PA, Augoustides JG, *et al.* Bivalirudin for cardiopulmonary bypass in the setting of heparin-induced thrombocytopenia and combined heart and kidney transplantation – diagnostic and therapeutic challenges. *J Cardiothorac Vasc Anesth* 2017; 31: 354–64.

Edwin F, Aniteye E, Tettey M, *et al.* Hypothermic cardiopulmonary bypass without exchange transfusion in sickle-cell patients: a matched-pair analysis. *Interact Cardiovasc Thorac Surg* 2014; 19: 771–6.

Estcourt LJ, Birchall J, Allard S, *et al.* Guidelines for the use of platelet transfusions. *Br J Haematol* 2017; 176: 365–94.

Hung M, Ortmann E, Besser M *et al.* A prospective observational cohort study to identify the causes of anaemia and association with outcome in cardiac surgical patients. *Heart* 2015; 101: 107–12.

Nickel KF, Long AT, Fuchs TA, Butler LM, Renne T. Factor XII as a therapeutic target in thromboembolic and inflammatory diseases. *Arterioscler Thromb Vasc Biol* 2017; 37: 13–20.

Ortmann E, Besser MW, Klein AA. Antifibrinolytic agents in current anaesthetic practice. *Br J Anaesth* 2013; 111: 549–63.

Rodeghiero F, Tosetto A, Abshire T, *et al.* ISTH/SSC bleeding assessment tool: a standardized questionnaire and a proposal for a new bleeding score for inherited bleeding disorders. *J Thromb Haemost* 2010; 8: 2063–5.

Royston D. Aprotinin; an economy of truth? *J Thorac Cardiovasc Surg* 2008; 136: 798–9.

Staibano P, Arnold DM, Bowdish DM, Nazy I. The unique immunological features of heparin-induced thrombocytopenia. *Br J Haematol* 2017; 177: 198–207.

Thachil J, Warkentin TE. How do we approach thrombocytopenia in critically ill patients? *Br J Haematol* 2017; 177: 27–38.

Chapter

37

Cardiac Surgery during Pregnancy

Savio J. M. Law and Sarah E. Round

Background

Cardiac disease has been the leading cause of overall maternal mortality in the UK since the 2002–2004 triennium. The maternal death rate from cardiac disease has increased from 1.65 per 100,000 maternities in the 1997–1999 triennium to 2.34 per 100,000 maternities in the 2013–2015 triennium. This is thought to be due to increasing maternal age, increasing levels of obesity and better recognition of cardiac pathology at autopsy.

The cardiac diagnoses from the women who died in 2009–2014 are shown in Table 37.1. Sudden arrhythmic cardiac death with a morphologically normal heart was the most common cause for death (31% of women who died from cardiac causes).

This was followed by ischaemic deaths (22%), myocardial disease/cardiomyopathy (18%), and aortic dissection (14%).

Several key areas for improvement have been identified in the recent review of maternal deaths due to cardiac disease. Pre-pregnancy counselling of women of child-bearing age with known cardiac disease is lacking and is a sensitive subject that is rarely broached by clinicians. Frequently, transitions from paediatric to adult cardiology services and massive changes in life circumstances at this age result in a lack or loss of follow-up. Logistical problems, such as the lack of co-location of obstetric and cardiac services, and the lack of access to cardiac investigations still need to be improved. In this high-risk maternity population, the management of signs and symptoms

Table 37.1 Sub-classification of cardiac deaths for whom information was available for an in-depth review (UK and Ireland, 2009–2014). (Reproduced with permission of Knight *et al.*, 2016)

Sub-classification	Number of deaths	Percentage of total (*n* = 153)*
Sudden arrhythmic cardiac death with a morphologically normal heart	47	31
Ischaemic deaths *Atherosclerosis (16), coronary dissection (11), other (7)*	34	22
Myocardial disease/cardiomyopathy *Dilated cardiomyopathy (4), LV hypertrophy with or without fibrosis (5), obesity cardiomyopathy (2), myocarditis (3), peripartum cardiomyopathy (9), hypertrophic obstructive cardiomyopathy (1), arrhythmogenic RV cardiomyopathy (2), other ventricular disease (1)*	27	18
Aortic dissection	21	14
Valvular heart disease *Valve disease (9), endocarditis (2)*	11	7
Others *Pulmonary arterial hypertension (6), undetermined cardiovascular disease (1)*	7	5
Essential hypertension	6	4
TOTAL	153	

* Excludes 36 late cardiac deaths for which no information was available.

Box 37.1 Normal physiological changes associated with pregnancy

Circulating volume

Blood volume ↑ 30-40%

Physiological anaemia (plasma ↑ 45%/erythrocytes ↑ 20%)

↓↓ Colloid osmotic pressure ⇒ ↑ risk of pulmonary oedema

Altered plasma protein binding of drugs

Neutrophilia

Hypercoagulable state

Cardiovascular

↑ Sympathetic tone ⇒ SV ↑ 30% + HR ↑ 15% ⇒ CO ↑ 50%

↑ Wall stress/contractility ➔ ↑ Myocardial O_2 consumption

CVP and PAWP unchanged (PVR and SVR ↓ 20%)

Systolic BP - unchanged

Diastolic BP – initially falls and then returns to normal at term

Aortocaval compression ⇒ ↓↓ CO

Increased vascularity of airway – especially nasal passages

Respiratory

Diaphragmatic splinting

↑ Minute ventilation, ↑ RR, ↑ V_T ↓ functional respiratory capacity

↓ $PaCO_2$, ↓ HCO_3^-, ↓ buffering capacity

Total body O_2 consumption ↑ 15–20%

Gastrointestinal

Delayed gastric emptying, constipation

Increased risk of gastro-oesophageal reflux

Genitourinary

↑ Renal blood flow and GFR

Increased risk of vesico-ureteric reflux/infection

Glycosuria (tubular transport maximum exceeded)

Proteinuria (up to 0.3 g d^{-1})

Metabolic & Endocrine

↑↑ Prolactin, adrenocorticotrophic hormone, cortisol

↓ Growth hormone

↑ Thyroid-binding globulin, T_4 and T_3 (free-T_4 near normal)

↑ Gastrin

Table 37.2 Timing of maternal deaths due to cardiac causes in relation to pregnancy. (UK and Ireland, 2009-2014). (Reproduced with permission from Knight *et al.*, 2016)

Time period of deaths in the pregnancy care pathway	Total (*n* = 153)* (frequency, %)
Antenatal period/still pregnant	24 (15)
Postnatal on day of delivery	32 (21)
Postnatal 1–42 days after delivery	52 (34)
Postnatal 43–91 days after delivery	18 (12)
Postnatal 92–182 days after delivery	12 (8)
Postnatal 183–273 days after delivery	9 (6)
Postnatal 274–364 days after delivery	6 (4)

* Excludes 36 late cardiac deaths for which no information was available.

suggestive of cardiorespiratory compromise should focus on making a diagnosis, rather than simply excluding a life-threatening diagnosis. In such circumstances, pregnancy or breast-feeding should not be the reason for failing to instigate potentially life-saving investigations or treatment.

Physiological Changes of Pregnancy

A number of the normal physiological changes cause exacerbation of coexisting cardiac disease (Box 37.1). The most significant changes are a 40% increase in intravascular volume by 32 weeks and a 40% increase in the CO. The CO increases further during labour and reaches its maximum immediately after delivery due to autotransfusion from the uterus and removal of the aortocaval compression by the foetus. These changes can lead to decompensation around the time of delivery and immediately afterwards.

Twenty-one per cent of maternal deaths occur on the day of delivery, while more than half of total maternal deaths due to cardiac causes occur during the period of the day of delivery to 42 days after delivery (Table 37.2).

Labour and Caesarean Section

Pregnant mothers with known and significant cardiac disease are at extremely high risk of dying and should be managed in a tertiary obstetric unit with on-site specialist cardiology and cardiac surgery services. These patients should receive specialist antenatal care from both obstetricians and cardiologists, ideally in a joint clinic. Plans for delivery should be discussed and jointly agreed upon by the multidisciplinary specialists – obstetricians, cardiologists, anaesthetists, haematologists and, potentially, cardiac surgeons. All reviews and plans should be communicated between specialists and clearly documented in the patient's hand-held notes.

Patients with milder cardiac disease may be allowed to continue their pregnancy until term and, if there are no signs and symptoms of deteriorating cardiac function, a normal vaginal delivery may be considered. Effective analgesia during labour is critical and epidural analgesia early in labour is recommended to alleviate the stress response during labour and delivery. A short second stage of labour is preferable. Blood loss following delivery must be managed aggressively, as severe haemorrhage will impose a further strain to an already compromised cardio-respiratory system.

A deterioration in cardiac function during pregnancy or another non-cardiac foeto-maternal problem may prompt earlier delivery by Caesarean section. Regional anaesthesia can be safely used for the majority of patients with cardiac disease undergoing Caesarean section when adequate assessment and monitoring has been undertaken. A combined spinal and epidural technique allows a gradual onset of block, with haemodynamic changes that are less pronounced than those associated with central neuroaxial blockade. Invasive BP monitoring is essential in perioperative management. Central venous access should be considered if vasopressor and inotropic support is anticipated.

In patients with poor cardiac function, inadvertent 'off-loading' of the heart, resulting from modest blood loss during Caesarean section, reduces the volume of autotransfusion that follows delivery and may be beneficial. Excessive haemorrhage leading to severe anaemia, hypovolaemia and spiralling coagulopathy is not usually tolerated and must be avoided.

Uterotonics commonly used in the peripartum period (e.g. oxytocin) may have profound, undesirable haemodynamic consequences in parturients with cardiac disease and should be used with caution. Avoiding uterotonics altogether risks the development of uterine atony, which may lead to continued bleeding.

Synthetic oxytocin is commonly used as a uterotonic agent following delivery. It stimulates uterine contraction and reduces post-partum haemorrhage from atony. Its use in Caesarean section is routine. Bolus administration will result in tachycardia, hypotension and a reduced CO. However, when given as an infusion, such effects can be minimized.

Ergometrine is an ergot alkaloid, which stimulates contraction of uterine and vascular smooth muscle. It is a second-line uterotonic, and is contraindicated in patients with eclampsia, pre-eclampsia, hypertension, cardiovascular and peripheral vascular disease. It can cause severe coronary artery vasoconstriction and myocardial ischaemia, and its use is associated with deaths of women with artherosclerotic coronary disease. It is present in Syntometrine®, which contains both synthetic oxytocin and ergometrine.

Carboprost is a synthetic analogue of prostaglandin $F_{2\alpha}$, with uterotonic properties. It is used for severe post-partum haemorrhage that is unresponsive to oxytocin and ergometrine. It causes smooth-muscle vasoconstriction and is contraindicated in patients with cardiac or respiratory disease.

Cardiac Surgery

Most cardiac disease in pregnant women can be managed without interventional procedures. However, the burden of haemodynamic changes in pregnancy may result in the deterioration of cardiac function and necessitate intervention. Indications for intervention can be broadly classified into the deterioration of a known cardiac condition during pregnancy (e.g. progressive aortic root dilatation in Marfan syndrome), deterioration of an undiagnosed cardiac condition before pregnancy (e.g. MS) or a new diagnosis (e.g. endocarditis, prosthetic valve thrombosis, type A aortic dissection).

Maternal mortality associated with CPB is relatively high (6%) but is comparable to that in the non-pregnant woman who undergoes a similar cardiac procedure. This is likely to be due to the urgent or emergency nature of such procedures. By contrast, the risks of foetal mortality (14–33%) and morbidity (including late neurological impairment) are significant. For this reason, cardiac surgery is only recommended for those who fail to respond to medical therapy or interventional procedures when cardiac disease is a threat to the maternal life.

The best period for cardiac surgery in pregnant women is between the 13th and 28th weeks of gestation. Surgery during the first trimester carries a higher risk of foetal malformation and, during the third trimester, there is a high incidence of pre-term delivery and maternal complications. At 26 weeks' gestation, foetal survival is generally ~80%, albeit with 20% having serious neurological impairment. Caesarean section before CPB may be considered if gestational age is >26 weeks. When gestational age >28 weeks, delivery before cardiac surgery should be considered. Prior to cardiac surgery, a full course of corticosteroids (at least 24 hours) should be administered to the mother to reduce the risk of neonatal mortality and morbidity.

MV disease is the commonest indication for cardiac surgery during pregnancy. The underlying pathology is usually stenosis secondary to chronic rheumatic heart disease, which although rare in developed countries, is still prevalent as a result of population migration. The symptoms of regurgitant lesions in pregnancy are often improved by the physiological reduction in the SVR. The symptoms of stenotic lesions, however, are worsened by the combination of an increased heart rate, circulating volume and CO. MS is not well tolerated during pregnancy and pre-pregnancy intervention is recommended when the valve orifice area is less than 1.5 cm^2. In such cases, the first intervention usually considered is percutaneous balloon valvotomy, which has a lower complication rate than open valve surgery. A significant number of these patients will, however, require subsequent valve replacement.

AS in women of child-bearing age is usually congenital in origin and places patients at an increased risk of both cardiac and obstetric complications. In the setting of haemodynamic deterioration that fails to respond to optimal medical therapy, balloon valvuloplasty may be a suitable option, providing a bridge to surgery after delivery. AV replacement may be unavoidable in some cases.

Patients who have previously undergone cardiac valve replacement present a multitude of problems. Biological prosthetic valves have accelerated deterioration necessitating early reoperation. Mechanical valves are associated with a high risk of maternal complications (e.g. valve thrombosis during pregnancy) and foetal abnormality secondary to warfarin therapy.

Progressive aortic dilatation and aortic dissection occurs mainly in women with connective tissue disease and bicuspid AV. The current recommendation is to consider prophylactic aortic surgery when aortic diameter is ≥50 mm, and increasing rapidly during pregnancy. When aortic dissection occurs, immediate surgery should be performed, and if the foetus is viable, consideration given to performing a Caesarean section immediately prior to cardiac surgery.

Anaesthetic Management

All women at more than 20 weeks pregnancy should be placed in a left lateral tilt to minimize the impact of aortocaval compression. As with all cardiac cases, invasive monitoring is best instituted before the induction of anaesthesia. TOE provides a better assessment of LV filling than CVP monitoring. The anaesthetist must be able to differentiate the normal TOE findings in the late stages of pregnancy (e.g. cardiac chamber enlargement, annular dilatation and valvular regurgitation) from pathological findings. The PAP is significantly overestimated when measured using TOE compared to values obtained at cardiac catheterization.

Many anaesthetic drugs and opioids readily cross the placenta and cause foetal depression and bradycardia. Although there is little evidence to suggest that any one drug is superior to another, propofol, thiopental, isoflurane, fentanyl and morphine have all been used safely for many years in obstetric anaesthesia. Non-depolarizing muscle relaxants are unable to cross the placenta. Both unfractionated and low-molecular-weight heparins do not cross the placenta and are non-teratogenic. In contrast, warfarin does cross the placenta and is teratogenic in the first trimester of pregnancy.

Cardiopulmonary Bypass

Foetal death during CPB is thought to be due to sustained uterine contractions resulting in uteroplacental hypoperfusion and foetal hypoxia. Triggers for uterine contractions include haemodilution, dilution of progesterone, non-pulsative blood flow, cooling and rewarming. Reduction in the maternal BP also causes a reduction in uteroplacental flow. Cardiotocography findings such as foetal bradycardia, reduced heart rate variability and late decelerations are all indicators of foetal hypoxia. It is therefore important to monitor the foetal HR throughout CPB.

The following strategies are thought to improve foetal outcome during CPB:

- Pump flow rate $> 2.5 \ l \ min^{-1} \ m^{-2}$
- Perfusion pressure > 70 mmHg
- Haematocrit $> 28\%$ to optimize O_2 carrying capacity
- Normothermia
- Pulsatile pump flow
- α-Stat blood-gas management
- Minimal CPB time

Key Points

- Cardiac disease is the leading indirect cause of maternal death in the UK.
- An increase in the average age of parturients is associated with an increase in the prevalence of pregnancy-associated cardiac disease.
- Decompensation is most likely to occur during and immediately after delivery.
- Cardiac surgery during pregnancy is sometimes unavoidable and is associated with significant morbidity and mortality.
- Whenever possible, cardiac surgery should be delayed until after delivery of a viable foetus.

Further Reading

Chandrasekhar S, Cook CR, Collard CD. Cardiac surgery in the parturient. *Anesth Analg* 2009; 108: 777–85.

Knight M, Nair M, Tuffnell D, *et al.* (eds.) on behalf of MBRRACE-UK. Saving Lives, Improving Mothers' Care – Surveillance of maternal deaths in the UK 2012–14 and lessons learned to inform maternity care from the UK and Ireland Confidential Enquiries into Maternal Deaths and Morbidity

2009–14. Oxford: National Perinatal Epidemiology Unit, University of Oxford; 2016. www.npeu.ox.ac.uk/downloads/files/mbrrace-uk/reports/MBRRACE-UK%20Maternal%20Report%202016%20-%20website.pdf

Pieper PG, Hoendermis ES, Drijver YN. Cardiac surgery and percutaneous intervention in pregnant women with heart disease. *Neth Heart J* 2012; 20: 125–8.

Regitz-Zagrosek V, Roos-Hesselink JW, Bauersachs J, *et al.* 2018 ESC

guidelines for the management of cardiovascular diseases during pregnancy. *Eur Heart J* 2018; 39: 3165–241.

Salaunkey K. Pregnancy and cardiovascular disorders. In Valchanov K, Jones N, Hogue CW (eds), *Core Topics in Cardiothoracic Critical Care*, 2nd edn. Cambridge: Cambridge University Press; 2018, pp. 408–17.

Yuan SM. Infective endocarditis during pregnancy. *J Coll Physicians Surg Pak* 2015; 25: 134–9.

Regional Anaesthesia

Trevor W. R. Lee

Cardiac surgery induces profound sympathetic nervous system and inflammatory responses. This so-called 'stress response' to surgery causes a multitude of adverse haemodynamic, metabolic, haematological, endocrine and immunological effects. In the setting of cardiac surgery, the attenuation of pain and sympathetic autonomic activity has many theoretical attractions. The introduction of high-dose opioid techniques into cardiac anaesthesia was based, in part, on the belief that they would inhibit the stress response. Failure to block the stress response completely, combined with equivocal evidence of clinical benefit and the need for prolonged postoperative mechanical ventilation, made the technique unpopular. The demonstration that thoracic sympathetic blockade improves the blood flow in severely diseased coronary arteries, the emergence of less invasive cardiac surgical techniques and economic pressures have prompted renewed interest in regional anaesthetic techniques.

Thoracic Epidural Anaesthesia

The first report of thoracic epidural anaesthesia (TEA) for analgesia *after* cardiac surgery appeared in 1976. It was not until 1987, however, that the first report of TEA *before* cardiac surgery was published. In most published series the interspaces between C_7 and T_1 and T_3 and T_4 have been used for TEA. The higher approaches are technically easier, although it should be borne in mind that the ligamentum flavum in the thoracic region is thinner and more delicate than in the lumbar region. Most practitioners use a midline approach, with the conscious patient sitting or lying. The method used to identify the epidural space varies. The avoidance of the 'asleep' epidural in this setting is more a function of retaining the ability to assess the efficacy of the block *before* induction of anaesthesia than a response to concerns about medicolegal implications of neurological injury.

Typical initial doses include 3 ml lidocaine 2% and 5 ml levobupivacaine 0.5% with or without fentanyl ~25 µg. repeated after 10 minutes, as necessary. Regardless of the epidural infusion regimen used, it is imperative that a bilateral T_1–T_5 dermatome block is achieved before proceeding. A continuous epidural infusion (e.g. levobupivacaine ~0.125% + fentanyl 1–5 µg ml^{-1} ± clonidine 0.5 µg ml^{-1} at a rate of 4–10 ml h^{-1}) is then started during surgery and usually continued for up to 3 days. The synergy between agents of different classes (i.e. opioids and local anaesthetics) permits the total dose and side effects of each to be reduced. Regular input from an acute pain management team maximizes epidural efficacy and allows early detection of adverse events. The 'pros' and 'cons' of TEA in cardiac surgery are shown in Box 38.1.

TEA is almost invariably used as an adjunct to general anaesthetic techniques, tailored to permit early recovery and neurological assessment. Recently some centres have been assessing the feasibility of using TEA alone in beating heart surgery. Apart from showing that *it is possible* to rise to this fresh challenge and the associated publicity, it is difficult to think of any other reason why anyone would want to routinely perform cardiac surgery on awake patients. The additional anxiety for both patients and staff is unnecessary, spontaneous respiration with open pleurae is physiologically undesirable, respiratory depression due to paralysis of the diaphragm or thoracic musculature may occur and TOE is impossible. Common sense suggests that the goals of anaesthesia for cardiac surgery should include the prevention of unanticipated patient movement during surgery.

The insertion of an epidural catheter prior to full anticoagulation is considered less taboo than in the past. Emerging evidence suggests that those most likely to benefit are patients with borderline pulmonary function, opioid addicts and patients likely to be

Box 38.1 The 'pros' and 'cons' of TEA and analgesia in cardiac surgery

Cardiac sympathetic blockade

Pro   Unmyelinated sympathetic neurones very sensitive to local anaesthetics

Blockade of sympathetic neurones from T_1 to T_5

Dilatation of severely diseased coronary arteries

↓ Incidence of postoperative arrhythmias

↑ Myocardial contractility - remains unproven

Con   Risk of hypotension

May inhibit sympathetic vasodilatation in normal coronary arteries

Attenuation of stress response

Pro   Local anaesthetics superior to epidural opioids alone

Attenuation of ↑ circulating catecholamine levels

BP and HR response to surgery blunted

Less effect on secondary metabolic, immune and haematological responses

Con   Unequivocal evidence of stress response attenuation difficult to obtain

Analgesia

Pro   Intense intraoperative and postoperative analgesia

Avoids adverse effects of parenteral narcotic analgesics

Early tracheal extubation and mobilization

Improved postoperative pulmonary function

Possible ↓ incidence of chronic pain syndromes

Con   Unilateral block or missed segments render technique ineffective

Motor and proprioception block may limit mobilization

---

incompletely revascularized by surgery. Recently published prospective studies suggest that TEA is associated with a lower incidence of postoperative respiratory tract infection, supraventricular dysrhythmias and renal dysfunction. No study yet published has had sufficient power to demonstrate any statistically significant reduction in perioperative mortality. Double-blind studies of TEA, with placement of a 'non-therapeutic' epidural catheter in control group patients, have not been undertaken.

Spinal Anaesthesia

The first report of spinal anaesthesia in cardiac surgery was published in 1980. In this report, as in the vast majority of subsequent publications, the agent used was preservative-free morphine sulphate. The potential benefits of spinal anaesthesia in cardiac surgery are the same as those for TEA, although the risk of epidural haematoma is probably less. Unlike TEA, however, spinal anaesthetic techniques in this setting have tended to be 'single shot' and opioid-based. The limited duration of drug action dictates that lumbar

puncture has to be performed shortly before heparinization. The major safety concerns, therefore, are respiratory depression and neuraxial bleeding, although pruritus, nausea, vomiting and urinary retention are usually more troublesome. The low lipid solubility of morphine results in the delayed onset of analgesia and unpredictable effects. Although some investigators have demonstrated superior postoperative analgesia, others have reported either no benefit or delayed recovery. This may explain the failure of intrathecal morphine to attenuate the stress response to surgery.

In contrast, published investigations of intrathecal local anaesthesia in cardiac surgery are scarce. In a retrospective study published in 1994, Kowalewski *et al.* reported that the combination of hyperbaric bupivacaine (30 mg) and morphine (0.5–1.0 mg) produced excellent postoperative analgesia compatible with early (same-day) tracheal extubation. Lee *et al.* demonstrated that general anaesthesia combined with intrathecal bupivacaine (37.5 mg) resulted in the significant attenuation of the stress response and improved the LV segmental wall motion (Box 38.2).

Box 38.2 Technique used for delivering a high or total-spinal anaesthesia (adapted from Lee *et al*, 2008)

- Patient pre-medicated with oral diazepam (0.1 mg kg^{-1}) or oral gabapentin (1.5 mg kg^{-1})
- IV volume repletion and loading accomplished with crystalloid 500 ml
- Lumbar spine is prepared and draped with the patient in the lateral decubitus position
- 25-gauge pencil point spinal needle is used to administer the intrathecal blockade
- Single-shot dose of 37.5–45 mg of hyperbaric bupivacaine 0.75%, in combination with 2–3 µg kg^{-1} (maximum total dose 300 µg) of preservative free spinal morphine injected into intrathecal space. Bevel of the spinal needle facing cephalad during injection may maximize local anaesthetic spread
- Operating table placed in <5° Trendelenburg, with the patient in supine position. A C8 or higher sensory block can take ~10 minutes to develop
- Small doses of IV phenylephrine and ephedrine are used to maintain a MAP of >65 mmHg
- General anaesthesia induced, after complete cardiac sympathectomy achieved, using IV propofol 0.5–1.0 mg kg^{-1} and rocuronium 0.6–1.0 mg kg^{-1}. IV narcotics may not be required for maintenance
- To ensure amnesia and hypnosis, general anaesthesia must be maintained at a minimum of 0.5–1.0 MAC
- Prior to chest closure, adjunctive analgesia can be provided using bilateral parasternal blocks
- Prior to emergence, the patient is given IV morphine or IV hydromorphone to achieve an RR between 15 and 20 bpm
- Trachea extubated in operating room immediately after procedure

When compared to patients who had a 'sham spinal', study patients had significantly lower serum levels of epinephrine, norepinephrine and cortisol, and a significantly enhanced preservation of atrial β-adrenoceptor function. Unfamiliarity with the technique and the perception of haemodynamic instability may limit the widespread adoption of high-dose intrathecal bupivacaine and intrathecal morphine by cardiac anaesthetists. Although haemodynamic instability is cited as one of the major risks of high spinal anaesthesia, the physiological responses to total sympathectomy can be managed with small, titrated doses of IV vasoconstrictors.

Lee *et al.* examined the impact of high spinal anaesthesia on the perioperative inflammatory response in 2016 (Figure 38.1). Patients receiving high spinal anaesthesia in addition to general anaesthesia, compared to general anaesthesia alone, had significantly increased anti-inflammatory biomarker serum concentrations (interleukin-10). This small study suggests that patients exposed to high spinal anaesthesia during cardiac surgery may obtain an incremental benefit up to 28 days after surgery.

Other clinical impacts of high regional anaesthesia for cardiac surgery may also include a reduction in postoperative delirium. In a retrospective, propensity-matched study, Petropolis *et al.* found that the incidence of postoperative delirium was significantly decreased in patients receiving high spinal anaesthesia when compared to controls.

High Spinal Anaesthesia and Organ Donor Harvest

In an animal model of donor organ harvest, Almoustadi *et al.* examined the effects of regional anaesthesia for cardiac surgery after brainstem death. Total spinal anaesthesia as a supplement to general anaesthesia in a large-animal model of heart donation after brainstem death resulted in reduced catecholamine release and improved cardiac function of the donor animal. Since haemodynamic collapse is often observed after brainstem death in humans, it is intriguing to consider that perhaps the administration of high spinal anaesthesia prior to organ harvest may be of some future benefit to donor organ functional preservation.

Risk of Neuraxial Bleeding

There is little doubt that the uptake of neuraxial techniques in cardiac anaesthetic practice has been slowed by 'the ill-defined risk of permanent paraplegia in a fully anticoagulated, unconscious patient'. For this reason, TEA and spinal anaesthesia remain in the hands of enthusiasts. Questions commonly asked by anaesthetists include those shown in Box 38.3.

It can be deduced from this list that the risks of neuraxial bleeding, epidural haematoma and permanent neurological injury are foremost in anaesthetists' minds. The absence of reported complications in relatively small prospective series (i.e. <1,000 patients) gives little cause for comfort – the so-called 'zero numerator' problem. While estimates vary from

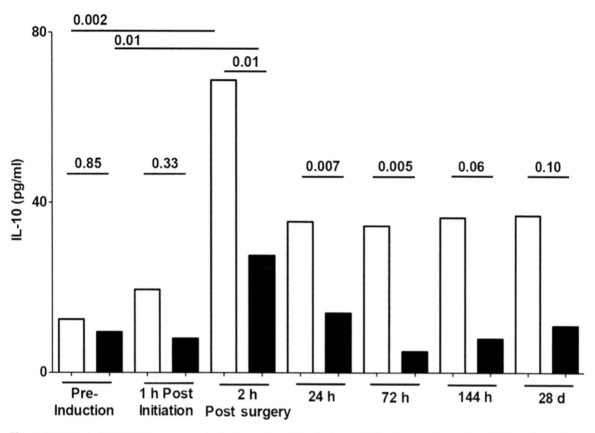

Figure 38.1 Interleukin-10 (IL-10) responses of patients receiving high spinal anaesthesia with general anaesthesia. Median values and P values are shown. High spinal plus general anaesthesia patients (open bars) versus general anaesthesia alone (solid bars) are shown. From Lee *et al*, *PLoS One* 2016; 11(3): e0149942.

Box 38.3 Questions frequently asked about the use of epidural anaesthesia in cardiac surgery

1. What is the incidence of epidural-associated spinal haematoma?
2. Do normal laboratory coagulation test results give comfort that clotting is normal?
3. Do antiplatelet agents increase the risk of spinal haematoma?
4. How should patients taking oral anticoagulants be managed?
5. What is the safest epidural insertion–heparin administration interval?
6. What is the appropriate response to a 'bloody tap' or 'dural tap'?
7. Is there an 'ideal' intervertebral space for epidural placement?
8. Does TEA make any difference to patient outcome?

1:1,500 to 1:150,000, data from neurologists and closed medicolegal claims analysis may provide a more accurate measure of the true incidence of epidural haematoma. In the context of the major risks of cardiac surgery (i.e. death and stroke), the risk of epidural-related paraplegia is very small.

In calculating the predicted risk, Ho *et al.* used existing published data to estimate the minimum and maximum risk of haematoma formation following instrumentation for cardiac surgery. The incidence of a clinically significant spinal haematoma was estimated to be between 1:3,600 and 1:220,000 after spinal anaesthesia and between 1:1,500 and 1:150,000 after TEA for cardiac surgery. In 2018, Horlocker *et al.* published guidelines on the use of neuraxial techniques in patients receiving antiplatelet agents and low-molecular-weight heparin (LMWH). Current recommendations suggest the avoidance of regional anaesthesia if potent

Table 38.1 Summary recommendations for the cessation of novel oral anticoagulants prior to neuraxial anaesthesia

Drug	Mechanism of action	Hold dose prior to block (days)
Clopidogrel	ADP receptor inhibitor	7
Ticlopidine	ADP receptor inhibitor	10
Ticagrelor	ADP receptor inhibitor	5–7
Rivaroxaban	Factor Xa inhibitor	3
Apixaban	Factor Xa inhibitor	3
Dabigatran	Direct thrombin inhibitor	5

antiplatelet drugs (e.g. thienopyridine derivatives) have been used within 7 days in the case of clopidogrel, or 10–14 days in the case of ticlopidine. Neuraxial anaesthesia is contraindicated in fully anticoagulated patients. In the event of a 'bloody tap', it is recommended that the institution of therapeutic heparinization be delayed by at least 1 hour, in order to reduce the relative risk of subsequent complications. Since 2010, with the introduction of new platelet adenosine diphosphate P_2Y_{12} inhibitors (e.g. ticagrelor), factor Xa inhibitors (e.g. rivaroxaban and apixaban) and direct thrombin inhibitors (e.g. dabigatran), perioperative management of antiplatelet therapy has become more complex. Table 38.1 summarizes current recommendations.

The greater risk of haematoma formation following TEA may explain the preference for spinal anaesthesia and analgesia for cardiac surgery in some institutions. The use of small-gauge needles and the avoidance of catheter insertion/removal are believed to reduce the risk of epidural haematoma after spinal anaesthesia.

Patient refusal, local or systemic infection, decompensated AS and coagulopathy are regarded as absolute contraindications to neuraxial blockade. In practice, coagulopathy means a platelet count of $<100 \times 10^9 \, l^{-1}$, an INR of >1.2 or an APTT of >45 seconds. Most patients undergoing elective cardiac surgery will be asked to discontinue aspirin and other antiplatelet agents 5–10 days before surgery. The magnitude of any additional epidural-related risk, directly attributable to concurrent antiplatelet therapy, is unknown. Oral anticoagulation should be stopped 3–4 days before surgery and normalization of the INR confirmed. Patients who cannot have their oral anticoagulation safely withdrawn before surgery should not have TEA. Opinion regarding the minimum safe interval between epidural catheter insertion and the administration of unfractionated heparin varies from 1 to 12 hours.

The optimal management of a bloody tap is unknown. Practices vary from the extreme; abandoning TEA and postponing surgery for 24 hours, to re-siting the epidural and continuing with the surgical procedure. The latter approach is based on the belief that blood clots in 10–12 minutes and that heparin is not thrombolytic. Due to the theoretical risk of bleeding following removal of the epidural catheter, this is usually performed after normalization of coagulation has been confirmed by laboratory tests. In patients receiving unfractionated heparin, the epidural catheter is typically removed not less than 4 hours after discontinuing the infusion or 1 hour before any dose of LMWH. In some centres, the institution of oral anticoagulation is delayed until after the epidural catheter has been removed.

The neurological sequelae that may accompany a spinal haematoma range from vague sensory and motor symptoms to dense paraplegia or even quadriplegia. The presence and extent of any neurological deficit may only be apparent after discontinuation of the block and removal of the epidural catheter. If there is any doubt, CT or MRI must be undertaken urgently and neurosurgical advice sought. Failure to make the diagnosis and institute management will rightly draw criticism.

Parasternal and Paravertebral Blockade

Although used routinely in some centres, parasternal blockade following cardiac surgery is poorly represented in the literature. Prior to skin closure, preservative free isobaric bupivacaine 0.25% with or without epinephrine (total volume 40–50 ml) is injected along the sternal borders, deep to the posterior intercostal membrane, to block the anterior cutaneous branches of the intercostal nerves for 6–10 hours. The technique may be considered in the patient with abnormal coagulation.

Paravertebral blockade is most commonly used to provide analgesia during and after thoracic surgery. Paravertebral blockade for cardiac surgery is used far less frequently. The paravertebral space lies just anterior to the parietal pleural of the lung, and posterior to the intercostal intimus muscle. Small-bore catheters are usually placed percutaneously, by 'walking' a large-bore epidural needle off the superior aspect of the transverse process of the thoracic vertebra (T_3–T_5). As with TEA, a 'loss of resistance' technique is used to identify the paravertebral space. Boluses of local anaesthetic (e.g. 5–10 ml bupivacaine 0.5%) are followed by an infusion (e.g. 6–8 ml h^{-1} bupivacaine 0.1%). A unilateral approach may be used for minimally invasive cardiac surgery via anterior short thoracotomy. Although continuous paravertebral blockade provides good analgesia and facilitates early tracheal extubation, difficulty in identifying and catheterizing the paravertebral space and a definite failure rate limit its applicability.

Key Points

- Cardiac sympathetic blockade, profound postoperative analgesia and attenuation of the stress response and alteration of the inflammatory response *may* improve patient outcome.

- The use of regional anaesthesia as a supplement to general anaesthesia for cardiac surgery may reduce postoperative delirium.

- The emergence of less invasive cardiac surgical procedures has prompted renewed interest in regional techniques.

- Although no longer taboo, the ill-defined risk of paraplegia in unconscious anticoagulated patients has deterred the majority of anaesthetists from using TEA in cardiac surgical patients.

- The optimal management strategy for the 'bloody tap' is unknown.

- Prospective, randomized, multicentre studies are required to demonstrate that TEA or spinal anaesthesia are superior to combined α and β adrenergic blockade.

Further Reading

Almoustadi WA, Lee TW, Klein J, *et al.* The effect of total spinal anesthesia on cardiac function in a large animal model of brain death. *Can J Physiol Pharmacol* 2012; 90: 1287–93.

Benzon HT, Avram MJ, Green D, Bonow RO. New oral anticoagulants and regional anaesthesia. *Br J Anaesth* 2013;111(Suppl 1): 196–113.

Cantó M, Sánchez MJ, Casas MA, Bataller ML. Bilateral paravertebral blockade for conventional cardiac surgery. *Anaesthesia* 2003; 58: 365–70.

Chaney MA. Intrathecal and epidural anesthesia and analgesia for cardiac surgery. *Anesth Analg* 2006; 102: 45–64.

Ho AM, Chung DC, Joynt GM. Neuraxial blockade and hematoma in cardiac surgery: estimating the risk of a rare adverse event that has not (yet) occurred. *Chest* 2000; 117: 551–5.

Horlocker TT, Vandermeulen E, Kopp SL, *et al.* Regional anesthesia in the patient receiving antithrombotic or thrombolytic therapy: American Society of Regional Anesthesia and Pain Medicine evidence-based guidelines (fourth edition). *Reg Anesth Pain Med* 2018; 43: 263–309.

Kowalewski RJ, MacAdams CL, Eagle CJ, Archer DP, Bharadwaj B. Anaesthesia for coronary artery bypass surgery supplemented with subarachnoid bupivacaine and morphine: a report of 18 cases. *Can J Anaesth* 1994; 41: 1189–95.

Lee TW, Kowalski S, Falk K, *et al.* High spinal anesthesia enhances anti-inflammatory responses in patients undergoing coronary artery bypass graft surgery and aortic valve replacement: randomized pilot study. *PLoS One* 2016; 11: e0149942.

Lee TWR, Jacobsohn E. Spinal anesthesia in cardiac surgery. *Tech Reg Anesth Pain Manag* 2008;12: 54–6.

Petropolis A, Maguire D, Grocott H, *et al.* High Spinal Anesthesia and Delirium Incidence After Cardiac Surgery. CCCF ePoster library. Oct 27, 2015; 117369. https://cccf.multilearning.com/cccf/2015/eposter/117369/andrea.petropolis.high.spinal.anesthesia.and.delirium.incidence.after.cardiac.html (accessed December 2018).

Svircevic V, van Dijk D, Nierich AP, *et al.* Meta-analysis of thoracic epidural anesthesia versus general anesthesia for cardiac surgery. *Anesthesiology* 2011; 114: 271–82.

Tabatabaie O, Matin N, Heidari A, *et al.* Spinal anesthesia reduces postoperative delirium in opium dependent patients undergoing coronary artery bypass grafting. *Acta Anaesthesiol Belg* 2015; 66: 49–54.

Chapter 39

Pain Management after Cardiac Surgery

Siân I. Jaggar and Helen C. Laycock

Introduction

Pain after cardiac surgery is common; 75% of patients recall experiencing moderate to severe pain on the cardiac ICU. This has significant physiological and psychological consequences, potentially leading to chronic pain, affecting up to 50% of patients. Adequate treatment is essential to recovery.

Basic Pain Physiology

Pain is 'an unpleasant sensory and emotional experience associated with actual or potential tissue damage or described in terms of such' (Association for the Study of Pain Taxonomy). It is an integrated process of peripheral and central events. Modulation and interpretation produce individual reactions, giving meaning to the stimulus–response relationship.

Nociceptors, peripheral projections of primary sensory neurones, are sensitive to physical and chemical stimuli, including heat and acid. These directly activate neuronal ion channels resulting in an action potential (AP). Additionally, inflammatory mediators produced following surgery indirectly sensitize nociceptors to subsequent stimuli, by reducing the AP generation threshold.

First-order neurones transmit APs to the dorsal horn (DH) of the spinal cord via:

- $A\beta$ fibres – conducting touch
- $A\delta$ fibres – causing sharp localized pain
- C fibres – producing dull, poorly localized pain

The majority of second-order neurones, transmitting impulses from the DH to the mid-brain, decussate before ascending spinothalamic pathways. Mid-brain fibres project to the sensory cortex where pain perception occurs. This is modulated by past experience and the balance between noxious and inhibitory impulses within the CNS and spinal cord. Pathological changes here are likely responsible for the development of chronic pain.

Causes of Pain Following Cardiac Surgery

Routine cardiac surgery produces a combination of somatic, visceral and neuropathic pain (Box 39.1):

Somatic pain: Superficial or deep, arising from skin, muscle and bone. Stimulating dermal nerve endings causes sharp, well-localized *superficial pain*. In contrast, *deep pain*, from muscles, is dull and poorly localized.

Visceral pain: From deep, internal tissues. Typically, diffuse and poorly localized pain, associated with autonomic disturbances (e.g. nausea, sweating). Afferents travel alongside autonomic projections; spinal-level convergence leads to referred pain in dermatomes of shared embryonic origin. Cardiac pathways specifically refer pain to the neck and arm

---

Box 39.1   Types and sources of pain following cardiac surgery

Somatic

Skin incisions

Drain and cannulation sites

Tissue retraction and dissection

Sternal and costal fractures and dislocations

Joint strain (sternoclavicular, acromioclavicular, costovertebral, cervicothoracic zygoapophyseal)

Visceral

Pericardium

Pleura

Myocardium (ischaemia)

Diaphragm

Neurological (from patient positioning, graft harvesting and sternal retraction)

Peripheral nerve injury (e.g. radial, saphenous)

Plexus injury (e.g. brachial)

Table 39.1 Effects of pain following cardiac surgery

System	Disadvantages
Cardiovascular	↑ Chronotropy ↑ Inotropy ↑ BP ↑ Cardiac work ↑ O_2 demand with ↓ supply, → ischaemia, dysrhythmias
Respiratory	↑ RR and ↓ tidal volume → ↑ work of breathing Atelectasis Impaired cough, retention of secretions ↑ Infection risk
CNS	Exhaustion, disorientation, agitation ↓ Satisfaction
Peripheral nervous system	↑ Incidence chronic pain
GI	Nausea, vomiting, anorexia
Other	Hypercoagulability → ↑ risk DVT and graft stenosis Poor wound healing Impaired glucose tolerance Altered immunological function → ↑ risk of infection Electrolyte imbalance → ↑ risk arrhythmias ↑ Length of stay
Psychological	Anxiety Depression Stress

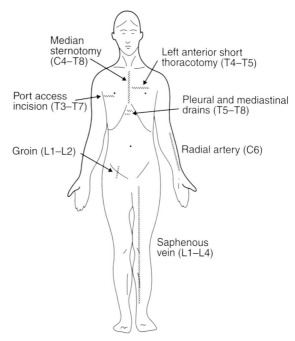

Figure 39.1 Cardiac surgical incisions and corresponding dermatomes

(e.g. vagus nerve, cervical sympathetic and upper five thoracic ganglia).

Neuropathic pain: Consequent upon neuronal tissue lesions (central or peripheral). Often accompanied by positive (e.g. allodynia, hyperalgesia) and/or negative symptoms (including loss of sensation: hypoaesthesia or hypoalgesia).

Common cardiac surgery incisions involve cervical, thoracic and lumbar dermatomes (Figure 39.1). Initially, pain is located within wound and drain sites. Over time it may become more generalized to trunk and limb, particularly following internal mammary artery (IMA) conduits.

The physiological and psychological consequences of pain following cardiac surgery are summarized in Table 39.1.

Acute Pain Management

Virtually all cardiac surgical patients experience pain from surgical incisions, medical devices and invasive procedures. As many have co-morbidities associated with chronic pain (e.g. DM, arthritis, heart failure), these must be considered in analgesic planning before surgery.

Regular pain assessment using validated tools improves patient outcomes, both alerting staff to its presence and allowing evaluation of interventions. Self-assessment tools (including numerical, verbal rating, visual analogue or descriptor scales) represent 'gold standard' pain evaluation, and these can be adapted for non-verbal patients. Those unable to self-report should be assessed with measures validated in ICU patients, such as the critical care pain observation tool.

Acute pain management should include:

Prevention: Attention to patient positioning, choice of incision(s) and operative technique minimizes the risk of postoperative pain. Placing the arms in internal, rather than external, rotation reduces the incidence of shoulder pain. Similarly, bony fractures and excessive sternal retraction, particularly during IMA harvesting, should be avoided. Endoscopic techniques for conduit harvesting may reduce incisional pain.

Patient and caregiver communication: Preoperative discussion regarding expectations and management plans is paramount. Deciding what is achievable and acceptable is especially important in individuals with pre-existing chronic pain; total absence of postoperative pain may be unrealistic. Agreed plans should be documented and communicated to all caregivers, ensuring consistent delivery.

Pharmacological management: Chronic postoperative pain is an emerging research field. It is thought to relate to neuronal plasticity and long-term neurophysiological change following acute pain. Thus, effective acute pain management enhances early comfort and reduces the risk of chronicity.

Moderate to severe nociceptive pain is best managed with opioids. Activation of central and peripheral opioid receptors inhibits release of, and response to, neurotransmitters. Additional benefits are associated with increased vagal tone. Various administration routes are available; however, patient-controlled administration provides better analgesia than nurse-controlled. When titrated intravenously, common drugs (e.g. remifentanil, fentanyl, morphine, oxyco-done) show similar efficacy; therefore, choice is based on patient co-morbidities and side effects. Side effects are often dose-related and can be reduced by titration to effect or choosing a different drug (opioid switching).

A 'multimodal' approach should be considered, using drugs synergistically to facilitate opioid sparing. Paracetamol is relatively safe in most patients. There is currently little place for NSAIDs in the early post-operative period. Their side-effect profile is concerning (risk of GI bleeding and renal insufficiency) and they are associated with an increased risk of death, re-infarction and cardiac failure in certain cardiac populations. Adjuncts for consideration where opioids and paracetamol are insufficient include α-agonists (e.g. clonidine), N-methyl-D-aspartate-receptor antagonists and α2δ ligands (e.g. gabapentin or pregabalin, which decrease acute pain scores and opioid consumption, and pain 3 months after surgery).

Central neuraxial blockade has failed to demonstrate any impact on either morbidity or mortality following cardiac surgery. Whilst meta-analysis of thoracic epidural analgesia suggests decreased postoperative complications, concerns about epidural haematoma formation limit its use. There is little convincing evidence to support wound infiltration or catheter-based regional nerve blocks in cardiac surgery; however, peripheral local anaesthesia may provide immediate postoperative analgesia.

Non-Pharmacological Interventions

These low-cost, simple measures enhance patient comfort more than expected:

- Attention to positioning, care of pressure areas, relieving tension on lines, drains and catheters
- Involving patients by providing information, enabling social interaction with friends/relatives
- Psychological interventions including active relaxation, guided imagery, music
- Physiotherapy reduces de-conditioning- and contracture-associated pain
- Transcutaneous electrical nerve stimulation (TENS) and acupuncture on occasion confer benefit

Whilst some lack an evidence base, they have few side effects and may be an effective adjunct to drug-based therapy.

Chronic Pain Management

Operative site pain persisting for more than 3 months is defined as chronic postoperative pain. The incidence following cardiac surgery approaches 50%, with the most frequent site being the sternum. Other sites include shoulders, back, neck and conduit harvest sites. Multi-site pain is common.

Chronic Sternotomy Pain

This is defined as 'new-onset, non-cardiac pain, of somatic, visceral and/or neuropathic origin after sternotomy'. Younger patients are at greater risk. Causes are multifactorial, resulting from:

- Surgical tissue destruction (e.g. rib fractures, intercostal nerve trauma)
- Scar formation
- Sternal or conduit harvest-site infection
- Presence of sternal wires
- Costochondral separation

Saphenous Neuralgia

Terminal sensory branches of the femoral nerve (L2–L4) supply the anteromedial leg, which is closely related to the great saphenous vein. Nerve continuity may be at risk during surgical procedures. Saphenous neuralgia describes a symptom complex comprising anaesthesia to light touch and pin prick, with hyperaesthesia and pain in the saphenous nerve distribution.

Overwhelming evidence suggests that severe acute postoperative pain is associated with a high incidence of chronic postoperative pain. Risk factors are shown in Box 39.2, although some patients simply seem more susceptible to acute and chronic pain.

Managing a cardiac surgical patient with chronic pain is no different to any chronic pain patient. The principal aims are to:

- Identify the type of pain (i.e. musculoskeletal or neuropathic)
- Exclude possible new diagnoses (e.g. recurrent angina, cervical spondylosis, myeloma)
- Formulate a treatment plan

A careful history should explore the symptoms, impact on the quality of life, exacerbating and relieving factors and the effect of previous therapies. Pharmacological therapy aims to avoid opioids (or minimize dose) and should include psychological support, physiotherapy and graded physical exercise. Adjuvant therapies include local anaesthetic infiltration, nerve blocks (e.g. intercostal), regional techniques (e.g. epidural) and complementary therapies (e.g. TENS, acupuncture).

Chronic Refractory Angina

Up to 10% of patients undergoing coronary angiography will have coronary anatomy that is not amenable to revascularization. Angina occurring despite maximal medical therapy is termed chronic refractory angina (CRA) – a neuropathic pain syndrome. Myocardial ischaemia leads to chronic elevation of sympathetic tone, producing a vicious cycle of myocardial oxygen imbalance and myocardial dystrophy. CRA patients require frequent hospitalization. Interventions include the modification of risk factors and the use of evidence-based stable angina therapies. Novel pharmacological interventions include late sodium current inhibition (ranolazine) and metabolic modulation (trimetazidine). Non-pharmacological therapies include laser revascularization (transmyocardial and percutaneous), high thoracic epidural analgesia and electrical spinal cord stimulation.

Key Points

- Cardiac surgical patients worry about death, disability and postoperative pain.
- An understanding of the pathophysiology of acute and chronic pain allows rational management strategies to be developed.
- Inadequate control of acute pain is associated with increased morbidity and mortality.
- Multimodal approaches to analgesia provide the best results.
- Spinal cord stimulation in CRA may reduce the frequency of hospital readmission and improve the quality of life.

Further Reading

Barr J, Fraser GL, Puntillo K, *et al.* Clinical practice guidelines for the management of pain, agitation, and delirium in adult patients in the intensive care unit. *Crit Care Med* 2013; 41: 263–306.

Gélinas C. Management of pain in cardiac surgery ICU patients: have we improved over time? *Intensive Crit Care Nurs* 2007; 23: 298–303.

Gélinas C, Fillion L, Puntillo KA, Viens C, Fortier M. Validation of the critical-care pain observation tool in adult patients. *Am J Crit Care* 2006; 15: 420–7.

Henry TD, Satran D, Jolicoeur EM. Treatment of refractory angina in patients not suitable for revascularization. *Nat Rev Cardiol* 2014; 11: 78–95.

Holdcroft A, Jaggar S (eds.). *Core Topics in Pain.* Cambridge: Cambridge University Press; 2005.

Lahtinen P, Kokki H, Hynynen M. Pain after cardiac surgery: a prospective cohort study of 1-year incidence and intensity. *Anesthesiology* 2006; 105: 794–800.

Mueller XM, Tinguely F, Tevaearai HT, *et al*. Pain location, distribution, and intensity after cardiac surgery. *Chest* 2000; 118: 391–6.

Reimer-Kent J. From theory to practice: preventing pain after cardiac surgery. *Am J Crit Care* 2003; 12: 136–43.

van Gulik L, Janssen LI, Ahlers SJ, *et al*. Risk factors for chronic thoracic pain after cardiac surgery via sternotomy. *Eur J Cardiothorac Surg* 2011; 40: 1309–13.

Chapter

40

Infection

Hannah McCormick and Judith A. Troughton

Knowledge of infections encountered in the setting of cardiac surgery, and their prevention and treatment, is essential for health professionals working in this area.

Endocarditis

The incidence ranges from three to seven cases per 100,000-person years. Recognized risk factors include age, pre-existing structural heart disease, prosthetic valves or devices and a history of endocarditis, with intravascular catheters or IV drug misuse also acknowledged.

Endocarditis may present acutely or indolently. Common features include fever and a new murmur.

Duke criteria (Box 40.1) are a useful method by which to attribute a likelihood of endocarditis.

Empirical regimens are based on the likely causative organisms (Box 40.2) and patient-specific factors such as colonization with resistant organisms. Antimicrobial treatment of endocarditis varies according to the pathogen, therefore culture is essential. Serological testing may be helpful for organisms which cannot be cultured (e.g. *Bartonella* species, *Coxiella burnetii* and *Brucella* species). If a causative organism

---

Box 40.1 Modified Duke criteria

Major
- Positive blood cultures:

  Two positive cultures with typical pathogen taken more than 12 hours apart, or majority of three or four taken less than 1 hour apart

- Single positive blood culture for *Coxiella burnetii* or anti-phase 1 immunoglobulin G titre >1,800
- Positive echocardiogram findings:

  Oscillating intracardiac mass on valve or supporting structures, in the path of regurgitant jets, or on implanted material in the absence of an alternative anatomic explanation

  Abscess

  A new partial dehiscence of prosthetic valve or new valvular regurgitation

  (TOE advised in patients with prosthetic valves)

- Evidence of endocardial involvement

Minor
- Predisposing factor
- Fever
- Positive blood culture that does not meet major criteria or serological evidence of infection
- Vascular phenomena:

  Embolic phenomena (arterial, pulmonary), conjunctival haemorrhage, Janeway lesions, mycotic aneurysm, intracranial haemorrhage

- Immunological phenomena:

  Glomerulonephritis, Osler's nodes, Roth spots, positive rheumatoid factor

Clinical diagnosis: Two major criteria, or one major criterion plus three minor criteria, or five minor criteria.

> **Box 40.2   Aetiology of endocarditis**
>
> *Streptococcus* spp.
> *Staphylococcus aureus*
> *Enterococcus* spp.
> Coagulase negative staphylococci
> HACEK (*Haemophilus* spp., *Aggregatibacter* spp.,
> *Cardiobacterium hominis, Eikenella corrodens,
> Kingella* spp.)
> Culture negative
> Fungi
> Polymicrobial
> Other

is not identified, antibiotic management is determined by epidemiological and risk factors that are specific to the individual patient; *16s* ribosomal RNA analysis of the tissue that is subsequently excised may be helpful.

Mycobacterium chimaera has recently been recognized as a cause of endocarditis amongst patients who have undergone open heart surgery. This organism is not detected by routine culture methods; therefore, specialist advice should be sought for patients with culture-negative prosthetic-valve endocarditis or endovascular graft infection.

The treatment duration for native-valve endocarditis varies from 2 weeks to 8 weeks, depending on the causative organism, and a minimum of 6 weeks for prosthetic-valve endocarditis.

A surgical consultation is advised for fungal infection, resistant organisms, prolonged bacteraemia, embolic events and left heart Gram-negative endocarditis. If surgery is performed during treatment, the duration of treatment does not change unless either an abscess is found or valve cultures are positive, in which case the day of surgery is counted as day one of treatment.

Guidelines on the management of endocarditis (American Heart Association 2015; European Society of Cardiology 2015) recommend a multidisciplinary team approach to treat patients with endocarditis, reflecting the many complications associated with this condition.

Prophylaxis against Endocarditis

Opinion is divided regarding the need for prophylaxis against infective endocarditis. NICE guidance (2008, updated July 2016) advises that prophylaxis is no

longer required for high-risk procedures and only needed if a surgical procedure is being carried out in an infected site. Several studies have suggested an increase in endocarditis incidence since 2008, though a causal relationship with the implementation of the NICE guidelines has not been established. In contrast to NICE, the European Society of Cardiology (2015) continues to recommend prophylaxis for procedures requiring manipulation of the gingival or periapical region, or perforation of the oral mucosa in patients defined as high risk.

Surgical Site Infections

Surgical site infections (SSIs) are one of the most common type of healthcare-associated infections in the UK. They usually occur within 30 days in the anatomical area where surgery occurred. SSIs can be:

- Superficial: limited to the skin and subcutaneous tissues
- Deep: involving muscle and fascia
- Organ/space: involving the anatomy opened or manipulated during the surgery e.g. bone, mediastinum, myocardium

Deep and organ/space SSIs include infections occurring up to 1 year after surgery, if an implant is in place.

The pathogens involved can be either endogenous (part of the patient's flora) or exogenous (from the physical environment or surgical team).

Factors contributing to the likelihood of an SSI include patient-related factors (e.g. age, nutritional state) and surgery-related factors (e.g. duration of surgery, presence of foreign material).

Surgical Prophylaxis

Antibiotic prophylaxis is an important measure in preventing a postoperative SSI. For effective prophylaxis, bactericidal concentrations of antibiotic must be attained in both the serum and target tissue from the time of incision until wound closure. SSI rates increase when prophylactic antimicrobials are given either too soon or too late; antimicrobial prophylaxis should be administered an hour or less before skin incision; as close to the time of incision as possible.

Prophylaxis is recommended for rhythm-management-device insertion, open heart surgery and interventional cardiac-catheter-device placement.

A single dose is sufficient for most types of surgical procedures although for cardiac surgery there is evidence to suggest that prolonging prophylaxis to 48 hours post surgery may reduce infections.

Whether or not a further intraoperative dose of antibiotic is required depends upon the duration of surgery, blood loss and the antibiotic half-life. Re-administration of the antibiotic during surgery should be within two half-lives, with some advising within one half-life.

There is lack of consensus as to the 'optimal' prophylaxis regimen but, as the most common pathogen is *Staphylococcus aureus*, regimens should ensure activity against this pathogen in line with local resistance profiles.

Additional cover for Gram-negative organisms can be provided by adding gentamicin to narrow-spectrum regimens such as glycopeptides or flucloxacillin.

Mediastinitis

Post-sternotomy mediastinitis is a serious complication with mortality of up to 47%. It is defined as any one of the following:

- Organism detected from mediastinal tissue or fluid
- Mediastinitis visualized at surgery
- Fever or chest pain or sternal instability in combination with either purulent discharge or mediastinal widening on imaging

Infection arises from the patient's own flora, contamination of the surgical field or secondary to sternal wound infections. The incidence ranges from 0.4% to 5%.

The commonest pathogens are Gram-positive organisms, principally *Staphylococcus aureus*. Infections caused by Gram-negative organisms are less frequent and have been associated with infections at other sites (e.g. pneumonia).

There is no universal agreement on risk factors or their relative contributions, but they include:

- Obesity
- Diabetes mellitus
- Previous sternotomy
- Prolonged operative time
- Infection at another site

Microbiological samples should include blood cultures, wound tissue or wound discharge. Management comprises surgical debridement in conjunction with broad-spectrum antibiotics, pending culture results.

The treatment duration depends upon the causative organism, involvement of the sternal bone and the response to therapy, but is likely to be weeks to months.

Sternal Osteomyelitis

This can be associated with mediastinitis or can present chronically, weeks to months after surgery with an unstable sternum or sinus tracts. Management involves both surgical debridement and prolonged antimicrobial therapy. It is important, therefore, to obtain high-quality samples (e.g. bone, tissue) prior to commencing treatment in order to target the causative organism with as narrow-spectrum therapy as possible.

Other Postoperative Infections
Infection of Implantable Devices

Implantable-device infection can present either in the early postoperative period or months to years later. The most common causative organisms are *Staphylococcus* species followed by *Streptococcus* species, *Enterococcus* species and Gram-negative organisms, but up to 15% of infections are culture-negative. Implantable-cardiac-device infection should be considered if a patient with a device has positive blood cultures with *Staphylococcus aureus* or multiple positive blood cultures with another micro-organism. Infection can involve any or all of the following: generator pocket, leads or heart valves. Optimal management requires removal of the entire device in conjunction with antibiotics. If removal is not possible, device retention can be attempted with 6 weeks of antibiotics, with subsequent consideration of lifelong suppression should this strategy fail.

Ventilator-Associated Pneumonia

Ventilator-associated pneumonia (VAP) is the onset of pneumonia in a patient who has been ventilated for 48 hours, although universal diagnostic criteria are lacking. VAP within the first 4 days of admission is generally caused by community-acquired organisms (e.g. *Streptococcus pneumoniae, Haemophilus influenzae*) while VAP developing after 4 days is caused by nosocomial organisms (e.g. *Staphylococcus aureus, Pseudomonas aeruginosa*). The antibiotic regimen should be tailored accordingly, with treatment duration around 7 days, depending upon clinical response.

'VAP care bundles' have been developed – a collection of interventions which, when applied together synergistically, reduce VAP incidence. Components include:

- Review of sedation and, if appropriate, stopped daily
- Daily assessment for weaning and extubation
- Patient in a semi-recumbent position (head at 30^0)
- Subglottic drainage of secretions if likely to be ventilated for more than 48 hours

Clostridioides difficile Infection

Clostridioides difficile disease has an attributable mortality of 8%. Risk factors include antibiotic exposure, proton pump inhibitors and previous *Clostridioides difficile* disease. The recommended treatment is oral metronidazole for mild or moderate disease and oral vancomycin for severe disease, as determined by leucocyte count, lactate concentration, renal function, BP, temperature, stool frequency and abdominal examination. Fidaxomicin is a new class of antibiotic which may decrease *Clostridioides difficile* recurrence. Treatment adjuncts include immunoglobulin and faecal transplant.

Antimicrobial Resistance and Stewardship

Infection with multi-resistant organisms can lead to poorer outcomes because of:

- Delayed appropriate therapy
- Susceptible antibiotics may be less efficacious than those to which the organism is resistant

- Toxicity of available antimicrobials

Antimicrobial stewardship and infection prevention and control interventions are the key strategies for preventing the emergence and spread of multi-resistant organisms. The 'Start Smart then Focus' toolkit (Public Health England) provides an outline for stewardship in secondary care. It promotes prompt initiation of antibiotic therapy, but emphasizes the need for both appropriate cultures prior to therapy and a review of the ongoing need, route of administration and type of antibiotic in light of clinical assessment and culture results after 48–72 hours.

The two main infection prevention and control strategies are:

- Early detection of resistant organisms or conditions, e.g. pre-emptive patient screening for MRSA
- Prevention of transmission, e.g. patient isolation, hand-washing

Key Points

- Opinion is divided regarding endocarditis prophylaxis.
- SSIs are one of the most common type of hospital-acquired infections; surgical prophylaxis is an important preventative measure.
- Infection prevention and control interventions and antimicrobial stewardship are important strategies for preventing the emergence and spread of bacterial resistance.

Further Reading

Baddour LM, Wilson WR, Bayer AS, *et al.* Infective endocarditis in adults: diagnosis, antimicrobial therapy, and management of complications: a scientific statement for healthcare professionals from the American Heart Association. *Circulation* 2015; 132: 1435–86.

Centre for Clinical Practice at NICE. Clinical guideline CG64. *Prophylaxis against Infective Endocarditis: Antimicrobial Prophylaxis against Infective Endocarditis in Adults and Children Undergoing Interventional Procedures.* London: National Institute for Health and Care Excellence (UK); updated July 2016.

Kohler P, Kuster SP, Bloemberg G, *et al.* Healthcare-associated prosthetic heart valve, aortic vascular graft, and disseminated *Mycobacterium chimaera* infections subsequent to open heart surgery. *Eur Heart J* 2015; 36: 2745–53.

National Collaborating Centre for Women's and Children's Health, commissioned by the National Institute for Health and Clinical Excellence. *Surgical Site Infection Prevention and Treatment of Surgical Site Infection.* London: RCOG Press; 2008.

Public Health England. Start smart then focus: antimicrobial stewardship toolkit for English hospitals. London: Public Health England; March 2015. www.gov.uk/government/publications/antimicrobial-stewardship-start-smart-then-focus (accessed December 2018).

Public Health England. Updated guidance on the management and treatment of *Clostridium difficile* infection. London: Public Health England; May 2013. www.gov.uk/ government/publications/ clostridium-difficile-infection- guidance-on-management-and- treatment (accessed December 2018).

Sandoe JAT, Barlow G, Chambers JB, *et al.* Guidelines for the diagnosis, prevention and management of implantable cardiac electronic device infection. Report of a joint working party project on behalf of the British Society for Antimicrobial Chemotherapy (BSAC, host organization), British Heart Rhythm Society (BHRS), British Cardiovascular Society (BCS), British Heart Valve Society (BHVS) and British Society for Echocardiography (BSE). *J Antimicrob Chemother* 2015; 70: 325–59.

Scottish Intensive Care Society Audit Group. *VAP Prevention Bundle Guidance for Implementation.* Edinburgh: NHS National Services Scotland; 2008.

Scottish Intercollegiate Guidelines Network (SIGN). *Antibiotic Prophylaxis in Surgery.* Edinburgh: SIGN publication no.104; 2008. Available from www.sign.ac.uk.

The Task Force for the Management of Infective Endocarditis of the European Society of Cardiology (ESC). 2015 ESC Guidelines for the management of infective endocarditis. *Eur Heart J* 2015; 36: 3075–128.

Index

abciximab, 262
abdominal examination, 8
abdominal surgery, 215
Abiomed Impella, 120
ablation procedures, cardiac, 136
absent pulmonary valve syndrome, 163
acid–base management, 42, 46
  cerebral protection, 196
  pharmacological effects, 200
activated clotting time (ACT), 40, 43
acute kidney injury (AKI), 61–4
  management, 64
  paediatric patients, 184
  prevention, 62
  risk factors, 63
acute lung injury (ALI), 59
acute renal failure (ARF), 61–4
acute respiratory distress syndrome
  (ARDS), 59
Adamkiewicz artery, 101
adrenaline. See epinephrine
adult congenital heart disease (ACHD),
  186–90
  anaesthetic management, 188–9
  antibiotic prophylaxis, 189
  blood management, 189
  classification, 186
  postoperative care, 189–90
  preoperative assessment, 187–8
after-drop hypothermia, 195
afterload, 55, 57
  paediatric patients, 182
air embolism (AE), 46, 210–12
  management, 211–12
  physical principles, 210–11
air entrainment
  CPB, 210
  ECMO, 220
air warmers, forced, 192
alfentanil, 26
α-stat blood-gas management, 42, 196
  paediatric patients, 150–1
  pH-stat management vs, 206–7
ε-aminocaproic acid, 152, 264
anaemia. See also haematocrit
  congenital haemolytic, 262
  dilutional, during CPB, 41, 207
  failure to wean from CPB, 47
  postoperative, 267

preoperative, 261
anaesthesia, 24–8
  checklist prior to surgery, 28
  during CPB, 42
  induction, 26
  maintenance, 28
  pregnancy, 272
  preparation for, 25
  transfer to operating room, 27–8
  vascular access, 25–6
anaesthetic agents
  ideal cardiac, 26
  pregnancy, 272
  preparation for use, 26
analgesia, postoperative. See
  postoperative pain management
anasarca, 7
andexanet alfa, 263
angina, 6
  aortic stenosis, 69
  chronic refractory, 283
antibiotics. See antimicrobials
anticoagulation
  AF, 58
  CPB, 40, 264
  ECMO, 219–20
  IABP, 48
  MV valve repair, 80–1
  off-pump coronary surgery, 93
  perioperative management, 262–3
  pregnancy, 272
  preoperative cessation, 24, 114–15
  regional anaesthesia and, 278
antifibrinolytics, 264
antimicrobials
  Clostridioides difficile infection,
    288
  endocarditis prophylaxis, 189, 286
  endocarditis therapy, 285–6
  heart transplant recipients, 128
  resistance and stewardship, 288
  surgical prophylaxis, 27, 286–7
antiplatelet agents, 262
  neuraxial blockade, 277
  preoperative cessation, 25, 262
antithrombin deficiency, 40
aorta
  atheroma, 65, 204
  cannulation, 2–3, 40–1

coarctation, 161–2, 171
  thoracic. See thoracic aortic surgery
aortic aneurysms, 99
  complications of surgery, 105–6
  descending aorta, 102–3
  indications for surgery, 99
  preoperative assessment, 100–1
aortic arch surgery, 101–2
aortic clamping/cross-clamping, 3, 41
  clamp-off, 4
  left heart bypass, 104
  minimally invasive surgery, 97
  off-pump surgery, 92
aortic disease
  imaging, 17–19, 101
  pregnancy, 272
  thoracic, 99–100
  TOE assessment, 258–9
aortic dissection, 99
  AR, 72
  classification, 99–100
  during CPB, 213
  indications for surgery, 1
  pregnancy, 272
  preoperative assessment, 100–1
  thrombolytic therapy, 263
  TOE assessment, 258–9
aortic interruption, 161
aortic pseudoaneurysms, 99
aortic regurgitation (AR), 71–3
  anaesthesia, 73
  grading of severity, 248
  investigations, 72–3
  mechanisms, 249
  pathophysiology, 72
  TOE assessment, 248
aortic root surgery, 101
aortic stenosis (AS), 69–71
  anaesthesia, 70–1
  grading of severity, 248–9
  investigations, 70
  pathophysiology, 69–70
  percutaneous interventions, 138, 140
  pregnancy, 272
  TOE assessment, 248–9
aortic valve (AV), 69
  balloon dilation, 140
  bicuspid, 69, 248
  TOE evaluation, 248

aortic valve replacement (AVR), 3
  minimally invasive, 5
  post-CPB hypertension, 71
  Ross procedure, 172–4
  transcatheter implantation, 5, 137–40
aortic valve surgery, 3, 69–73
  anaesthesia, 70–1, 73
  key points, 73
  surgical approach, 73
aortography, 21–2
apex beat, 8
apixaban, 263, 278
aprotinin, 152, 264
argatroban, 264
arrhythmias
  adult congenital heart disease, 188
  after MV repair, 81
  CPB termination, 42–3, 46
  CVP waveforms, 225
  device-based therapy, 131
  electrophysiological procedures,
    134–6
  mapping, 136
  paediatric patients, 183
  postoperative, 55, 58
arrhythmogenic right ventricular
    cardiomyopathy (ARVC),
    111–12
arterial BP monitoring, 223–4
  artefacts, 47
  underdamping and overdamping,
    223
arterial cannulae, 33
  cerebral perfusion, 101
  removal, 53–4
arterial cannulation, 25
  BP monitoring, 223
  CPB, 40–1, 43
arterial oxygen content (CaO$_2$), 226
arterial shunts, 154–5
arterial switch procedure, 177–8
arteriovenous fistula, haemodialysis
    patients, 64
arteriovenous oxygen content
    difference, 20, 211
aspirin, 25, 262
atelectasis, 53, 59
atherosclerosis, aortic, 65, 204
atracurium, 26
atrial fibrillation (AF)
  ablation procedures, 136
  after MV repair, 81
  DC cardioversion, 135
  MV disease, 76–8, 81
  postoperative, 52, 58
  TOE assessment, 255
atrial septal defect (ASD), 156
  percutaneous closure, 141
  surgical closure, 156–7

TOE assessment, 254–5
atrial septostomy, balloon
  PHT, 113
  transposition of the great arteries,
    147, 177
atrioventricular (AV) block, 12
  indications for pacing, 132
  VSDs, 180
atrioventricular septal defects
    (AVSDs), 156, 158–9
auditory evoked potentials (AEPs), 233
auscultation, 8–10

balloon aortic valve dilation, 140
balloon atrial septostomy. See atrial
    septostomy, balloon
balloon pulmonary angioplasty, 116
base excess, 42
benzodiazepines, 201
Bernoulli equation, 239
bidirectional cavopulmonary shunt
    (BCPS), 160
bivalirudin, 264
biventricular support devices, 118
Blalock–Taussig (B-T) shunt, modified,
    147, 154–5
  pulmonary atresia, 172
bleeding. See haemorrhage/bleeding
blood donation, preoperative
    autologous, 261
blood flow
  effects of CPB, 199
  myocardial oxygen supply, 30
blood pressure (BP)
  invasive monitoring, 223
  paediatric patients, 145
blood transfusion
  adult congenital heart disease, 189
  after aortic surgery, 105
  coagulopathies, 264
  during CPB, 207
  paediatric patients, 182
blood-gas management, 42, 206–7
bloody tap, 278
Boyle's law, 210–11
bronchospasm, CPB termination, 46
bubble oxygenators, 210
bubble traps, 38
bupivacaine, hyperbaric, 275–6

Caesarean section, 270–1
calcium
  coronary, scoring, 16
  pharmacological use, 52
CaO$_2$ (arterial oxygen content), 226
carboprost, 271
carcinoid heart disease, 87–9
carcinoid syndrome, 87
cardiac ablation procedures, 136

cardiac allograft vasculopathy, 129
cardiac arrest. See also resuscitation
  AV surgery, 71
  CPB for resuscitation, 216–17
  MS, 77
  postoperative, 55, 67
  therapeutic hypothermia, 191–2
cardiac catheter laboratory procedures
  DC cardioversion, 135–6
  electrophysiological, 134–6
  mapping and ablation, 136
  rhythm management, 131–4
  structural heart disease, 137–42
cardiac catheterization, 20
cardiac disease
  maternal deaths, 269–70
  physical signs, 7–10
  pregnancy and delivery, 270–1
  symptoms, 6–7
cardiac index (CI), 20, 45
  neonates, 145
cardiac magnetic resonance imaging
    (CMR), 18–20
  adult congenital heart disease, 188
  coronary artery disease, 17, 19
  valvular disease, 19
cardiac masses, 19–20, 255–6
cardiac output (CO). See also low
    cardiac output state
  CPB, 41
  measurement, 20, 226
  postoperative optimization, 52, 55
  shock, 228
cardiac resynchronization therapy
    (CRT), 131–2
cardiac rhythm. See also arrhythmias
  during CPB, 42–3
  management devices, 131–4
cardiac surgery, 1–5, See also
    cardiopulmonary bypass
  early postoperative care, 50–4
  minimally invasive (MICS), 5, 94–7
  myocardial protection, 3, 30–3
  off-pump, 4–5, 91–4
  operative principles, 2–4
  patient selection, 1–2
  pregnancy, 271–3
  risk assessment, 2
  setting up, 2–3
cardiac tamponade
  haemodynamic parameters, 228
  postoperative, 57–8
  TOE assessment, 256
cardiogenic shock
  critical, 119–20
  haemodynamic parameters, 228
cardiomyopathies, 107–12
cardioplegia, 3, 32–3, See also deep
    hypothermic circulatory arrest

cardioplegia (cont.)
  AV surgery, 3
  delivery, 33–4
  minimally invasive surgery, 95
  myocardial protection, 30
  normothermic versus hypothermic,
    205
cardioprotection. *See* myocardial
    protection
cardiopulmonary bypass (CPB), 30–44
  air embolism, 45–6, 210–12
  anaesthesia, 42
  anticoagulation, 40, 264
  blood transfusion, 207
  blood-gas management, 42, 206–7
  cannulation, 40–1
  cardiac rhythm, 42–3
  circuit. *See* cardiopulmonary bypass
    circuit
  coming off, 4
  communication, 39–40
  conduct, 39–43
  controversies, 203–8
  de-airing, 4
  decannulation, 43
  deep hypothermic circulatory arrest,
    192–7
  descending aorta surgery, 102–3
  drug pharmacokinetics, 199–200
  emergencies, 208
  femoro-femoral, 215
  haematocrit, 41, 207
  haemodynamic management, 41–2
  haemostasis and closure, 43
  hypothermia, 42, 192–7
  inadequate flow, 212–13
  inadequate oxygenation, 212
  initiation, 41
  metabolic management, 42
  mini, 39, 207–8
  minimally invasive surgery, 95–7
  myocardial protection, 30–3
  non-cardiac applications, 215–17
  normothermia versus hypothermia,
    205
  off-pump surgery conversion to, 93
  paediatric patients, 150–2
  pregnancy, 272–3
  preparation for, 40
  pressure versus flow, 203–5
  prothrombotic risk, 263
  pulsatile flow, 205–6
  resuscitation using, 216–17
  setting up, 2–3
  temperature management, 191–8
  ventilation and oxygenation, 208
  weaning. *See* weaning from CPB
cardiopulmonary bypass circuit, 33–9
  air entrainment, 210

  components, 33–8
  filters and bubble traps, 38–9
  mini, 39, 207–8
  safety standards, 39
  sequestration of drugs, 200
cardiotomy suction, 39
cardiovascular complications, 55–8
cardiovascular monitoring, 223–8
cardioversion
  CPB weaning, 46
  DC, 135–6
  postoperative arrhythmias, 52, 55, 58
carotid sinus hypersensitivity, 132
Carpentier classification, 248
catheter-based procedures. *See* cardiac
    catheter laboratory procedures
cavopulmonary shunt, bidirectional,
    160
cell salvage, 39
central shunt, 154
central venous access
  aortic surgery, 103
  cardiac surgery, 25–7
  CVP monitoring, 224
  heart transplantation, 127
  paediatric cardiac anaesthesia, 150
  rhythm-management-device
    implantation, 134
central venous oxygen saturation
    (ScvO$_2$), 228
central venous pressure (CVP). *See also*
    right atrial pressure
  CPB, 41, 46–7
  monitoring, 224–5
  shock, 228
  waveforms, 224–5
centrifugal pumps, 35, 194
CentriMag® ventricular assist device,
    119–20
cerebral artery blood flow velocity
    (CBFV), 234
cerebral autoregulation, 203–5
cerebral ischaemia, EEG changes,
    230–1
cerebral oxygenation monitoring, 102,
    233–5
cerebral perfusion, 101–2
  CPB perfusion pressure and,
    203–4
  intermittent, 197
  monitoring, 102, 233–5
  retrograde, 101–2, 197, 211–12
  selective antegrade, 101–2, 197
cerebral protection
  aortic arch surgery, 101–2
  deep hypothermic circulatory arrest,
    196–7
  paediatric patients, 150–1
cerebrospinal fluid (CSF) drainage, 104

cerebrovascular disease, pre-existing,
    204
CHARGE association, 163
Charles' law, 210–11
CHD. *See* congenital heart disease
chest drains, removal, 53
chest pain, 6
chest radiography (CXR), 14
cholecystitis, postoperative, 60
chordae tendinae, 75
chronic refractory angina, 283
chronic thromboembolic pulmonary
    hypertension (CTEPH), 113–16
chylothorax, postoperative, 184–5
clonidine, 25
clopidogrel, 262, 278
Clostridioides difficile infection, 288
coagulation testing, 264
coagulopathy
  blood product replacement, 264
  heart transplant recipients, 127–8
  paediatric patients, 152
  postoperative, 53, 267
coarctation of the aorta (CoA), 161–2,
    171
cognitive dysfunction, postoperative,
    64, 66–7
cold agglutinins, 262
colour flow Doppler (CFD), 239
communication, 39–40, 282
complement activation, during CPB,
    263
computed tomography (CT), 15–18
computed tomography angiography
    (CTA)
  aortic disease, 18, 101
  coronary artery disease, 15–18
congenital heart disease (CHD), 145,
    154–80, *See also* paediatric cardiac
    anaesthesia
  adult, 186–90
  anaesthesia, 148–50
  closed cardiac surgery, 148
  cyanotic, 148
  failure to wean from CPB, 47
  outcome of surgery, 185
  pathophysiology, 149
  postoperative care, 181–5
  postoperative problems, 182–5
  surgical strategy, 147–8
constrictive pericarditis, 109, 111
  restrictive cardiomyopathy versus,
    111
  TOE assessment, 256
continuous haemodiafiltration, 64
continuous veno-venous
    haemofiltration (CVVHF), 64
continuous wave Doppler (CWD), 239
contractility, paediatric patients, 182

contrast echocardiography, 14
COPS protocol, 105
cor triatriatum, 176
coronary angiography, 21–2
  aortic disease, 101
  intravascular ultrasound versus, 22–3
  non-invasive, 17
coronary artery bypass graft (CABG) surgery
  conduit harvesting, 2
  indications, 1
  off-pump (OPCAB), 4–5, 91–4
  operative principles, 3
coronary artery calcium scoring, 16
coronary artery disease (CAD)
  angiography. See coronary angiography
  cardiac magnetic resonance, 17, 19
  CT, 15–16, 18
  exercise ECG, 11–13
  indications for surgery, 1
  intravascular ultrasound, 22–3
  non-invasive imaging, 17
coronary blood flow (CBF), 30
coronary computed tomography angiography (CTA), 15–18
coronary fistulae/sinusoids, 172
coronary perfusion, PHT, 114
Corrigan's sign, 8
CPB. See cardiopulmonary bypass
creatinine kinase MB (CK-MB), 57
creatinine, serum, 63
cryoablation, 136
cryohydrocytosis, 262
cryoprecipitate, 264
CvO₂ (mixed venous oxygen content), 226
cyanosis, 8
  adult congenital heart disease, 187–8
  CHD, 148
  differential, ECMO, 219
  Fallot's tetralogy, 163
  total anomalous pulmonary venous drainage, 176

dabigatran, 263, 278
DC cardioversion, 135–6
de Musset's sign, 7
de-airing, 4, 211–12
DeBakey classification, 99–100
deep hypothermic circulatory arrest (DHCA), 192–7, See also cardioplegia; hypothermia
  anaesthesia, 193–4
  aortic surgery, 101
  circulatory arrest, 195

cooling, 195
CPB modifications, 194–5
failure to wean from CPB, 46
indications, 193
neurological monitoring, 197, 231–2
neurosurgery, 216
paediatric cardiac surgery, 150–1
postoperative care, 197
rewarming, 195–6
surgical aspects, 194
delirium, postoperative, 64, 66–7, 276
depth-of-anaesthesia (DOA) monitoring, 26–7, 233
descending thoracic aorta surgery, 102–5
desflurane, 201
Di George syndrome (22q11 deletion), 148, 163, 179
diabetes mellitus, 65, 204
diagnostic tests, 11–23
diastolic dysfunction, LV, 243
diathermy, pacemaker/ICD recipients, 134
dilated cardiomyopathy (DCM), 108–9
dimensionless index (DI), 248
direct antiglobulin test, 262
direct-acting oral anticoagulants (DOACs), 24–5, 263, 278
distal limb ischaemia, 219
dobutamine, 151
dopamine, 63, 151
Doppler ultrasound, 239
Down syndrome, 158
drugs
  pharmacological effects of CPB, 199–201
  preoperative cessation, 24–5
dual source computed tomography (DSCT), 15–16
ductus arteriosus (DA), 170
  closure, 145–6, 170
  dependent circulation, 146, 154
  patent (PDA), 146, 170
Duke Activity Status Index (DASI), 7
Duke criteria, endocarditis, 285
Duroziez's sign, 9
dyspnoea, 6
dysrhythmias. See arrhythmias

echocardiography, 13–14
  contrast, 14
  stress, 13
  transoesophageal. See transoesophageal echocardiography
  transthoracic (TTE), 13

ECMO. See extracorporeal membrane oxygenation
Eisenmenger syndrome, 187
ejection fraction (EF)
  3D right ventricular, 245
  left ventricular, 242
elderly, CPB perfusion pressure, 204
electrical power failure, 213
electrocardiography (ECG), 11–13
  abnormalities, 12
  ambulatory, 13
  atrial, 183
  exercise, 11–13
  implantable recorders, 13
  intraoperative, 28
  limitations to resting, 11
  perioperative myocardial infarction, 57
electroencephalography (EEG), 231–2
  deep hypothermic circulatory arrest, 230–3
  depth-of-anaesthesia monitoring, 26, 233
electrolyte management
  CPB, 42, 46
  paediatric patients, 181–2
  postoperative, 52
electromagnetic interference (EMI), 134
electron beam computed tomography (EBCT), 15–16
electrophysiological disorders, 135
electrophysiological procedures, 134–6
embolus filters, 263
emergencies, CPB, 208
emphysema, 216
end-diastolic volume index, 20
endo-aortic balloon clamp, 97
endocarditis, infective, 285–6
  aetiology, 286
  after MV surgery, 81
  AR, 72
  Duke criteria, 285
  MR, 78
  prophylaxis, 189, 286
  TOE assessment, 256
endotracheal tubes, paediatric, 150
end-systolic pressure–volume relationship (ESPVR), 55
enflurane, 201
epidural anaesthesia
  neuraxial bleeding, 276
  paediatric cardiac surgery, 150
  thoracic, 26, 274–5, 282
epidural haematoma, 276–8
epinephrine
  paediatric patients, 151

epinephrine (cont.)
postoperative cardiac arrest, 55
ventricular assist device insertion, 121–3
ε-aminocaproic acid, 152, 264
eptifibatide, 262
ergometrine, 271
etomidate, 26
EuroSCORE (European System for Cardiac Operative Risk Evaluation), 2
evoked potentials, 104–5, 233
exercise electrocardiography (exECG), 11–13
exertional syncope, 7
extracorporeal life support, after paediatric cardiac surgery, 182–3
extracorporeal membrane oxygenation (ECMO), 218–20
cannulation, 219
cardiogenic shock, 119
equipment, 218–19
management, 219–20
outcomes, 220
paediatric patients, 182–3
patient selection, 218
weaning, 220

factor VIIa, recombinant, 264
factor VIII deficiency, 263
factor IX deficiency, 263
Fallot's tetralogy, 163–4
anatomy, 163
physiology, 147, 163
surgery, 163–4
family, 54, 148
fast-tracking, 50
fatigue, 7
femoral arterial cannulation, 219
femoral vein cannulation, 224
femoro-femoral cardiopulmonary bypass, 215
fentanyl, 26, 150, 274
fibrinogen concentrate, 264
fibrinolysis, 264
filters, CPB circuit, 38
flow index, effect of hypothermia, 46
flow rate, CPB pump, 41–2
inadequate, 212
perfusion pressure and, 203–5
fluid management
aortic surgery, 105
off-pump surgery, 93
paediatric patients, 181–2
postoperative, 52–3
fluid warming, 192
Fontan procedure, 165–6
postoperative management, 165

surgery in adulthood, 186, 190
foramen ovale
closure, 145
patent. See patent foramen ovale
fractional area change, right ventricular (RVFAC), 245
fractional flow reserve (FFR), 22
fractional shortening (FS), 243
fresh frozen plasma (FFP), 264
functional status, 6
fundal examination, 8
furosemide, 52–3

gadolinium diethylene triamine pentaacetic acid (Gd-DTPA), 19
gastric tube, 27
gastrointestinal (GI) complications, 59–61
gastrointestinal (GI) haemorrhage, 60–1
gastrointestinal (GI) perforation, 60
Glenn procedure, 160
global longitudinal strain (GLS), 243
glucose management, 42, 197
glyceryl trinitrate (GTN), 52, 151
greater radicular artery (of Adamkiewicz), 101

haematocrit, 41
correction prior to weaning, 47
deep hypothermic circulatory arrest, 196
minimum acceptable, 207
haematology, 261–7
intraoperative care, 263–7
postoperative problems, 267
preoperative care, 261–3
haemodialysis patients, 64
haemodilution
cerebral protection, 196
during CPB, 41
pharmacokinetic effects, 199
haemodynamics
CPB, 41–2
off-pump coronary surgery, 93
postoperative, 51–2, 55
shock, 228
haemofilters, 194
haemofiltration, intraoperative, 64
haemoglobinopathies, 262
haemolytic anaemia, congenital, 262
haemophilia, 263
haemoptysis, 6
haemorrhage/bleeding
blood product replacement, 264
failure to wean from CPB, 47
GI, 60–1

neuraxial, 276–8
postoperative, 53, 267
haemostasis
aortic surgery, 105
paediatric cardiac surgery, 152
post-bypass, 4, 43, 196
preoperative considerations, 261
handover (to ICU), 50–1
paediatric patients, 181
Harlequin syndrome, 219
heart block, 12, 132
after paediatric cardiac surgery, 183
VSDs, 180
heart failure
acute, mechanical circulatory support, 119–20
carcinoid heart disease, 87–8
cardiac resynchronization therapy, 131–2
diastolic dysfunction, 243
dilated cardiomyopathy, 108–9
heart transplantation, 125–6
paediatric patients, 146, 148
VSDs, 118
heart rate (HR)
after paediatric cardiac surgery, 182
paediatric patients, 145
heart sounds, 9
heart transplantation, 125–9
anaesthesia, 126–7
antimicrobial therapy, 128
bridge to, 118–21
early complications, 128
immunosuppression, 128
late complications and morbidity, 128–9
organ donor harvest, 276
patient selection, 125–6
reperfusion and weaning from CPB, 127–8
HeartMate 3, 121
HeartMate II LVAD, 121–2
HeartMate PHP, 120
HeartMate VE/XVE LVAD, 121
HeartWare HVAD, 121–2
heat conservation, 92–3, 191
heat exchangers, 38
heat loss, 191
Henry's law, 210–11
heparin (unfractionated heparin; UFH)
alternatives, 264
CPB, 40
ECMO, 219–20
IABP, 48
off-pump coronary surgery, 93
pharmacokinetic interactions, 199
preoperative management, 25, 263
resistance, 40
reversal, 43

heparin-induced thrombotic
    thrombocytopenic syndrome
    (HITTS), 40, 267
hepatic dysfunction, 60
history, clinical, 6–7
humidification, 192
5-hydroxyindoleacetic acid (5-HIAA),
    88–9
hyoscine hydrobromide, 25
hyperglycaemia, 52
hyperkalaemia, 52
hypertension
    CPB perfusion pressure, 204
    postoperative, 52, 71
hyperthermia, postoperative, 181
hypertrophic obstructive
    cardiomyopathy (HOCM), 107–8
    pathophysiology, 107
    surgical complications, 47
hypokalaemia, 52
hypomagnesaemia, 52
hypoplastic left heart syndrome
    (HLHS), 167–8
    Fontan procedure, 165
    Norwood procedure, 167–8
hypotension
    AV surgery, 71, 73
    artefactual, during CPB, 47
    carcinoid heart disease, 89
    MV surgery, 77, 79
    pharmacokinetic effects, 199
    postoperative, 51
    postural, 7
hypothermia, 191–7, See also deep
    hypothermic circulatory arrest
    after-drop, 195
    aortic surgery, 101
    cerebral protection, 196
    during CPB, 42, 192–7
    failure to wean from CPB, 46
    inadvertent, 181
    myocardial protection, 30, 33
    normothermia versus, 205
    paediatric cardiac surgery, 150–1
    pathophysiology, 51, 193
    pharmacological effects, 199–201
    postoperative rewarming, 51
    therapeutic, cardiac arrest, 191–2
hypovolaemic shock, 228

IABP. See intra-aortic balloon pump
ICU. See intensive care unit
idarucizumab, 263
ileus, postoperative, 60
imaging, cardiovascular, 14–20
immunosuppression, 128
implantable-cardioverter defibrillators
    (ICDs), 131
    DC cardioversion, 135

explantation, 132–3
    implantation, 131–3
    perioperative management, 133
implantable device infection, 287
implantable ECG recorders, 13
induction of anaesthesia, 26
    paediatric surgery, 149–50
    procedures following, 27–8
infection, 285–8
    after MV repair, 81
    postoperative, 286–8
infection prevention and control
    interventions, 288
inferior vena cava (IVC)
    interruption, 160
    renal tumours involving, 216
inhalational anaesthetics. See volatile
    anaesthetics
inotropic agents
    paediatric patients, 151
    weaning from CPB, 47
insulin, 52
intensive care unit (ICU)
    early postoperative care, 51–2
    family involvement, 54
    fast-tracking, 50
    first postoperative day, 54
    paediatric patient transfer, 153, 181
    postoperative complications, 53,
        55–67
    spinal cord perfusion, 105
    transfer, admission and handover,
        50–1
    VADs, 123–4
INTERMACS patient profiles, 118
internal jugular vein (IJV) cannulation,
    25–6, 224
intra-aortic balloon pump (IABP).
    See also ventricular assist devices
    critical cardiogenic shock, 119
    failure to wean from CPB, 48–9
    indications, 49
intrathecal pressure (ITP), 104–5
intravascular ultrasound (IVUS), 22–3
intravenous anaesthesia, 42
invasive diagnostic tests, 20–3
iron deficiency, 261
ischaemia reperfusion injury (IRI), 31
ischaemic conditioning, 31
ischaemic heart disease (IHD). See
    coronary artery disease
ischaemic postconditioning, 31
ischaemic preconditioning (IPC), 31–2
isoflurane, 201
isoproterenol (isoprenaline), 151

jugular bulb oxygen monitoring, 234
jugular vein pressure levels and
    waveforms, 8

jugular venous oxygen saturation
    (SjvO$_2$), 234
junctional ectopic tachycardia, 183

Kawashima operation, 160
ketamine, 149
Kussmaul's sign, 8

labour, 270–1
Laplace's law, 55
laryngeal nerve injury, 184
left anterior hemiblock, 12
left atrial appendage (LAA)
    occlusion, 142
    thrombus, 255
left atrial hypertrophy, 12
left atrial myxoma, 255–6
left atrial pressure (LAP)
    elevated, 75–6, 78
    estimation, 226
left bundle branch block (LBBB), 12
left coronary artery, anomalous, 163
left heart bypass (LHB), 102–4
left heart catheterization, 20–2
left internal mammary artery (LIMA),
    2–3
left posterior hemiblock, 12
left ventricular aneurysms, 110
left ventricular assist devices (LVADs),
    118
    long-term, 119
    postoperative care, 123–4
    preoperative assessment, 120–1
    short-term, 118–19
left ventricular diastolic function, 243
left ventricular dysfunction
    postoperative, 55
    TOE assessment, 243
left ventricular ejection fraction
    (LVEF), 242
left ventricular end-diastolic pressure
    (LVEDP)
    AR, 72
    AS, 69–70
    estimation, 226
    mitral regurgitation, 78
left ventricular end-diastolic volume
    (LVEDV), 243
left ventricular end-systolic volume
    (LVESV), 243
left ventricular hypertrophy (LVH), 12,
    69, 72
left ventricular internal dimension
    (LVID), 243
left ventricular outflow tract (LVOT)
    obstruction
    hypertrophic cardiomyopathy, 107
    management, 108
    MV repair, 80–1

left ventricular pressure, 20
left ventricular pressure–volume loops, 57
  AR, 72
  AS, 70
  MR, 78
  MS, 76
left ventricular systolic function, 243
  regional, 243–4
  strain imaging, 243
left-to-right shunts, 20, 147
leucocyte depleting filters, 38
Levine's sign, 6
levobupivacaine, 274
lidocaine, 274
liver transplantation, 216
long saphenous vein (LSV), 2
loop diuretics, 63
lorazepam, 25
low cardiac output state (LCOS)
  after Fallot's tetralogy surgery, 163–4
  after paediatric cardiac surgery, 181–3
  post-bypass, 45
low-molecular-weight heparin (LMWH), 263
lung
  auscultation, 9
  isolation, pharmacokinetic effects, 200
lung fields, examination, 8
lung transplantation, 216
lupus anticoagulant, 263
lymphoma, 262

magnesium sulphate, 52
magnetic resonance imaging (MRI)
  cardiac. See cardiac magnetic resonance
  pacemaker/ICD interference, 134
magnets, application of, 134
maintenance of anaesthesia, 28
major aorto-pulmonary collateral arteries (MAPCAs), pulmonary atresia with, 172–3
mannitol, 63
mapping, electrophysiological, 136
masses, cardiac, 19–20, 255–6
maternal deaths, cardiac disease, 269–70
mattress, heated, 192
mean arterial pressure (MAP)
  acute kidney injury, 62–3
  aortic surgery, 104
  CPB, 41–2, 46–7, 203–4
  invasive monitoring, 223
  postoperative management, 55

mechanical circulatory support (MCS), 118–24, See also ventricular assist devices
  failure to wean from CPB, 47–9, 120
  long-term, 119–21
  short-term, 119–20
median sternotomy, 2
mediastinal surgery, 216
mediastinitis, post sternotomy, 287
membrane oxygenators, 37–8, 210
mesenteric ischaemia, 60–1
metaraminol, 93
methadone, 25
midazolam, 26
milrinone, 151
mini cardiopulmonary bypass (mini CPB), 39, 207–8
minimally invasive cardiac surgery (MICS), 5, 94–7
  anaesthesia, 95–7
  MV, 75
  postoperative care, 97
  preoperative assessment, 94–5
  types, 94
minimally invasive extracorporeal circulation (MiECC) techniques, 39
MitraClip® system, 140–1
mitral regurgitation (MR), 78–81
  anaesthesia, 78
  Carpentier classification, 248
  catheter-based therapies, 140–1
  grading of severity, 250–1
  pathophysiology, 78
  persistent, 80
  surgery, 79
  TOE assessment, 79, 248–50
mitral stenosis (MS), 75–8
  after MV repair, 80
  anaesthesia, 77
  catheter-based therapies, 140–1
  investigations, 76–7
  pathophysiology, 75–6
  pregnancy, 272
  surgical options, 77–8
  TOE assessment, 250
mitral valve (MV), 75
  myxomatous degeneration, 78
  orifice area (MVA), 75–6
  pressure gradient, 75–6
  systolic anterior motion. See systolic anterior motion of anterior MV leaflet
  TOE evaluation, 248
mitral valve clipping, 140–1
mitral valve commissurotomy, balloon, 141

mitral valve surgery, 3–4, 75–81
  anaesthesia, 77–8
  catheter-based procedures, 140–1
  failure to wean from CPB, 47
  minimally invasive, 5
  MV repair, 79–80
  MV replacement, 80
  pregnancy, 272
mitral valvotomy, percutaneous transeptal, 77–8
mixed venous oxygen content (CvO_2), 226
mixed venous oxygen saturation (SvO_2), 226–8
  during CPB, 42
  paediatric cardiac anaesthesia, 151
  shock, 228
  variables affecting, 228
modified ultrafiltration, 152
monitoring
  cardiovascular, 223–8
  deep hypothermic circulatory arrest, 193–4
  heart transplantation, 127
  neurological. See neurological monitoring
  off-pump surgery, 92
  paediatric cardiac anaesthesia, 150
  postoperative transfer to ICU, 50–1
  pregnancy, 272
  vascular access, 25–6
morphine, 25, 275–6
motor evoked potentials (MEPs), 104–5, 233
mouth examination, 8
Müller's sign, 8
multidetector row computed tomography (MDCT), 15–18
murmurs, cardiac, 8–9
muscle relaxants. See neuromuscular blocking drugs
Mycobacterium chimaera, 38, 286
myocardial hibernation, 30–1
myocardial infarction (MI), acute
  cardiogenic shock, 228
  ECG changes, 12
  perioperative, 47, 55–7
myocardial ischaemia, 12
  exercise ECG, 12
  intraoperative, 28, 30–2
  postoperative, 51–2
  reperfusion injury, 31
myocardial oxygen delivery, 30
myocardial oxygen demand, 30
myocardial perfusion imaging, 15
myocardial protection, 3, 30–3
  cardioplegia, 30, 32–3

ischaemic conditioning, 31
myocardial stunning, 30–1, 45
myocardial viability assessment, 15, 19
myxomas, 255–6

nail beds, examination, 8
near infrared spectroscopy (NIRS),
    235–6
    aortic surgery, 102
    paediatric cardiac anaesthesia, 151–2
neck examination, 8
necrotizing enterocolitis, 184
neonates
    cardiopulmonary interactions, 147
    coarctation of the aorta, 161
    duct-dependent circulation, 146,
        154
    normal physiology, 145
    systemic and pulmonary
        circulations, 146–7
    transitional circulation, 145–6
neuraxial blockade, central, 274–8,
    282
neurological complications, 64–7
    aortic surgery, 104–6
    cardiac ablation procedures, 136
    CPB perfusion pressure and, 204
    deep hypothermic circulatory arrest,
        195
    diagnosis, 65–6
    management, 66–7
    neuraxial blockade, 276–8
    normothermia versus hypothermia,
        205
    paediatric cardiac surgery, 184
    prevention, 65
    risk factors, 65
neurological monitoring, 230–7
    aortic surgery, 102, 104–5
    cerebral perfusion and oxygenation,
        233–5
    deep hypothermic circulatory arrest,
        197, 231–2
    neuronal function, 230–3
neuromuscular blocking drugs
    effects of CPB, 201
    induction, 26–7
neuropathic pain, 280–1
neuroprotection. See also cerebral
    protection
    air embolism, 212
    aortic surgery, 101–2, 104–5, 197
    paediatric patients, 150–1
neurosurgery, 215–16
New York Heart Association (NYHA)
    functional capacity classification,
        6
nitric oxide (NO), inhaled
    paediatric patients, 152, 155, 184

ventricular assist device insertion,
    123–4
nitrous oxide (N_2O), 149
nociception, 280
non-compaction cardiomyopathy
    (NCC), 110
non-invasive diagnostic tests, 11
non-steroidal anti-inflammatory drugs
    (NSAIDs), 51, 282
norepinephrine, paediatric patients,
    151
Norwood procedure, 167–8
novel oral anticoagulants. See direct-
    acting oral anticoagulants
nuclear cardiology, 14–15
nutrition, postoperative, 182

obesity, DC cardioversion, 135
observation, clinical, 7–8
octreotide, 89
oedema, 7, 70
off-pump cardiac surgery, 4–5, 91–4
off-pump coronary artery bypass
    (OPCAB), 4–5, 91–4
    anaesthetic management, 92–3
    conversion to on-pump, 93
    history, 91
    outcome, 94
    postoperative care, 93
    rationale, 91–2
    surgical approach, 91–2
Ohm's law, 30
oliguria, 53
operating room
    arrival of patient, 25
    transfer to, 27–8
    transfer to ICU from, 50–1
opioids
    effects of CPB, 201
    induction of anaesthesia, 26–7
    postoperative analgesia, 51, 282
optical coherence tomography, 23
oral anticoagulants, direct/novel, 24–5,
    263, 278
osteomyelitis, sternal, 287
oxygen administration
    air embolism, 211
    preanaesthesia, 25
oxygen consumption (VO_2), 226
oxygen delivery (DO_2), 226
oxygen demand, 226
oxygen extraction ratio (O_2 ER), 226
oxygen, myocardial supply and
    demand, 30
oxygenation
    during CPB, 208
    inadequate, during CPB, 212
oxygenators
    changeout during CPB, 212

CPB, 37–8
ECMO, 218
failure during CPB, 212
oxytocin, 271

pacemakers, permanent (PPMs), 131
    classification, 131
    DC cardioversion, 135
    explantation, 132–3
    implantation, 131–3
    perioperative management, 133
pacing, temporary epicardial, 131
    AVR, 71, 73
    heart transplantation, 127
    intraoperative, 43
    off-pump surgery, 93
    postoperative, 51, 54
paediatric cardiac anaesthesia,
        145–53, See also congenital heart
        disease
    conduct of, 148–50
    CPB, 150–2
    drug doses, 151
    induction, 149–50
    outcome of surgery, 185
    post-bypass management, 152
    postoperative care, 181–5
    premedication, 148–9
    preoperative assessment, 148
    principles, 145–8
    transfer to intensive care, 153
    vascular access and monitoring, 150
pain
    assessment, 281
    physiology, 280
    postoperative. See postoperative pain
palpation, 8
palpitations, 7
pancreatitis, acute, 60
pancuronium, 26–7
papillary fibroelastoma, 256
papillary muscle
    dysfunction, 78
    rupture, 80
paracetamol, 51, 282
paraplegia, 104–6, 278
parasternal blockade, 278–9
paravalvular leaks (PVLs)
    grading of severity, 253
    percutaneous closure, 141
    transcatheter aortic valve
        implantation, 138
paravertebral blockade, 279
patent ductus arteriosus (PDA), 146,
    170
patent foramen ovale (PFO), 254
    percutaneous closure, 141
    total anomalous pulmonary venous
        drainage, 176

percussion, 8
percutaneous balloon mitral valvotomy (PBMV), 141
percutaneous septal closure, 141
percutaneous therapies. *See* cardiac catheter laboratory procedures
perfusion pressure, CPB, 203–5
pericardial disease
anaesthesia, 110
imaging, 18–20
TOE assessment, 256–8
pericardial tamponade. *See* cardiac tamponade
pericarditis, constrictive. *See* constrictive pericarditis
peritoneal dialysis, 64
paediatric patients, 181–2, 184
persistent PHT of the newborn, 145, 147
pharmacodynamics, effects of CPB, 200
pharmacokinetics, effects of CPB, 199–200
phenylephrine, 151
phosphodiesterase (PDE) inhibitors, paediatric patients, 151
phrenic nerve injury, 136, 184
pH-stat acid–base management, 42
α-stat management vs, 206–7
cerebral protection, 196
paediatric patients, 150–1
pharmacokinetic effects, 200
PHT. *See* pulmonary hypertension
physical examination, 7–10
plasma protein binding, during CPB, 199
platelet counts, 261
platelet transfusion, 53, 261
pneumonia, ventilator-associated (VAP), 287–8
polycythaemia, 188
positive end-expiratory pressure (PEEP), 51
positron emission tomography (PET), 14–15, 17
postoperative care. *See also* intensive care unit
fast-tracking, 50
first day, 53–4
minimally invasive surgery, 97
off-pump coronary surgery, 93
paediatric, 181–5
routine early, 50–4
postoperative complications, 53, 55–67
haematological, 267
paediatric patients, 182–5
postoperative pain, 280–3
acute, 281–2
adverse effects, 281

causes, 280–1
chronic, 282–3
minimally invasive cardiac surgery, 97
prevention, 281–2
postoperative pain management, 51, 281–2
aortic surgery, 105
chronic, 282–3
minimally invasive cardiac surgery, 97
multimodal approach, 282
non-pharmacological, 282
postural hypotension, 7
prasugrel, 262
praecordium, examination, 8
prednisolone, for thrombocytopenia, 261
pregnancy, 269–73
cardiac disease, 270–1
cardiac surgery, 271–3
physiological changes, 270
preload, 46
paediatric patients, 182
postoperative optimization, 55, 57
premedication, 25
preoperative assessment, 24–5
pressure half-time (PH-T), 76
pressure support ventilation (PSV), 51
pre-syncope, 7
primary graft dysfunction, 128
propofol
anaesthesia, 26, 28
pharmacology during CPB, 200
postoperative sedation, 51
prostacyclin I$_2$ (PGI$_2$), 264
prostaglandin E$_2$ (PGE$_2$), 146
prosthetic heart valves
carcinoid heart disease, 89
malfunction, failure to wean from CPB, 47
paravalvular leaks. *See* paravalvular leaks
pregnancy, 272
TOE evaluation, 253
transcatheter aortic implantation, 137
protamine, 43
Protek Duo catheter, 120
prothrombin complex concentrate (PCC), 264
proximal isovelocity surface area (PISA), 77
pulmonary angioplasty, balloon, 116
pulmonary artery (PA)
banding, 171, 177
catheterization, 26, 225, 227
iatrogenic injury, 116, 225
sarcomas, 256

pulmonary artery floatation catheter (PAFC), 26, 225, 227
pulmonary artery pressure (PAP), 20, 113
measurement, 225
waveform, 227
pulmonary artery wedge pressure (PAWP), 55
measurement, 225
PHT, 113
pulmonary atresia, 172–3
pulmonary blood flow (PBF)
balancing. *See* pulmonary:systemic blood flow balance
CHD, 147–8
drug pharmacokinetics, 200
optimization, univentricular heart, 175
truncus arteriosus, 179
pulmonary circulation
balancing. *See* pulmonary:systemic blood flow balance
duct-dependent, 146, 154
perinatal changes, 146
pulmonary embolism, massive, 228
pulmonary hypertension (PHT), 113–16
adult congenital heart disease, 187
chronic thromboembolic (CTEPH), 113–16
classification, 113
failure to wean from CPB, 47
investigations, 20–1
management, 113–16
mitral stenosis, 76
paediatric cardiac surgery, 183–4
persistent, of newborn, 145, 147
postoperative, 152
RV pathophysiology, 113–15
truncus arteriosus surgery, 179
VSDs, 180
pulmonary oedema, reperfusion, 116
pulmonary regurgitation (PR), 86–7, 253
pulmonary stenosis (PS), 85–6, 251
pulmonary thromboendarterectomy (PTE), 114–16
pulmonary valve (PV), 85
absent, 163
carcinoid heart disease, 87–8
Ross procedure, 172–4
TOE evaluation, 251–3
pulmonary vascular disease, 113–16
pulmonary vascular resistance (PVR), 20, 113
CPB, 46–7
neonates, 145, 147
partitioning, 20
right-sided valve surgery, 85–7

pulmonary vasodilators, 114
pulmonary:systemic blood flow balance (Q_P:Q_S)
    adult congenital heart disease, 187
    arterial shunt procedures, 154–5
    measurement, 20
    neonates, 146–7
    Norwood circulation, 167–8
    postoperative care, 181–2
    PA banding, 171
pulse, 8
pulsed-wave Doppler (PWD), 239
pulsus alternans, 8
pulsus biferiens, 8
pumps, blood, 35
    failure, 213

Qp:Qs. See pulmonary:systemic blood flow balance

radial artery, cannulation, 25
radiant heaters, 192
radiofrequency ablation, 134, 136
recurrent laryngeal nerve injury, 184
regional anaesthesia, 274–9
    Caesarean section, 271
    paediatric cardiac surgery, 150
regional cerebral tissue oxygen saturation (rSO_2), 102, 235
regional wall motion abnormalities (RWMAs), 243–4
ReliantHeart aVAD, 121
REMATCH trial, 118
remifentanil, 26
remote ischaemic preconditioning (RIPC), 32
renal failure. See also acute kidney injury
    heart transplant recipients, 129
    postoperative, 61–4
    pre-existing, 63–4
renal replacement therapy (RRT), 64
    paediatric patients, 181–2, 184
renal tumours, IVC, 216
reperfusion injury, 31, 116
respiratory complications
    CPB termination, 46
    postoperative, 53, 58–9
respiratory failure
    ECMO, 218
    postoperative, 53, 58–9
respiratory rate (RR), 8, 145
restrictive cardiomyopathy, 109, 111
resuscitation. See also cardiac arrest
    CPB for, 215–17
    postoperative cardiac arrest, 55, 67
retrograde cerebral perfusion (RCP), 197

aortic surgery, 101–2
    massive air embolism, 211–12
Reveal® implantable cardiac monitoring (ICM) systems, 13
rewarming, 192
    deep hypothermic circulatory arrest, 195–6
    postoperative, 51
    rates, 42
rheumatic heart disease, 78, 82, 141
RIFLE classification, 61
right atrial cannulation, for CPB, 2–3
right atrial hypertrophy, 12
right atrial pressure, 20, 225
    measurement, 225–6
    tricuspid disease, 82, 84
    waveforms, 224–5
right bundle branch block (RBBB), 12
right heart catheterization, 20–1
right ventricle (RV)
    ejection fraction (RVEF), 245
    fractional area change (RVFAC), 245
    free wall strain, 245
    function, TOE assessment, 244–5
    hypertrophy, 12
    PHT, 113–15
    pressure, 20, 227
right ventricular (RV) dysfunction/failure
    after pulmonary thromboarterectomy, 116
    carcinoid heart disease, 87–8
    grading, 245
    paediatric patients, 152
    postoperative, 56–7
    TOE assessment, 244–5
    VADs, 121, 123
right ventricular assist devices (RVADs), 118
    indications, 119, 123
right ventricular outflow tract (RVOT) obstruction
    Fallot's tetralogy, 163–4
    pulmonary atresia, 172
risk assessment, cardiac surgery, 2
rivaroxaban, 263, 278
rocuronium, 26
roller pumps, 35
Ross procedure, 172–4
Ross–Konno procedure, 174
rSO_2 (regional cerebral tissue oxygen saturation), 102, 235

S' velocity, tricuspid annulus, 245
saphenous neuralgia, 282–3
sarcomas, cardiac, 256
SAVE (Survival After Veno-arterial ECMO) score, 218
scars, surgical, 7

scintigraphy, 14–15
screen filters, CPB circuit, 38
$ScvO_2$ (central venous oxygen saturation), 228
sedation, postoperative, 51, 105
seizures, 7
selective antegrade cerebral perfusion, 101–2, 197
sensory evoked potentials (SEPs), 233
septal closure, percutaneous, 141
serotonin, 88–9
shock, haemodynamic parameters, 228
shunt fraction. See pulmonary:systemic blood flow balance
shunts
    bidirectional cavopulmonary (BCPS), 160
    Blalock–Taussig. See Blalock–Taussig (B–T) shunt, modified
    diagnostic evaluation, 20
    left-to-right, 20, 147
    systemic arterial to pulmonary, 147, 187
    unrestricted, adult congenital heart disease, 187
sickle cell disease, 262
single photon emission computed tomography (SPECT), 14, 17
single ventricle circulation. See univentricular circulation
sinus node dysfunction, 132
$SjvO_2$ (jugular venous oxygen saturation), 234
skin, examination, 7–8
sodium nitroprusside, 151
somatic pain, 280
somatosensory evoked potentials (SSEPs), 105, 233
spherocytosis, hereditary, 262
spinal anaesthesia, 275–6
    neuraxial bleeding, 276–8
    organ donor harvest, 276
spinal cord
    function monitoring, 104–5, 233
    injury/ischaemia, 104
    protection, 104–5, 197
spinal cord perfusion pressure (SCPP), 104–5
spinal haematoma, 276
spongiform cardiomyopathy, 110
stabilizer devices, off-pump coronary artery surgery, 91
Stanford classification, aortic dissection, 100
sternal closure, delayed, 152
sternal osteomyelitis, 287
sternotomy
    chronic pain after, 282
    J-shaped upper partial (mini), 73

sternotomy (cont.)
median, 2
postoperative mediastinitis, 287
Stokes–Adams attacks, 7
stomatocytosis, hereditary, 262
strain imaging
left ventricle, 243
right ventricle, 245
stress echocardiography, 13
stress imaging, cardiac, 15
stress response, surgery, 274
stroke
CPB perfusion pressure and, 204
diagnosis, 65–6
LA appendage occlusion, 142
perioperative, 64–7
previous history, 65
thrombolytic therapy, 263
subclavian flap angioplasty, 161
subclavian vein (SCV) cannulation,
25–6, 224
sufentanil, 26
surgical site infection, 286–7
SvO₂. *See* mixed venous oxygen
saturation
Syncardia Total Artificial Heart, 118,
121, 123
synchronized intermittent mandatory
ventilation (SIMV), 51
syncope, 7
AS, 69
exertional, 7
Syntometrine®, 271
systemic arterial to pulmonary shunts,
147, 187
systemic circulation
balancing. *See* pulmonary:systemic
blood flow balance
duct-dependent, 146, 154
systemic inflammatory response
syndrome (SIRS), 62
measures to reduce, 264–7
paediatric patients, 182
systemic vascular resistance (SVR), 20
CPB, 41, 45–7
measurement, 226
neonates, 147
shock, 228
systolic anterior motion of anterior MV
leaflet (SAM), 80–1, 107

tachyarrhythmias, paediatric patients,
183
tachycardia, postoperative, 52
Takotsubo cardiomyopathy, 110–11
tamponade. *See* cardiac tamponade
temazepam, 25
temperature. *See also* hypothermia
after-drop, 195

cerebral metabolism and, 196
measures for maintaining, 191
monitoring, 27, 42, 102
regulation, 191
temperature management, 191–8
EEG monitoring, 231–2
paediatric patients, 150
tetralogy of Fallot. *See* Fallot's tetralogy
thermodilution method, 226
thienopyridines, 24
thiopental, 26
thoracic aortic surgery, 99–106
anaesthesia, 101–5
aortic arch, 101–2
aortic root and ascending aorta, 101
complications, 105–6
descending aorta, 102–5
pathology, 99–100
postoperative care, 105–6
pregnancy, 272
preoperative preparation, 100–1
spinal cord perfusion, 104–5
thoracic epidural anaesthesia, 26,
274–5, 282
neuraxial bleeding risk, 276
pros and cons, 275
thoracic surgery, non-cardiac, 215–16
Thoratec pVAD, 120
thrombocytopenia, 261
thromboelastography (TEG), 265
thrombolytic agents, 263
thrombophilia, 263
thrombosis, postoperative, 185
thrombus, intracardiac, 255
ticagrelor, 262, 278
ticlopidine, 278
tirofiban, 25, 262
TOE. *See* transoesophageal
echocardiography
total anomalous pulmonary venous
drainage (TAPVD), 147, 176
Total Artificial Heart, Syncardia, 118,
121, 123
total cavopulmonary connection
(TCPC). *See* Fontan procedure
tracheal intubation, 27
tranexamic acid (TXA), 152, 264
transcatheter aortic valve implantation
(TAVI), 5, 137–40
anaesthesia, 139–40
devices and techniques, 137
echocardiography, 140
patient selection, 138
procedural risks, 137
transcranial Doppler (TCD), 233
transfusion. *See* blood transfusion
transitional circulation, 145–6
transoesophageal echocardiography
(TOE), 239–41

adult congenital heart disease, 189
aortic disease, 258–9
ASDs, 254–5
basic views, 240
cardiac masses, 255–6
complications, 239
indications, 239
LA appendage occlusion, 142
MV clipping, 140–1
off-pump surgery, 92
paediatric patients, 152
percutaneous septal closure, 141
pericardial disease, 256–8
physical principles, 239
pregnancy, 272
probe insertion, 27
valvular heart disease, 248–53
VAD insertion, 121, 123
ventricular function, 242–7
transposition of the great arteries
(TGA), 177–8
arterial switch procedure, 177–8
balloon atrial septostomy, 147, 177
PA banding, 171, 177
transpulmonary gradient (TPG), 160
transthoracic echocardiography (TTE),
13
Traube's sign, 9
tricuspid annular plane systolic
excursion (TAPSE), 244
tricuspid annulus, S′ velocity, 245
tricuspid regurgitation (TR), 83–5
carcinoid heart disease, 87
grading of severity, 251
TOE assessment, 251
tricuspid stenosis (TS), 82–3, 251
tricuspid valve (TV), 82
carcinoid heart disease, 87
surgery, 83–5
TOE evaluation, 251
troponin I, 57
truncus arteriosus (TA), 179
tubing, CPB circuit, 33
tumours, cardiac, 255–6

22q11 deletion (Di George syndrome),
148, 163, 179

ultrasound, physics, 239
univentricular circulation
arterial shunts, 154–5
bidirectional cavopulmonary shunt,
160
Fontan procedure, 165–6
postoperative care, 181–2
pulmonary artery banding, 171
staged palliation, 175
urinary catheterization, 27, 54
urine output, 41, 45, 63

urological surgery, 216
uterotonics, peripartum, 271

VACTERL syndrome, 163
VADs. *See* ventricular assist devices
valvular heart disease
  imaging, 18–19
  indications for surgery, 2
  percutaneous procedures, 137–41
  pregnancy, 272
  prosthetic valves. *See* prosthetic heart
    valves
  TOE assessment, 248–53
vascular access, 25–7
  adult congenital heart disease, 189
  aortic surgery, 101–3
  CPB, 40–1
  heart transplantation, 127
  minimally invasive surgery, 95–6
  paediatric cardiac anaesthesia, 150
vasoconstrictors, paediatric patients,
    151
vasopressin, 151
vecuronium, 26
vegetations, 256
venous cannulae, 33, 95
venous cannulation
  CPB, 41, 43
  minimally invasive surgery, 95–6
  preoperative, 25
venous oximetry, 226–8
venous reservoir, CPB, 34
ventilation, mechanical
  after induction, 27

during CPB, 208
ECMO, 220
neonates with CHD, 147
paediatric patients, 181
post-bypass failure, 46
postoperative continuation, 51
weaning from, 51
ventilator-associated pneumonia
    (VAP), 287–8
ventricular aneurysms, 110
ventricular assist devices (VADs),
    118–24, *See also* intra-aortic
    balloon pump (IABP)
  bridge to recovery, 118–19
  bridge to transplantation, 118–21
  design, 118
  destination therapy, 118–21
  implantation, 121–3
  indications and patient selection,
    118
  long-term, 119
  paediatric patients, 183
  postoperative care, 123–4
  preoperative assessment, 120–1
  short-term, 119–20
ventricular dysfunction
  postoperative, 52, 55–7
  TOE assessment, 242–7
  weaning from CPB, 45
ventricular dysrhythmias,
    postoperative, 183
ventricular fibrillation (VF), 30, 42–3
ventricular function, TOE assessment,
    242–7

ventricular pseudoaneurysms, 110
ventricular septal defects (VSDs), 180
  percutaneous closure, 141
  PA banding, 171
  pulmonary atresia with, 172–3
  surgical closure, 180
  transposition of the great arteries,
    177
ventricular septum, 180
ventricular tachycardia (VT),
    postoperative, 42–3
ventricular thrombus, 255
ventriculography, 21–2
vents, CPB, 39, 95–7
visceral pain, 280–1
vocal cord palsy, 184
volatile anaesthetics, 28, 201
  cardioprotection, 32
  during CPB, 42
  paediatrics, 149
  pharmacology during CPB, 201
VSDs. *See* ventricular septal defects

warfarin, 114–15, 262–3
'waterhammer' pulse, 8
weaning from CPB, 43, 45–9
  causes of failure, 45
  correctable problems, 45–7
  ECMO for failure, 219
  heart transplantation, 127–8
  mechanical support, 47–9, 120
  non-correctable problems, 47
  paediatric patients, 151–2
  pharmacological support, 47